Nursing Laboratory and Diagnostic Tests

DeMYSTiFieD

Nursing Laboratory and Diagnostic Tests
DeMYSTiFieD

Jim Keogh, DNP, RN-BC

Second Edition

New York   Chicago   San Francisco   Athens   London   Madrid
Mexico City   Milan   New Delhi   Singapore   Sydney   Toronto

Nursing Laboratory and Diagnostic Tests Demystified, Second Edition

1 2 3 4 5 6 7 8 9   LCR   22 21 20 19 18 17

ISBN 978-1-259-85953-3
MHID 1-259-85953-3

This book was set in Minion Pro by Cenveo® Publisher Services.
The editors were Susan Barnes and Kim J. Davis.
The production supervisor was Richard Ruzycka.
Production management was provided by Neha Bhargava, Cenveo Publisher Services.
The index was prepared by Susan Hunter.
LSC Communications was printer and binder.

This book is printed on acid-free paper.

Library of Congress Cataloging-in-Publication Data

Names: Keogh, James Edward, 1948- author.
Title: Nursing laboratory and diagnostic tests demystified / Jim Keogh.
Description: Second edition. | New York : McGraw-Hill Education, [2017] |
    Includes index.
Identifiers: LCCN 2017000596 (print) | LCCN 2017001753 (ebook) | ISBN
    9781259859533 (pbk. : alk. paper) | ISBN 1259859533 (pbk. : alk. paper) |
    ISBN 9781259859540 (ebook) | ISBN 1259859541 (ebook)
Subjects: | MESH: Nursing Diagnosis—methods | Clinical Laboratory Techniques
    | Nursing Care—methods
Classification: LCC RB37 (print) | LCC RB37 (ebook) | NLM WY 100.4 | DDC
    616.07/5—dc23
LC record available at https://lccn.loc.gov/2017000596

Contents

This book is dedicated to Anne, Sandy, Joanne, Amber-Leigh Christine, Shawn, Eric, and Amy, without whose help and support this book could not have been written.

Introduction

"We need to take a sample of your blood."

These words can make a patient cringe grabbing their arms in a subtle attempt to product against the prodding, poking and eventually the pinch that precedes the outpouring of blood—not a pleasant experience for some. And then what follows can be traumatic...." put pressure on the gauge until it stops bleeding." Somehow the band aide that eventually covers the site isn't as soothing as it was when you were a child.

And then anxiety sets in waiting for the dreaded test results. Friends and family members are kind enough to share advice that they found online, in a magazine, and from television—and from those television commercials too. Test results are know immediately on TV medical shows or at least after the next commercial. In real life it can take days or weeks of anticipation and worry.

Not knowing makes medical tests scary. It starts with the patient telling the practitioner about aches, pains, and annoying discomforts. This is followed by a series of seemingly unrelated questions from the practitioner as the practitioner pieces together pieces of the puzzle in her mind. And then just when the patient expects a prescription for medication to make it all better, the practitioner says. "I'd like to run a few tests."

"My God, I have cancer." The thought of the worse runs through her mind. Like a deer in headlights she freezes giving the practitioner a miscue. Silence implies that she has no future questions and the practitioner moves on to the next patient. This is also the cue for the nurse to step in to help put the patient at ease by anticipating the questions that the patient probably wants answered.

In this book you will learn about common medical tests. You will learn

- What they are
- Why they are ordered
- How they are performed
- How the patient should prepare for those tests
- How long it takes to receive test results
- How to understand those test results

Consider this book as a book of answers to questions that patients want answered even though they might not be able to ask those questions at the moment.

A Look Inside

Medical tests can be challenging to learn unless you follow the step-by-step approach that is used in Medical Testing Demystified. Topics are presented in an order in which many students like to learn them—starting with basic components and then gradually moving on to those that are a little more complex to understand.

Each chapter follows a time-tested formula that explains the topic in an easy-to-read style. You can then compare your knowledge with what you are expected to know by taking chapter tests and the final exam. There is little room for you to go adrift.

Chapter 1 Understanding Laboratory Tests

There is more to laboratory test than high, low, and normal ranges. Laboratory tests give the practitioner a unique way to look into the body without actually opening the body. Laboratory tests usually measure something in a sample taken from the body such as blood, urine, and other fluids or at times even a tissue sample. The measurement may be an amount of that something in the sample or simply the presence—or absence—of that something. In this chapter you will learn the foundation of medical tests.

Chapter 2 Hematology Tests

Hematology laboratory tests are one of the most commonly ordered laboratory tests used by the practitioner to study blood, blood diseases, and organs that form blood. Hematology tests count the number of white and red blood cells and platelets, measure the time necessary for blood to clot and the capability of blood to carry oxygen throughout the body. The practitioner can also use hematology tests to determine whether the patient has inflammation or an infection. This chapter explores hematology tests.

Chapter 3 Electrolytes

Electrolytes are chemicals that help generate an electrical impulse that contracts muscles, move fluids within the body, maintain stability of cells, and enable cells to generate an electrical charge. The concentration of electrolytes within the body is on constant change and the balance is maintained by the kidneys. Cells in the kidney monitor the amount of sodium, potassium, and fluid in the bloodstream. Hormones from the kidneys (renin), adrenal gland (aldosterone), and the pituitary gland (antidiuretic hormone) are used to adjust the electrolytes balance. You will learn about electrolytes and electrolyte tests in this chapter.

Chapter 4 Arterial Blood Gases Tests

Gas exchange in the alveoli and the network of capillaries in the walls of the lungs replaces carbon dioxide on hemoglobin in blood with oxygen. The arterial circulation system then distributes the oxygenated hemoglobin throughout the body. Disorders can lead to an ineffective gas exchange resulting in the pH of the patient's blood to fall outside the normal pH range of 7.35 to 7.45. The patient's blood may become acidic or alkalic. Arterial blood gases tests are discussed in this chapter.

Chapter 5 Liver Blood Tests

The liver detoxifies blood, produces clotting factors, and metabolizes medication and nutrients. The liver synthesizes albumin, which maintains blood volume and clotting factors, and synthesizes, stores, and metabolizes fatty acids and cholesterol. Fatty acids are used for energy by the body. The liver stores and metabolizes carbohydrates. Carbohydrates are converted into glucose for energy. These tests are discussed in this chapter.

Chapter 6 Cardiac Enzymes and Markers Tests

Cardiac cells contain enzymes and other substances. Cardiac cells rupture when there is damage to cardiac muscle. As a result, substances once inside the cardiac cells are released into the bloodstream. A practitioner who suspects that a patient has had an acute coronary syndrome or cardiac ischemia will likely order the cardiac enzymes test and the cardiac markers test. The cardiac enzymes test determines the level of cardiac enzymes in the patient's bloodstream. The cardiac markers test measures other substances in addition to cardiac enzymes that are produced if the heart is damaged or under stress. You will learn about these tests in this chapter.

Chapter 7 Serologic Tests

The patient's immune system reacts to bacteria, viruses, and foreign substances that are recognized as alien to the body referred to as an antigen. The reaction creates antibodies. An antibody is a protein called an immunoglobulin that is triggered in the presence of the antigen in the patient's blood. The antibody chemically combines with the substance and metabolizes the substance into components that can be excreted safely by the body.

In this chapter you will learn about common serologic tests.

Chapter 8 Endocrine Tests

The endocrine system is an organization of glands that create, store, and release hormones to regulate metabolism, moods, growth, and other functions of the body. Glands increase or decrease hormone production based on the level of hormones in the blood. Hormones act as chemical messengers that signal other glands and organs to react in a specific manner. These tests are discussed in this chapter.

Chapter 9 Tumor Markers

An uncontrollable growth of abnormal cells in the body is called a tumor. A tumor that is unable to spread to other parts of the body is called benign (noncancerous) and remains in one location. Although a benign tumor does not spread, the size of the tumor may affect nearby areas such as pressuring a nerve or compressing a blood vessel. A tumor that is able to spread to other parts of the body is called malignant (cancerous) and can invade surrounding tissues and travel throughout the body using the lymphatic and circulatory systems. This is referred to as metastasized. Cells in a malignant tumor do not have chemical properties to anchor the cells to the original site. In this chapter you will learn about these tests.

Chapter 10 Pregnancy, Infertility and Genetic Tests

Pregnancy tests determine if the patient is pregnant based on hormone levels in her blood such as the low or high levels of prolactin (increase lactation), hCG (produced after the placenta is implanted), and AFP (a substance made by the liver of the fetus). Infertility tests are ordered by the practitioner to assess why the patient is unable to become pregnant. Genetic testing is ordered by the practitioner before the patient becomes pregnant and at the request of the patient to determine if he/she and his/her partner is a carrier of a genetic disease. If genetic testing is positive, then genetic counseling is usually done to help the patient and his/her partner make an informed decision about becoming pregnant. Genetic testing is also ordered early in the pregnancy especially if the pregnancy was unplanned. Results of genetic testing indicate if the fetus will develop a genetic disease. In this chapter you are introduced to these tests and learn what they are, how they are performed, how to prepare the patient for the test, and how to interpret the test result.

Chapter 11 Simple X-ray Imaging

Simple X-ray imaging is a cost-effective noninvasive radiological test that enables the practitioner to view inside the body. Although a simple X-ray provides a primitive view when compared with a CT scan and an MRI, these images provide sufficient information in some cases to rule out a diagnosis, make a diagnosis or serve as justification for ordering more expensive imaging tests such as a CT scan or an MRI. Radiology imaging based on X-rays is founded on the principle that X-rays are absorbed by dense objects and pass through lesser dense objects. Dense objects such as bone appear white on the X-ray image, lesser dense objects such as air appear black, and fluid and fat appear as a lighter shade of gray. In this chapter you will learn about simple X-ray imaging.

Chapter 12 Computed Tomography Scan

A computed tomography (CT, CAT) scan is a radiology imaging test that creates detailed images of structures within the body using a doughnut-shaped X-ray machine. The patient lies within the doughnut-shaped scanner and an X-ray beam rotates around the patient creating an image that represents a thin slice of the patient. Each rotation takes less than a second. All sliced images are stored on a computer. The computer is used to reassemble sliced images of the patient enabling the healthcare provider to identify any abnormalities.

Typically, the healthcare provider will print the image of any slices that indicate an abnormality, which is then saved with the patient's chart.

You will learn about different types of CT scans in this chapter.

Chapter 13 Magnetic Resonance Imaging and Positron Emission Tomography Scan

Magnetic resonance imaging (MRI) is a radiology imaging test that uses pulsating radio waves in a magnetic field to produce an image of inside the patient's body. The patient lies on his/her back on a table. A coil is placed around the area of the patient that is being scanned and a belt is placed around the patient to detect breathing. The table moves into the magnetic field and the belt triggers the MRI scan so that breathing does not interfere with capturing the image. A positron emission tomography (PET) scan is a nuclear medicine test that creates a roadmap of blood flow in the patient's body, enabling the healthcare provider to visualize abnormal blood flow to the patient's tissues and organs. In this chapter you learn about MRI and PET medical tests.

Chapter 14 Ultrasound Scan

An ultrasound scan creates an image of organs and structures inside the body using sound waves similar in concept to the way in which ship crews are able to identify underwater objects while on the surface of the water. High-frequency sound waves are transmitted by a transducer that is placed on the patient's skin. Sound waves penetrate the skin, bounce off organs and structures in the patient's body, and are detected by the transducer. In this chapter you will learn about different kinds of ultrasound scans.

Chapter 15 Cardiovascular Tests and Procedures

Cardiovascular tests are performed to assess the patient's heart and vascular system to determine if the blood is adequately being pumped and flowing throughout the patient's body. These tests measure cardiac contraction, the risk for coronary artery disease, and are used to identify blockage to coronary arteries and blood vessels of the extremities. When a blockage is identified, the healthcare provider can perform one of several procedures to restore blood flow. The blockage might be surgically removed or pressed against the wall of the blood vessel and held in place by a stent. Alternatively, the healthcare provider may surgically bypass the blocked blood vessels using a vein from the patient's leg or by using an artificial blood vessel. In this chapter you will learn about these tests and procedures.

Chapter 16 Female and Maternity Tests and Procedures

Female patients routinely undergo breast and cervical examinations for signs of cysts, growths, abnormal tissue, structural abnormalities, and infection. In this chapter you will learn about tests and procedures that are performed to test for disorders and repair of disorders. When a mammogram reveals a suspicious growth, the healthcare provider usually orders a breast ultrasound to closely examine the growth and then possibly a breast biopsy. If the tissue sample is cancerous, the healthcare provider may perform a mastectomy. A mastectomy may be performed even if there is no sign of breast cancer. The patient may decide to have her breasts altered for therapeutic or cosmetic reasons. There are a number of tests used to examine the vulva, vagina, cervix, uterus, and fallopian tubes. Many of these tests enable the healthcare provider to take a tissue sample or perform a biopsy on abnormal tissue. If the tissue sample is identified to be cancerous, the cancerous organ is removed. There are several tests that are performed during pregnancy and shortly after childbirth to assess the health of the fetus and newborn. In a high-risk pregnancy, the healthcare provider might perform a chorionic villus sampling or amniocentesis early on in the pregnancy to determine if the fetus has a genetic disorder or other health issues. You will learn about these tests and procedures in this chapter.

Chapter 17 Tests for Males

There are a number of medical tests and procedures that are specifically designed to diagnose and treat disorders that affect men. There are a group of tests and procedures focused on fertility. When a man is unable to impregnate a woman, the healthcare provider orders tests to assess if there is an underlying problem with the man's reproductive organs. The initial test is a semen analysis that assesses the man's semen and sperm. Depending on the results, a testicular scan or testicular ultrasound is ordered to determine if there is a structural disorder. One such structural disorder is varicocele, which is a large vein that blocks blood flow to the testicles. This is relieved by performing a varicocele repair. The healthcare provider may follow up with a testicular examination or an erectile dysfunction test. If the erectile dysfunction test returns positive results, the healthcare provider may perform a penile implant procedure where a device is inserted to cause an erection. Some men desire to become infertile by having their vas deferens cut or blocked by a vasectomy. This prevents sperm from mixing with semen, resulting in no sperm in the ejaculate. A vasectomy in some instances can be reversed by performing a vasovasostomy. Men are susceptible to developing an enlarged prostate gland, which could be caused by prostate cancer. Prostatic cancer cells are in part fueled by testosterone, which is produced by the testicles. The healthcare provider might perform an orchiectomy, which is the surgical removal of one or both testicles. This reduces the level of testosterone in the patient's body. Alternatively, the healthcare provider may perform a prostatectomy, which is the removal of the prostate gland. However, this procedure may leave the patient with erectile dysfunction and urinary incontinence. In this chapter, you will learn about these tests and procedures.

Chapter 18 Lung, Chest, Abdominal, Urinary Tract Tests and Procedures

When there are suspected disorders of the upper gastrointestinal tract, the thyroid gland, the liver, gallbladder, kidneys, spleen, the urinary tract and other organs in the upper part of the body, the healthcare provider is likely to order a number of tests to uncover the underlying problem. Some tests enable the healthcare provider to look down the esophagus to examine the stomach, duodenum, and the bile and pancreatic ducts and to take a biopsy or, in some cases, to remove an obstruction. Other tests enable the healthcare provider to scan the liver, spleen, gallbladder, and kidneys by using contrast material to highlight the structure of the organ. Images of the organ are captured with a camera and studied to uncover diseases and disorders. There are also procedures that the healthcare provider can perform to temporarily or permanently repair a problem. It can be to remove a cancerous thyroid gland, remove a tumor from the bladder, or fix urinary incontinence. The lungs exchange carbon dioxide and oxygen in the hemoglobin in red blood cells. In order to do so effectively, the lungs must be able to expand and retract and blood must flow freely to the lungs. When the patient experiences signs and symptoms of lung disorder and disease, the healthcare provider tests the lungs and orders procedures to evaluate the respiratory system. The healthcare provider can examine the respiratory tract using bronchoscopy and removes samples of suspicious tissue for microscopic examination. The capacity and function of the lungs are measured using several pulmonary function tests. Blood flow to the lungs is monitored by a lung scan and by performing a pulmonary angiogram to identify restriction or blockage of blood flow to the lungs. This is also performed using CT imaging. The patient may experience difficulty breathing when excess fluid builds in the plural space, inhibiting the expansion of the lung. A thoracentesis is sometimes performed, which removes the excess fluid. Diseases such as lung cancer can destroy part of or the entire lung, requiring the healthcare provider to surgically remove a portion (wedge resection), lobes of the lung (lobectomy), or the entire lung (pneumonectomy). You will learn about these and other tests and procedures in this chapter.

Chapter 19 Skin, Muscle, and Bone Tests

Skin is the largest and the most visible organ in the body and is susceptible to wrinkles, blemishes, growths including both non-melanoma and melanoma, and infection. Healthcare providers perform an assortment of tests and procedures to diagnose and treat skin conditions. Aching bones and muscles might be from a cause other than over exercising. It could be a sign of an underlying disorder that needs immediate medical attention. Healthcare providers are able to assess the reason for the patient's discomfort by testing the patient's bones and muscles.

Healthcare providers have an assortment of tests and procedures that are used to investigate signs of a disorder. You will be learning about these in this chapter.

Chapter 20 Sinus, Ears, Nose, Throat (ENT) Tests and Procedures

Snoring is annoying to those who have to listen to it and can also be a symptom of something more ominous such as obstructed sleep apnea. The healthcare provider can fix this problem by performing an uvulopalatopharyngoplasty or radiofrequency palatoplasty that focus on the underlying cause of snoring. There can be a number of reasons why a patient has a headache. One common cause is sinusitis. The healthcare provider can perform a number of tests to assess the sinus, including a sinus endoscopy, sinus X-ray, and a sinus aspiration where a sample of sinus is sent to the laboratory for a culture and sensitivity test. If problem is a blockage of the sinus rather than an infection, the healthcare provider might perform sinus surgery to remove the blockage. Decreased hearing can be caused by a number of factors, including a buildup of cerumen in the ear canal, disorders of the eardrum, or a neurological problem. The healthcare provider can perform tympanometry and audiometric tests to determine the cause of hearing loss. These and other tests and procedures are discussed in this chapter.

Chapter 21 Vision Tests and Procedures

Light rays pass through the cornea, the pupil, and lenses which focus the ray of light on to the retina located at the back of the eye. When light rays are not properly focused on the retina, the patient is unable to see clearly. Light rays focused in front of the retina cause myopia (nearsightedness), enabling patients to better see things near them than at a distance. Light rays focused behind the retina cause hyperopia (farsightedness), enabling patients to see things at a distance better than up close. When light rays are irregularly bent, images are blurred resulting in astigmatism. In this chapter you will learn about tests that are used to diagnose problems with sight and disorders that can lead to loss of vision. You will also learn about procedures that can be performed to treat vision disorders.

chapter 1

Understanding Laboratory Tests

LEARNING OBJECTIVES

1. Labs a Part of a Workup
2. What Is Working—and Not Working?
3. Hematologic System
4. White Blood Cells
5. Red Blood Cells
6. Platelets (Thrombocytes)
7. Liver
8. Pancreas
9. Kidneys
10. Cardiovascular
11. Electrolytes
12. Acid-Base Balance
13. Imaging: X-rays, MRI, CT Scans

1

KEY WORDS

Alanine aminotransferase	Eosinophils
Albumin	Glucagon
Alkaline phosphatase	Glycogen
Aspartate aminotransferase	Insulin
Basic metabolic panel	Leukocytes
Basophils	Lipase
Bile	Lipid panel
Bilirubin	Lymphocytes
Blood urea nitrogen	Monocytes
Cardiac biomarkers	Neutrophils
Cardiac panel	Pancreatic panel
Chem 14	Prothrombin
Chem 7	Thrombocytes
Chymotrypsin	Troponin
Complete metabolic panel	Trypsin
Creatinine	von Willebrand factor
Electrolyte panel	Workup

There is more to laboratory test than high, low, and normal ranges. Laboratory tests give the practitioner a unique way to look into the body without actually opening the body. Laboratory tests usually measure something in a sample taken from the body such as blood, urine, and other fluids or at times even a tissue sample. The measurement may be an amount of that something in the sample or simply the presence or absence of that something.

That something is usually a chemical unless the test is an imaging test such as an X-ray, MRI, or CT scan in which structures within the body are representated. The chemical can be hormones, enzymes, antibodies or other elements normally—or not normally—found in the body. Sometimes these chemicals are contained in cells. If you find the chemical in blood, then there is a possibility that blood cells have ruptured letting the contents of the cell flow into the bloodstream. Subsequently, there is routine rupture of few cells releasing the chemical into the bloodstream maintaining the normal range of chemicals in the blood. However, a high amount of the chemical in the blood out of cell rupture shows abnormal range.

Each measurement unto itself is meaningless but gives the practitioner a clue as to what is happening inside the patient's body. Laboratory results may give the practitioner a direction to follow looking for additional clues. The practitioner may go down one path ordering additional tests or exclude a path because the laboratory results ruled out the likelihood that there are more clues down that road.

In this chapter you will learn the science that forms the foundation for laboratory tests. You will learn how laboratory tests provide clues as to what might be going on inside the patient's body. At the end of this chapter you will have insights into the science behind many laboratory tests that will help you understand and explain to your patients specific laboratory tests that are presented throughout this book.

1. Labs a Part of a Workup

A workup is a medical investigation performed by the practitioner based on symptoms presented by the patients and signs that the practitioner discovers during the practitioner's physical assessment of the patient. Signs and symptoms are possible clues of an underlying problem. However, more clarity is needed before the practitioner decides on a course of treatment.

The practitioner must decide which of hundreds of possible tests should be ordered to provide the clarity that will lead the practitioner to formulate a treatment plan. The practitioner must balance the inconvenience, risks, and expense with the value the test results will provide to further understand the possible cause of the patient's complaint.

Some signs and symptoms combined with the patient's history may indicate the patient may have a serious disease that warrant a full workup requiring blood tests and body scans. However, other signs and symptoms do not point to a serious disease. For example, an annoying cough that came on suddenly within the past 2 weeks is likely caused by a virus. The practitioner could order a full workup of blood tests and body scans; however, the patient may be placed in more harm with exposure to radiation then the benefits the test results will have in diagnosing the problem. The practitioner may treat the cough with over-the-counter medication and wait a few weeks to see if the cough resolves itself.

2. What Is Working—and Not Working?

The practitioner usually orders a group of laboratory tests called a panel to quickly assess the patient's status—what is working and what is not working.

FIGURE 1–1 · Complete metabolic panel (CMP).

The tests are complete blood count (CBC), basic metabolic panel (Chem 7), complete metabolic panel (Chem 14), and other similarly grouped laboratory tests. The number represents the number of laboratory test in the group. The tests are usually ordered as part of the patient's annual physical or when the patient first enters the hospital to give a snap-shot of his condition and serve as a baseline for comparison to future laboratory tests.

Although laboratory test results are listed in a report, sometimes it is easier to use notation to arrange results in a logical format that helps to understand the results. Results are copied from the laboratory report into the notation form. Figure 1–1 shows the notation for the metabolic panel. The top notation form is for the basic metabolic panel (BMP). The BMP panel is a blood test that consists of seven measurements: sodium, potassium, chloride, carbon dioxide, blood urea nitrogen, creatinine, and glucose. The bottom notation is combined with the basic metabolic panel to form the complete metabolic panel (CMP). The additional tests are total bilirubin, total protein, aspartate aminotransferase (AST), alanine aminotransferase (ALT), alkaline phosphatase (ALP), and albumin.

Figure 1–2 shows notation for the complete blood count (CBC). The CBC consists of four measurements: white blood cells, hemoglobin, hematocrit, and platelets. The notation form associates measurements that are sometimes

FIGURE 1–2 · Complete blood count (CBC).

related and helps to compare related laboratory results. For example, there is a relationship between sodium and potassium, and a relationship between blood urea nitrogen and creatinine, and between chloride and carbon dioxide.

Blood contains many elements that are measured by a laboratory test. A sample of blood is removed from the patient's vein—a sample from the artery is taken to measure blood gases—and placed in a glass test tube using phlebotomy. The test tube is spun in a centrifuge that separates components of blood based on density. RBC is the densest component of blood and stays at the bottom of the test tube. WBC and platelets are less dense than RBC but more dense than plasma. As a result, WBC and platelets are sandwiched between RBC and plasma in the test tube. The least dense component plasma sits at the top of the test tube at the end of the centrifuge process. CMP panel components are found in plasma (see Figure 1–3).

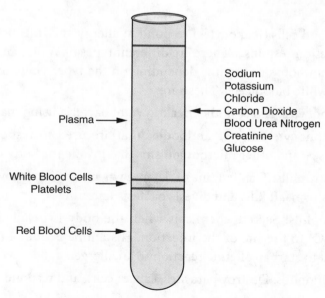

FIGURE 1–3 · CMP panel components.

Routine laboratory tests are processed and analyzed by a biochemistry analyzer. The sample is placed into the analyzer. The analyzer automatically assesses the sample and generates a computerized report. The report is usually electronically stored in the patient's electronic medical record and in other related systems. It is then transmitted to the clinical area and the practitioner for evaluation.

3. Hematologic System

The hematologic system produces and transports blood throughout the body. It consists of plasma, red blood cells, white blood cells, protein and other substances that keep the body stable. The hematologic system:

- Maintains the acid-base balance (pH)
- Maintains the fluid and electrolyte balance
- Transports glucose, oxygen, and hormones
- Distributes antibodies and other cells that protect the body
- Clots leakage of blood
- Helps regulate temperature

4. White Blood Cells

White blood cells (leukocytes) respond to allergy and infection as part of the inflammation response. There are different types of WBCs and their life span varies from hours to months depending on the type. There are five different types of white blood cells. These are:

- Monocytes: Assist in the breakdown of bacteria using macrophages.
- Lymphocytes: Create antibodies that are used to respond to bacteria, viruses, and other microorganisms that invade the body.
- Neutrophils: The first line of defense when the body is invaded by microorganisms. It kills and digests bacteria and fungi.
- Basophils: Secrete chemicals when the body is invaded alerting other WBCs to the site of the infection. Histamine is one of those chemicals used to start an allergic reaction to an allergen.
- Eosinophils: Destroy parasites, cancer cells, and respond to allergens.

A differential WBC count measures the percentage of each type of WBC in the sample of blood. Measurements are percentage of WBC in the blood sample. A high WBC count may indicate an immune response—the patient has an indication. High levels of specific types of WBC give a clue to the type of infection. However, a high WBC may also indicate myelodysplastic syndrome or myeloproliferative disorder, which is the abnormal production of blood cells by the bone marrow. A low WBC count may indicate that the patient's immune system is compromised and requires support to prevent infections. This can happen as a result of chemotherapy, radiation therapy, or disease such as HIV. Leukemia and lymphoma can also cause low WBC count.

5. Red Blood Cells

Red blood cells carry oxygen and carbon dioxide using an iron-rich protein called hemoglobin. Hemoglobin develops in bone marrow cells and gives the RBC its red color. Hemoglobin transports oxygen to tissues where oxygen is exchanged for carbon dioxide. Hemoglobin then travels to the lungs where carbon dioxide is exchanged for oxygen. Glucose also binds to hemoglobin enabling glucose to be transported to cells throughout the body. Glucose forms a cover over hemoglobin. The thickness of the coating indicates the amount of glucose in blood over the previous 3 months as measured by the glycohemoglobin (A1c) test.

Red blood cells have a life span of approximately 120 days; afterwards the RBC dies and hemoglobin decomposes. Iron is returned to bone marrow by proteins called transferrins. The remaining components of hemoglobin forms bilirubin. Bilirubin is excreted into bile and leaves the body as feces. Bilirubin gives feces the yellow-brown color.

The complete blood count measures the number of red blood cells in a micro liter of blood. Low oxygen levels in the blood from disease or from environmental conditions such as being in high altitudes may cause the body to compensate and increase the number of red blood cells giving the body more opportunities to bind with oxygen. Red blood cell stimulating drugs can also increase the number of red blood cells. These are commonly referred to as performance-enhancing drugs. Dehydration may increase the number of red blood cells. Even if the number of red blood cells is within normal range, the concentration of blood may increase. You will read about other conditions that cause an increase in red blood cells in Chapter 2.

A low red blood cell count can be caused by a number of factors such as less production of red blood cells, blood loss, or the body is destroying red blood cells at a faster pace. Iron deficiency is a common cause of low red blood cell count. Iron is ingested as food or taken as a supplement. A decrease in iron intake, an inability to absorb iron, or excessive bleeding lowers the level of iron in the body and as a result lowers the number of red blood cells.

6. Platelets (Thrombocytes)

Platelets are disc-shaped cells, half the size of a red blood cell. Approximately 70% of platelets are found in plasma and the remaining are stored in the spleen. Platelets have a life span of 10 days after which platelets are destroyed in the spleen and the liver. When bleeding occurs, platelets form a temporary patch over the leak and remains until the body replaces the tissue.

The lining of blood vessels is comprised of endothelial cells. Below the lining is collagen. A rupture of the lining exposes blood to collagen. Platelets are attracted to collagen. Platelets are able to adhere to collagen through the use of a protein called von Willebrand factor (VWF) that is stored in and released by endothelial cells of the lining. The von Willebrand factor attaches to receptors on collagen cells and platelets.

Platelets then change into a ball shape with long arms. The arms attach to other platelets and clotting proteins that are in plasma. Platelets contain granules that are secreted into the bloodstream when platelets change shape. Chemicals in granules signals other platelets to the site and form a platelet plug called a platelet aggregation that temporarily covers the break in the blood vessel's lining.

The platelet aggregation is not long lasting. A fibrin clot needs to be formed to provide a longer lasting coverage for the break that stops bleeding. A fibrin clot is created by proteins in plasma called clotting factors. There are 12 clotting factors each identified as a Roman numeral. Clotting factors form threads of protein called fibrin that is weaved over the platelet plug. The fibrin clot is removed by the body when new tissue mends the tear in the lining.

7. Liver

The liver filters blood that arrives from the digestive tract. Chemicals are detoxified and medication is metabolized. Filtered blood is then sent to the rest of the body while waste is secreted as bile that returns to the intestines where it is excreted as feces and urine. The liver, with the help of vitamin K, produces proteins important in blood clotting. The liver converts fat into energy and produces a yellowish, brown, or green fluid called bile. Bile is collected in the bile ducts before passing to the duodenum where bile is used to break down and absorb fats. The liver metabolizes carbohydrates into glucose. The liver also removes and stores glucose in the form of glycogen. Glycogen is then broken down and released into the blood whenever blood glucose levels are low. The liver stores vitamins and minerals such as iron releasing it into the blood when levels are low.

The liver function panel is used to assess how well the liver is functioning. Two enzymes that are measured are alanine aminotransferase (ALT) and aspartate aminotransferase (AST). ALT is found inside liver cells. A number of liver cells die as part of normal metabolism. Enzymes contained in those cells enter plasma and are measured as part of the liver function panel. A high amount of ALT in plasma indicates that an abnormal amount of liver cells are dying. AST is normally found in the kidneys, muscle tissue, pancreas, cardiac cells, liver cells, and red blood cells.

Alkaline phosphatase (ALP) is an enzyme found mostly in bile-secreting living cells but is also found in kidneys, bones, and intestine. ALP is commonly used to measure liver and gallbladder function. It can also help to assess for vitamin D deficiency or unusual bone growth. A high level may indicate that the flow of bile out of the liver is blocked suggesting there is a blockage in the gallbladder.

Bilirubin is a brownish-yellow substance produced when old red blood cells are broken down in the liver. Bilirubin is found in bile (fluid in the gallbladder) and is removed in feces. Bilirubin gives feces its color. Excess bilirubin also causes the yellowish color of jaundice. There are two forms of bilirubin that circulates in blood. These are indirect bilirubin also called unconjugated bilirubin and direct bilirubin known as conjugated bilirubin. Indirect bilirubin cannot be dissolved in water—referred to as insoluble. The liver converts indirect bilirubin to direct bilirubin so that bilirubin can dissolve in water—referred as soluble—and excreted in feces. The bilirubin test measures total bilirubin (both indirect and direct bilirubin) levels in blood. Subtracting direct bilirubin from total bilirubin indicates the value for indirect bilirubin. A high level of bilirubin may indicate that gallstones (crystallized substances in bile) are blocking bile in the gallbladder leading to swelling and pain.

Albumin is a protein produced by the liver that prevents leaking of fluids from blood vessels. Albumin also carries hormones, medication, and enzymes throughout the body assisting in tissue repair and nutrition.

Ammonia is formed when bacteria in the intestine break down protein. Ammonia is carried by the bloodstream to the liver where the liver converts ammonia to urea. Urea is then excreted in urine. Liver disease such as cirrhosis of the liver or severe hepatitis can lead to high ammonia levels in blood resulting in loss of brain function called hepatic encephalopathy.

Prothrombin is a protein made by the liver and found in plasma that is transformed into thrombin by clotting factor X. Thrombin then transforms fibrinogen into fibrin that combines with platelets to form a blood clot. Prothrombin time test (PT) measures how long it takes blood to clot. The result can be measured as the international normalized ratio (INR), which is a way to standardize the results regardless of which testing method was used by the practitioner. Thromboplastin is an enzyme released by damaged cells that convent prothrombin to thrombin. Partial thromboplastin time (PTT) is a test that measured thromboplastin to assess the time required for blood to clot.

8. Pancreas

The pancreas is part of the digestive system and secretes enzymes into the duodenum through the pancreatic duct to break down food. Enzymes are produced in the exocrine cells. The pancreas also produces insulin and glucagon. Insulin is a hormone produced in the islets of Langerhans. Glucagon is a hormone secreted by pancreatic alpha cells.

Enzymes secreted by the pancreas are:

- Trypsin is an enzyme that breaks down proteins.
- Chymotrypsin is an enzyme that breaks down proteins.
- Amylase is an enzyme that breaks down carbohydrates into simple carbohydrates that can be utilized by the body.
- Lipase is an enzyme that breaks down fats into fatty acids and cholesterol.
- Insulin is a hormone that moves glucose from plasma into cells throughout the body providing cells with energy. Insulin assists the liver to store glucagon.
- Glucagon is a hormone secreted by the pancreas when there are decreased blood glucose levels. Glucagon causes glycogen, which is stored in the liver, to break down into glucose causing an increase in blood glucose levels.

The pancreatic panel is a group of blood tests used to assess pancreatic function (see Chapter 2). These tests are:

- Serum lipase: A high level indicates acute pancreatic disease such as acute pancreatitis.

- Serum amylase: A high level may indicate chronic pancreatic disease.
- Serum glucose: A high or low value may indicate problems with insulin or glucagon production.

9. Kidneys

The kidneys excrete waste and excess fluid, maintain electrolyte levels, and produce hormones that regulate blood pressure, influence creation of red blood cells, and help to maintain vitamin D level. Kidneys contain millions of filters called nephrons. Glomerulus makes up the filtered portion of the nephron that filters plasma. Blood cells, minerals, and proteins returned to the bloodstream through tubules in the nephron. Excess fluids and waste product pass through the filter eventually becoming urine that is excreted from the body. Normal urine volume in a 24-hour period is between 800 to 2,000 mL presuming the person intakes 2 L of fluid during that period.

Creatinine: Creatinine is a waste product found in blood when muscle tissue breaks down usually through normal activity. Nephrons remove creatinine from blood where it is excreted in urine. A high level of creatinine may indicate a problem with nephrons; however, high creatinine levels may be normal if the person has recently exercised heavily. A 24-hour urine sample is also used to measure creatinine clearance—the amount of creatinine that was excreted in urine for the 24-hour period. High levels of creatinine may indicate the nephrons are failing to properly filter blood.

Blood Urea Nitrogen (BUN): The liver produces ammonia after metabolizing proteins. Ammonia contains nitrogen. Nitrogen combines with oxygen, hydrogen, carbon, and other elements. The resulting product is called urea. Urea is a waste product that is in blood. Nephrons remove urea from blood and urea is excreted in urine. High levels of blood urea nitrogen may indicate the nephrons are failing to properly filter blood.

10. Cardiovascular

Blood tests to assess the cardiovascular system are typically organized into two groups. These are the cardiac panel, sometimes referred to as cardiac biomarkers and the lipid panel. The cardiac panel is used to assess the heart and the lipid panel is used to assess cholesterol in blood vessels. The practitioner will also order other blood test such as the complete blood count and an electrocardiogram in addition to the cardiac panel and the lipid panel to assess the patient's heart and vessel.

The cardiac panel consists of:

- Troponin: Troponin is a protein in muscle cells and is released into plasma when muscles cells are damaged. The higher the troponin level, the more the damage to the muscles including the heart. Troponin levels rise between 4 and 6 hours following damage and remain elevated for a week. This enables the practitioner to detect a myocardial infarction that occurred days before the patient presented. However, only the primary myocardial infarction is detectable with troponin. Subsequent myocardial infarctions that occur during days after the first are not detectable with troponin. There are two types of troponin that are measured. Troponin I noted as TnI or cTnI measures troponin from cardiac cells. Troponin T noted as CTnT or TnT measures troponin from cardiac cells but also may be cross-reactive with troponin from damaged cells from muscles other than cardiac muscle cells. As a result, Troponin T can be positive without cardiac muscle damage. Troponin T can be elevated as a result of a myocardial infarction or as a result of any muscle damage. Troponin I is elevated as a result of a myocardial infarction or other types of cardiac muscle damage.

- High-sensitivity troponin (hs-troponin) test: A relatively new high-sensitivity troponin test measures lower levels of troponin. This test assists the practitioner to differentiate between angina and a myocardial infarction.

- Creatine kinase (CK): Creatine kinase is an enzyme found in skeletal muscle cells, brain cells, and cardiac cells. Strenuous exercise, trauma, and inflammation can cause creatine kinase to be elevated. The troponin test has replaced the creatine kinase because the troponin test is more specific for damage to the heart. However, the creatine kinase test remains an acceptable substitute. The practitioner typically orders a total creatine kinase test to measure the amount of creatine kinase in plasma. The amount of creatine kinase reflects not only cardiac muscle damage but also damage to any muscle. CK levels can be found 4 to 8 hours after damage and peaks between 12 and 24 hours returning to normal in 3 or 4 days. Creatine kinase MB (CK-MB) measures creatine kinase from cardiac cells and is detectable 3 to 6 hours after reports of chest pain and peaks in 12 to 24 hours returning to normal in 2 to 3 days. Levels may rise again or remain high for longer if the patient experiences another myocardial infarction. The laboratory reports CK-MB as a ratio to total creatine kinase because CK-MB is normally at a low level in plasma. A ratio of 2.5:3 indicates damage to the heart.

- Myoglobin: Myoglobin is a protein found in cardiac and skeletal muscles. Myoglobin enters plasma when either cardiac or skeletal muscle cells rupture. The myoglobin test is less frequently used to detect heart damage; however, the practitioner may use the myoglobin test as an early assessment of a myocardial infarction.

The lipid panel consists of tests that measures lipids in the blood in the form of cholesterol. Lipids are fatty acids. Cholesterol is waxy fatlike substance found in cells throughout the body mostly made by the liver. It is used to produce hormones, assist in digestion, and has many other functions in the body. Cholesterol cannot be dissolve in blood; therefore, cholesterol must be carried through the bloodstream by lipoprotein. Lipoprotein is a substance made up of lipid and proteins. There are two types of lipoproteins. These are low-density lipoprotein (LDL) and high-density lipoprotein (HDL). Low-density lipoprotein (LDL) is referred to as LDL cholesterol and high-density lipoprotein (HDL) is referred to as HDL cholesterol.

LDL cholesterol sticks to the smooth lining of blood vessels and is absorbed for use by cells. HDL cholesterol removes excess LDL cholesterol. There is a balance between LDL cholesterol and HDL cholesterol that prevents LDL cholesterol from blocking blood vessels leading to atherosclerosis. A low HDL cholesterol level or high LDL cholesterol creates an unbalance that may lead to blocked blood vessels. The lipid panel assesses these levels.

There are four tests in the lipid panel:

- Total cholesterol: Total cholesterol is the sum of cholesterol in the blood—both LDL cholesterol and HDL cholesterol.

- Low-density lipoprotein (LDL cholesterol): A high level of LDL cholesterol relative to the level of HDL cholesterol can lead to accumulation of plaques (fatty deposits) in arteries resulting in decreased blood flow leading to atherosclerosis.

- High-density lipoprotein (HDL cholesterol): HDL cholesterol attaches to the LDL cholesterol removing the LDL cholesterol from the lining of blood vessels thereby keeping blood flowing. HDL cholesterol carries LDL cholesterol to the liver where LDL cholesterol is destroyed.

- Triglycerides: Triglycerides are lipids found in blood and stored in adipose cells (fat cells). Hormones release triglycerides between meals to main energy levels in the body. A poorly balanced diet may result in ingesting more calories than is burned by the body especially more car-bohydrates and fats than the body needs. As a result, there is a high level of triglycerides. Think of cholesterol as lipids needed to build cells and for other functions of the body. Think of triglycerides as excessive calories.

There are other tests ordered by the practitioner that may not be part of the lipid panel. These are:

- Non–high-density lipoprotein cholesterol: This test measures the differ-ence between total cholesterol and HDL cholesterol. The difference is non–high-density cholesterol. Non–high-density cholesterol includes LDL cholesterol along with intermediate-density lipoprotein and very low density lipoprotein. Patients who have myocardial infarction do not have high LDL cholesterol but do have high non–high-density cholesterol; therefore, some practitioners feel high non–high-density cholesterol is a better marker for risk of myocardial infarction.

- Lipoprotein (a) or Lp(a): This is a type of LDL cholesterol whose level is determined by genes and not by the patient's lifestyle. The practitioner may order the Lipoprotein (a) test for a patient whose family history indicates early onset heart disease or sudden death. A high lipoprotein (a) indicates there might be a risk of heart disease but it does not measure the risk.

- Plasma ceramides: Ceramides are lipids that play a role in how cells respond to stress and signal inflammation. The plasma ceramides test measures the level of ceramides in plasma. A high level of ceramides may indicate that the patient is at risk for an adverse cardiovascular even related to unstable plaque in the blood vessels. High levels are also associ-ated with insulin resistance.

- Natriuretic peptides (brain natriuretic peptide (BNP): Natriuretic peptide is a protein that is produced by the heart and helps the body eliminate fluids, dilates blood vessels, and assists with excretion of sodium in urine. High levels of BNP are secreted when there is damage to the heart in an attempt to reduce strain on the heart. A high level of BNP may indicate unstable angina, heart failure or that a patient has suffered a myocardial infarction. Since normal level varies by age, gender, and weight, the prac-titioner may order a baseline BNP level as part of a normal examination. The practitioner may order the BNP test to identify if shortness-of-breath is due to heart failure or another underlying cause. Some laboratories using a variation of BNP called the N-terminal BNP for the same purpose.

- High sensitivity C-reactive protein (CRP): This test measures inflammation in the body that may be caused by a cardiovascular disorder or from a different course. C-reactive protein is a protein that the liver produces as part of the inflammatory response. A high level indicates there is inflammation in the body but doesn't identify the location or what caused the inflammation. Inflammation plays a role in atherosclerosis. This test is administered twice—two weeks apart for patient who reports symptoms of heart disease. Statin medications used to lower cholesterol may lower the CRP levels.

11. Electrolytes

Electrolytes are minerals found in the body that carry an electric charge and must be in the proper proportions in bodily fluids to ensure that the body functions such as muscles and nerves operate properly. Electrolytes maintain the balance between fluid levels inside and outside the cell. An increase in electrolytes within the cell causes fluids to enter the center. Decreasing electrolytes within the cell causes fluids to leave the cell. Electrolytes also carry electrical impulses across cells to promote cell activity such as contracting muscles. Electrolytes are paired based in it interaction. Potassium and sodium is an electrolyte pair with sodium outside the cell and potassium inside the cell. Sodium draws fluid into the cell and potassium moves fluid out of the cell to form a sodium-potassium pump. Fluid exiting the cell contains waste products from the cell. Calcium and magnesium is another electrolyte pair where calcium activates nerves and magnesium blocks calcium enabling nerves to relax. Changes in one influence the other in the pair.

An electrolyte panel is a group of tests that measures electrolytes in plasma. The more commonly tested electrolytes are:

Calcium: Calcium plays critical role in muscle contraction, blood clotting, cardiac functions, and transmission of nerve impulses. Calcium is stored in bones and teeth.

Magnesium: Magnesium is used in chemical reactions in the body to maintain normal nerve and muscle functions such as cardiac contractions. Magnesium also plays a critical role in regulating blood sugar and maintaining blood pressure. Magnesium is found in bones and in cell tissues.

Sodium: Sodium regulates fluid in the body and plays a critical role in transmission of nerve impulses. Sodium is found outside the cell.

Potassium: Potassium plays a critical role in muscle contraction including cardiac muscles, function of the kidney and digestion. Potassium also plays a role in transmission of nerve impulses. Potassium is found inside cells. Excess potassium is eliminated by the kidneys in urine and some is eliminated in sweat. The kidneys regulate potassium. Aldosterone from the adrenal gland stimulates the kidneys to eliminate potassium. Potassium can be lost as a result of an over intake of caffeine and sugary drinks, alcohol, and diuretic medication.

Phosphate: Phosphate is critical for protein synthesis used for cell growth and repair. Phosphate is also used by the body to metabolize carbohydrates and lipids. Phosphate is stored in bones and teeth. Phosphate is absorbed from the small intestine.

Chloride: Chloride helps to keep a balance of fluids in the body and helps to maintain the acid-base balance. Chloride is found outside the cell.

An imbalance of electrolytes can occur by having too much or too little of an electrolyte. This commonly occurs as the result of loss of fluids due to vomiting, diarrhea, or sweating. Kidney disease, malabsorption disorders, and medications can also lead to an electrolyte imbalance. An electrolyte imbalance is reversed by either removing the excess electrolyte or replacing the missing electrolyte to a level that balances electrolytes in the body.

12. Acid-Base Balance

The degree of acidity (acid) or alkalinity (base) of the blood may have a sever effect on organs. The body's acid-base balance mechanism ensures that the acidity/alkalinity is within normal range. Acid-base balance is measured using the pH scale. The pH scale ranges from zero, which is strong acidity, to 14, which is strong alkaline (base). A pH scale of 7.0 is considered neutral. The body maintains blood close to 7.40. The pH range of 7.35 to 7.45 is considered normal range. The acid-base balance is measured by performing the arterial blood gas test.

Acidity increases with either the intake of or production of acidic compounds and decreases with the elimination of acidic compounds. An increase in acidity causes a decrease in alkalinity (base) and a decrease in acidity causes an increase in alkalinity. The lungs, kidneys, and buffer systems are involved in maintaining the acid-base balance.

The lungs control the blood pH by managing carbon dioxide. Carbon dioxide is an acid waste created when cells metabolize oxygen. Retention of carbon dioxide in blood causes an increase in acidity in blood. This increase signals the brain to increase the speed and depth of breathing to exhale carbon dioxide thereby reducing the acidity of blood. Conversely, speed and depth of breathing may decrease retaining carbon dioxide to compensate if the blood becomes too alkaline.

Kidneys assist in maintaining the acid-base balance by excreting or retaining acid or alkaline substances. Adjustments made by the kidneys are gradual while adjustments made by the lungs are rapid. The body's natural buffer system increase or decrease acids (carbonic acid) and alkaline (bicarbonate) in the body.

There are two types of acid-base disorders. Acidosis is when there is too much acid or too little base in blood resulting in the decrease in blood pH. Alkalosis is when there is too much base or too little acid leading to an increase in blood pH. Acidosis and alkalosis develops as a result of an underlying cause. Acid-base balance normally returns once the underlying cause is addressed.

The underlying cause is categorized as metabolic or respiratory. Metabolic acidosis and metabolic alkalosis is the result of an imbalance caused by failure of the kidneys to excrete acids or alkaline substances to maintain the acid-base balance. Respiratory acidosis and respiratory alkalosis is the result of an imbalance caused by failure of the lungs to exhale carbon dioxide or inhale and absorb oxygen.

13. Imaging: X-rays, MRI, CT Scans

Practitioners can "see" inside the body by using imaging technology. Imagining technology may use X-rays or magnets and radio waves to "peek" inside the body and generate quality images on a computer screen that enables the practitioner to assess the condition of internal organs. There are three commonly used imaging technologies. These are X-rays, magnetic resonance imaging (MRI), and computerized tomography (CT).

An X-ray is a type of radiation that is generated by an X-ray machine. Some X-rays directed at the body pass through the body and other X-rays are blocked by dense objects such as bone. Most X-ray images are generated on the computer and not on film. Dense objects appear as white or gray on the X-ray because they block the X-ray. Dark areas on the X-ray indicate that X-rays successfully passed through the body. The practitioner orders an X-ray to assess for fractures, bone degeneration, dislocations, and possibly tumors.

MRI uses radio waves and strong magnets to create images of inside the body. The magnet creates a magnetic field that lines protons in the body. Short burst of radio waves are targeted on protons. The MRI scanner picks up the radio waves and information is sent to a computer that generates a three-dimensional image of inside the body. The MRI is used to identify injury to soft tissues including joints, tendons, and ligaments.

Computerized tomography (CT) creates multiple two-dimensional images of the body from different angles using X-ray technology. A computer assembles these cross-sectional images into a three-dimensional image of inside the body. CT scans are used to identify injuries to the head, chest, spine, abdomen, and pelvis and can identify characteristics of tumors.

The practitioner may order an imaging test with contrast to enhance the image of a specific structure within the body. The patient is administered the contrast agent before the image is taken. There are two types of contrast agents. Radiopaque contrast agents (dyes) can be seen on X-rays and CT scans. The contrast agent can be injected into veins, taken by mouth, or inserted through the rectum. Some patients may experience an allergic reaction to the contrast agent especially iodinated contrast agent.

Paramagnetic contrast agents are substances that change the magnetic properties of particles to increase the contrast between different tissues resulting in a clearer image. There are no side effects of paramagnetic contrast; however, patients with severe kidney disease who undergo dialysis should not undergo paramagnetic contrast MRI since this may cause nephrogenic systemic fibrosis, which is a life threatening disease.

QUIZ

1. **What is the primary function of eosinophils?**
   A. Destroy parasites, cancer cells, and respond to allergens
   B. The first line of defense when the body is invaded by microorganisms
   C. Create antibodies that are used to respond to bacteria and viruses
   D. Assist in the breakdown of bacteria using macrophages

2. **What is Glycogen?**
   A. An enzyme produced by the liver
   B. Glucose produced by the pancreas
   C. A form of glucose stored in the liver
   D. Produced by liver cells when liver cells die

3. **What is the function of albumin?**

   A. Prevents fluid from leaking from blood vessels
   B. Carries hormones in blood
   C. Carries medication throughout the body
   D. All of the above

4. **How is ammonia formed in the body?**

   A. This is the byproduct of protein metabolism by a virus.
   B. This is the byproduct of protein metabolism by bacteria.
   C. This is the byproduct of metabolism of bacteria by a virus.
   D. This is the byproduct of bacteria metabolism by protein.

5. **What is creatinine?**

   A. Creatinine is the result of ingesting large amounts of food that contain potassium.
   B. Creatinine is the result of ingesting large amounts of food that contain magnesium.
   C. The liver produces Creatinine after metabolizing proteins.
   D. Creatinine is a waste product found in blood when muscle tissue breaks down.

6. **What is troponin?**

   A. A protein in muscle cells that is released into plasma when muscle cells are damaged
   B. A protein in pancreatic cells that is released into plasma when pancreatic cells are damaged
   C. Is a form of lipid
   D. Is a form of cholesterol

7. **What type of cholesterol level is determined by genes and not by the patient's lifestyle?**

   A. Ceramides
   B. Lipoprotein (a)
   C. BNP
   D. CRP

8. **Carbon dioxide is a/an**

   A. Base
   B. Alkalinity
   C. Alkaline
   D. Acid

9. **Why is a contrast agent used in imaging?**
   A. To enhance the image
   B. To outline specific structures in the body
   C. To outline specific tissues in the body
   D. All of the above

10. **When do troponin levels rise following damage to the heart?**
   A. Between 4 and 6 hours
   B. Between 6 and 12 hours
   C. Between 1 and 4 hours
   D. Between 12 and 16 hours

ANSWERS

1. A. Destroy parasites, cancer cells, and respond to allergens.
2. C. A form of glucose stored in the liver.
3. D. All of the above.
4. B. This is the byproduct of protein metabolism by bacteria.
5. D. Creatinine is a waste product found in blood when muscle tissue breaks down.
6. A. A protein in muscle cells that is released into plasma when muscle cells are damaged.
7. B. Lipoprotein (a).
8. D. Acid.
9. D. All of the above.
10. A. Between 4 and 6 hours.

chapter **2**

Hematology Tests

LEARNING OBJECTIVES

1. Amylase
2. Blood Alcohol
3. Blood Glucose
4. Blood Type Test
5. Blood Urea Nitrogen
6. Chemistry Screen
7. Cholesterol and Triglycerides Tests
8. Cold Agglutinins
9. Complete Blood Count (CBC)
10. C-peptide
11. C-Reactive Protein (CRP)
12. Creatinine and Creatinine Clearance
13. D-xylose Absorption Test
14. Ferritin
15. Folic Acid
16. Gastrin

17. Glycohemoglobin (GHb)

18. Iron (Fe)

19. Lactic Acid

20. Lead

21. Lipase

22. Partial Thromboplastin Time (PTT)

23. Prothrombin Time (PT)/INR

24. Reticulocyte Count

25. Schilling Test

26. Sedimentation Rate (SR)

27. Serum Osmolality

28. Serum Protein Electrophoresis (SPE)

29. Total Serum Protein

30. Toxicology Tests (Tox Screen)

31. Uric Acid in Blood

32. Vitamin B_{12}

KEY WORDS

ABO	Fasting blood glucose (FBG) test
Agglutinins	Ferritin
Albumin	Fibrinogen
Ammonia	Gastrin
Antidiuretic hormone (ADH)	Globulin
Antigens	Heparin
Blood creatinine level test	HgbAIC test
Blood group antigens	High-density lipoprotein (HDL)
Coumadin	Insulinoma
C-reactive protein	Intrinsic factor
Creatine	Lactic acid
Creatine phosphate	Low-density lipoprotein (LDL)
D-xylose	Malabsorption
Erythrocyte indices	Nitrogen
Fasting blood glucose (FBG)	Oral glucose tolerance test

Oral glucose tolerance test (OGTT)	2-hour postprandial blood sugar test
Osmolality	Rh factor
Parietal cells	Rouleaux formation
Partial thromboplastin time (PTT)	Thromboplastin
Phlebitis	Total cholesterol
Proinsulin	Toxin
Prothrombin time (PT)	Transferrin protein
Purine	Triglycerides
Random blood glucose (RBG)	Urea
Reticulocyte	Very low-density lipoprotein (VLDL)
Rh antigen	

Hematology laboratory tests are one of the most commonly ordered laboratory tests used by the practitioner to study blood, blood diseases, and organs that form blood. Hematology tests count the number of white and red blood cells and platelets, measure the time necessary for blood to clot, and the capability of blood to carry oxygen throughout the body. The practitioner can also use hematology tests to determine whether the patient has inflammation or an infection.

Hematology laboratory tests are also used to assess two pancreatic endocrine hormones secreted by the islet cells in the pancreas. These are insulin and glucagon. Both are secreted based on blood glucose levels. When blood glucose is elevated, the pancreas secretes insulin, which causes glucose to cross the cell membrane allowing it to be used for energy, resulting in a decrease in blood glucose. When blood glucose levels are low, the pancreas secretes glucagon, which signals the liver to release stored glucose into the blood, resulting in an increase in blood glucose. Other cells such as muscles also release glucose in response to glucagon. Blood glucose must be maintained within a narrow range, which occurs naturally with the secretion of insulin and glucagon. However, failure of islet cells to properly function, caused by diseases such as diabetes, can result in high levels of blood glucose (hyperglycemia) or low levels of blood glucose (hypoglycemia).

Hematology laboratory tests are also used to assess kidney function. Metabolic waste is carried by the blood to the kidneys. The glomerulus in the kidneys acts as a filter to remove waste from the blood, which is collected in a renal tubule as urine. Metabolic waste such as sodium, potassium, and phosphorus can be reused by the body and is returned to the blood by the kidneys.

The remaining waste is excreted as urine. Renal failure occurs when the glomerulus no longer filters waste from the blood. This can occur suddenly (acute renal failure) in response to illness, medications, accidents, and poisons. It can also happen slowly (chronic kidney disease) from illnesses such as diabetes and high blood pressure. Chronic kidney disease can lead to end-stage renal disease, where all or nearly all the renal functions are permanently destroyed.

Renal function is measured in percentages. A person with two healthy kidneys has 100% renal function. Likewise, a person with one healthy kidney and one kidney with total renal failure is said to have 50% renal function. A person will experience health problems if he/she has 25% or less renal function. Dialysis is typically ordered for a patient with less than 15% renal function.

Lipids are compounds used to store energy, to develop cell membranes, and are elements of vitamins and hormones. Lipids combine with proteins to form lipoproteins. Common lipoproteins in the body are cholesterol and triglycerides. Cholesterol is released into the bloodstream mostly by the liver and other organs, although some cholesterol is ingested in food. Two types of cholesterol are high-density lipoprotein (HDL) and low-density lipoprotein (LDL).

There is a balance between LDL and HDL. LDL is distributed to cells throughout the body through the bloodstream. Excess LDL is removed by HDL from the blood and transported to the liver, where LDL is metabolized into bile acids and excreted from the body. An imbalance occurs when too much LDL is in the blood, leading to accumulation of LDL on the artery walls, which causes a narrowing of the arteries that leads to a blockage.

In this chapter you will learn about commonly performed hematology tests. You will also learn about glucose tests and tests used to determine renal function and lipid metabolism in this chapter.

1. Amylase

Amylase is an enzyme that breaks down starch into sugar. Amylase is produced by salivary glands and the pancreas. The amylase test measures the amount of amylase in the blood. There is normally a low level of amylase in blood unless the salivary glands or pancreas is blocked or damaged.

What Is Being Measured?

- Amylase level in blood

How Is the Test Performed?

- Refrain from eating or drinking, except water, for 2 hours before the test.
- Avoid drinking alcohol for 24 hours before the test.
- See "How to Collect Blood Specimen From a Vein" in Appendix A.

Rationale for the Test

- Screen for
  - Pancreatic disease
  - Pancreatitis
  - Inflammation of the salivary glands
- Assess
  - Treatment for pancreatic and salivary gland disease

Nursing Implications

- Assess if the patient
  - Refrained from eating and drinking, except water, 2 hours before the test
  - Drank alcohol 24 hours before the test
  - Has taken codeine, morphine, diuretics, Coumadin, Indocin, aspirin, or birth control pills, since these can affect the test results
  - Has chronic kidney disease, since this can cause high levels of amylase
  - Liver or pancreatic damage, since this can affect the test results

> **NURSING ALERT**
>
> The healthcare provider is likely to order a lipase test along with the amylase test. Lipase is an enzyme that is produced only by the pancreas. The amylase test may also be performed with the creatinine test to help the healthcare provider diagnose pancreatitis.

Understanding the Results

- Test results are available within 3 days. The laboratory determines normal values based on calibration of testing equipment with a control test. Test results are reported as high, normal, or low based on the laboratory's control test.

- Generally the normal range is 60 to 180 U/L.
- High levels may indicate
  - Pancreatitis
  - Pancreatic cancer
  - Mumps
  - Bowel infarction
  - Inflammation of the salivary glands
  - Cystic fibrosis
  - Diabetic ketoacidosis
  - Gallstones
  - Stomach ulcer
  - Macroamylasemia
  - Ectopic pregnancy
- Low levels may indicate
  - Preeclampsia
  - Advanced cystic fibrosis
  - Severe liver disease
  - Macroamylasemia

NURSING ALERT

High values are normal for older adults and pregnant women. The patient may have chronic pancreatitis even if there is a low amylase level. Children have very little amylase until they reach their first birthday and then their amylase increases to the normal adult level.

Teach the Patient

- Explain
  - Why blood sample is taken.
  - The function of amylase and the meaning of abnormal values.

- That the patient must refrain from eating or drinking, except water, for 2 hours before the test and avoid drinking alcohol for 24 hours before the test.
- That the patient should tell the healthcare provider if they are taking codeine, morphine, diuretics, Coumadin, Indocin, aspirin, or birth control pills, since these can affect the test results.

2. Blood Alcohol

Alcohol depresses the central nervous system (CNS) when large amounts of alcohol enter the blood. Alcohol is absorbed within a few minutes and peaks within an hour. Food decreases absorption of alcohol. Alcohol is mostly metabolized by the liver and excreted in urine and by breathing. The blood alcohol test measures the level of alcohol in the blood.

> **NURSING ALERT**
>
> A taximeter that measures alcohol levels in the patient's breath is another test to determine the level of alcohol consumed by the patient.

> **NURSING ALERT**
>
> The patient's signed consent may be required before the test is administered because the result of the blood alcohol test can have legal repercussions for the patient. Consult the healthcare facility's policies regarding administering the blood alcohol test.

What Is Being Measured?

- Alcohol level in the blood

How Is the Test Performed?

- See Appendix A "How to Collect Blood Specimen."

Rationale for the Test

- Screen for
  - Intoxication
  - The underlying cause of altered mental status (AMS)
  - Ingested alcohol

Nursing Implications

- The result of the blood alcohol test represents the level of alcohol at the time the test was administered and cannot predict the amount of alcohol consumed by the patient because alcohol continues to be metabolized by the liver.
- Assess if the patient
  - Has taken sedatives, kava, ginseng, or antihistamines, since these can enhance the sedative effect of alcohol.
  - Has diabetic ketoacidosis.
  - Ingested methanol or isopropyl alcohol.
  - Has vital signs. Alcohol ingestion can depress respiration and the central nervous system.
- Assess if the insertion site was cleaned with alcohol, since this can affect the test results.
- Take safety precautions, since the patient may have impaired reaction time and decreased vision.
- The speed in which alcohol is metabolized is influenced by
  - The proof of each drink. The higher the proof, the higher the blood alcohol level.
  - The patient's weight. Blood alcohol level decreases as weight increases, since additional weight represents increased water that dilutes the alcohol.
  - The number of drinks the patient ingested each hour. It takes approximately an hour to metabolize a drink. The greater the number of drinks per hour, the higher the blood alcohol level.
  - The patient's age. The older patient will have a higher blood alcohol level than a young patient who consumed the same quantity of alcohol because the older patient's metabolism is slower.

- The amount of food ingested by the patient. The higher the ingestion of food, the lower the blood alcohol level, since the food can absorb some alcohol.
- Women have a higher blood alcohol level than men because they have less water than men in their body.
- The use of mixers such as club soda increases the absorption of alcohol, resulting in a higher blood alcohol level.
- Quick assessment
  - 0.03 to 0.059 blood alcohol level
    - Talkativeness
    - Decrease in inhibition
    - Decrease in alertness, coordination, and concentration
  - 0.06 to 0.1 blood alcohol level
    - Decrease in reflexes, peripheral vision, depth perception, and reasoning
    - Blunted feelings
    - Impaired sexual pleasure
  - 0.11 to 0.20 blood alcohol level
    - Staggering
    - Slurred speech
    - Decreased reaction time
    - Emotional swings
    - Over expression
  - 0.21 to 0.29 blood alcohol level
    - Blackout of memory
    - Stupor
    - Loss of consciousness
    - Impaired sensations
  - 0.30 to 0.39 blood alcohol level
    - Decrease in breathing
    - Decrease in heart rate
    - Severe depression
    - Unconsciousness
    - Risk of death

- Greater than four blood alcohol level
  - Death

Understanding the Results

- Test results are available quickly. The laboratory determines normal values based on calibration of testing equipment with a control test. Test results are reported as high, normal, or low based on the laboratory's control test.
- Normal range: 0.0
- Abnormal level: Greater than 0.0
- Intoxication (National Highway Traffic Safety Administration): 0.08 g/dL or 80 mg/dL or 17 mmol/L

Teach the Patient

- Explain
  - Why blood sample is taken.
  - That the patient consent is needed to administer the test unless ordered by legal authorities. Check your healthcare facility's policy.
  - The test result.

NURSING ALERT

The Clinical Institute Withdrawal Assessment (CIWA) should be performed what a patient is at risk for alcohol withdrawal. CIWA measures pulse and blood pressure and determines if the patient is experiencing nausea/vomiting; tactile disturbances; tremors; visual/auditory disturbances; sweating; anxiety/agitation; and disorientation. The assessment is performed regularly to identify when withdrawal systems appear and track the severity of withdrawal systems until withdrawal symptoms are absent.

---

3. Blood Glucose

Glucose is the source of energy for cells and is transported into cells by insulin. As blood glucose levels rise following ingestion of food, the pancreas releases insulin to move the glucose from blood into cells. The blood glucose tests measure the level of glucose in the blood. There are four blood glucose tests:

- Oral glucose tolerance test (OGTT): This test measures the blood glucose levels at specific time intervals after the patient ingests a glucose drink. The OGTT is ordered to screen for gestational diabetes and to confirm positive results of other blood glucose tests.
- Two-hour postprandial blood sugar test: This test measures blood glucose levels 2 hours after the patient ingests food.
- Fasting blood glucose (FBG) test: This test measures blood glucose levels after the patient has fasted for 8 hours. The FBG test is the initial test for diabetes.
- Random blood glucose (RBG): This test measures blood glucose levels several times a day regardless of food intake.

> **NURSING ALERT**
>
> Glucose levels can also be measured in urine; however, this is not used to diagnose or monitor glucose levels. The healthcare provider may order the glycohemoglobin (GHb) blood test, which is used to monitor blood glucose levels for the previous 120 days.

What Is Being Measured?

- Glucose levels in blood

How Is the Test Performed?

- FBG test requires the patient to fast for 8 hours before the test is administered. Insulin and other diabetes medications are withheld until the test is administered.
- Two-hour postprandial test requires the patient to eat a normal meal 2 hours before the test is administered.
- Oral glucose tolerance test requires the patient to fast 8 hours before the test. Ingesting water is permitted. A blood sample is taken to be used as a baseline. The patient ingests a glucose drink. A blood sample is taken in hourly intervals for 3 hours.
- See Appendix A "How to Collect Blood Specimen."

> **NURSING ALERT**
>
> The blood glucose test for diagnosing diabetes must be repeated on two different days.

Rationale for the Test

- Screen for
  - Diabetes
  - Hypoglycemia
  - Assessment of the treatment for diabetes

Nursing Implications

- Assess if the patient
  - Is ill. Illness can increase blood glucose levels and affect the test result.
  - Smokes, since this can affect the test result.
  - Uses caffeine, since this can affect the test result.
  - Is experiencing stress, since this can affect the test result.
  - Has eaten or fasted according to procedures for the blood glucose test.
  - Has taken Dyrenium, Dyazide, Dilantin, Lasix, niacin, Inderal, Esidrix, Hydro Par, Oretic, prednisone, or birth control pills, since these medications may affect the test result.

Understanding the Results

- Blood glucose test results are available in 2 hours. The laboratory determines normal values based on calibration of testing equipment with a control test. Test results are reported as high, normal, or low based on the laboratory's control test.
- Normal blood glucose range
  - FBG test: 70 to 99 mg/dL
  - Two-hour postprandial blood sugar test: 70 to 145 mg/dL
  - RBG test: 70 to 125 mg/dL

- High blood glucose may indicate
  - Diabetes
    - FBG test: Greater than 125 mg/dL
    - Two-hour postprandial blood sugar test: Greater than 199 mg/dL
    - RBG test: Greater than 199 mg/dL and the presence of symptoms of diabetes
  - Prediabetes
    - FBG test: 100 to 125 mg/dL
  - Acromegaly
  - Cushing syndrome
  - Stroke
  - Myocardial infarction
  - That the patient has taken corticosteroid medication
- Low blood glucose may indicate
  - Hypoglycemia (FBG less than 40 mg/dL)
  - Insulinoma/insulin-producing tumor
  - Hypothyroidism
  - Addison disease
  - Kidney failure
  - Malnutrition
  - Cirrhosis
  - Anorexia
  - That the patient has taken insulin or other diabetes medication

Teach the Patient

- Explain
  - Why the blood sample is taken.
  - The dietary restriction required by the test if any.
  - That the healthcare provider may ask the patient to stop taking Dyrenium, Dyazide, Dilantin, Lasix, niacin, Inderal, Esidrix, Hydro Par, Oretic, prednisone, or birth control pills for 2 weeks prior to the test.

4. Blood Type Test

Blood is identified by an antigen on the surface of red blood cells. Major types of these antigens are blood group antigens and Rh antigen. There are four types of blood group antigens that are determined by performing the ABO test.

- Type A: Has the A antigen and antibodies in plasma against B antigen.
- Type B: Has the B antigen and antibodies in plasma against A antigen.
- Type O: Has neither the A antigen nor the B antigen and antibodies in plasma against A antigen and B antigen.
- Type AB: Has both the A antigen and the B antigen and no antibodies in plasma against A antigen and B antigen.

Red blood cells may have the Rh antigen attached to them, sometimes called the Rh factor, and is determined by the Rh test.

- Rh positive (+): The Rh antigen is presented on the red blood cells.
- Rh negative (−): The Rh antigen is not presented on the red blood cells.

A patient's blood type is described as a combination of blood group antigen and Rh antigen by using the blood type letter(s) followed by a plus (+) or minus (−) sign, indicating if the Rh antigen is present. For example, type A means that the patient has the A antigen but doesn't have the Rh antigen attached to the red blood cells.

NURSING ALERT

The test will also examine minor antigens that, attached to red blood cells, can cause an adverse blood transfusion reaction.

What Is Being Measured?

- Blood group antigens on red blood cells
- Rh antigens on red blood cells

How Is the Test Performed?

- See Appendix A "How to Collect Blood Specimen."

Rationale for the Test

- Assess
  - Blood compatibility for a blood transfusion and organ transplant
  - If a pregnant woman is Rh positive or negative

Nursing Implications

- Assess the patient for conditions that might affect the test results.
  - The patient has taken methyldopa, levodopa, or cephalexin. These medications can cause a false Rh positive test result.
  - Recent X-ray with contrast.
  - Bone marrow transplant.
  - A blood transfusion in the previous 3 months.
  - Has or has had cancer or leukemia.

Understanding the Results

- The result is available in an hour.
- The following chart lists blood type compatibility between a recipient (the patient) and a donor.

Blood Transfusion Compatibility Chart	
Recipient	Donor
A–	A– O–
A+	A– A+ O– O+
B–	B– O–
B+	B– B+ O– O+
AB–	AB– O–
AB+	AB– AB+ A– A+ B– B+ O– O+
O–	O–
O+	O– O+

> **NURSING ALERT**
>
> It was once thought that type O negative is the universal blood donor, meaning that a patient can receive O negative blood regardless of the patient's blood type. Type AB positive is the universal recipient. It is now understood that these blood types contain antibodies that can cause a transfusion reaction. Before any transfusion, a sample of the recipient's blood is cross-matched (mixed) with the donor's blood in the laboratory to determine compatibility.

Teach the Patient

- No special preparation is needed for the test.
- Explain how the test is performed.
- Explain the conditions that can negatively affect the test results.

5. Blood Urea Nitrogen

Ammonia is formed when bacteria in the intestines break down protein. Ammonia is then converted by the liver into the waste product urea, which is excreted by the kidneys in urine. Urea contains nitrogen. The blood urea nitrogen (BUN) test measures the level of nitrogen in the blood derived from urea.

> **NURSING ALERT**
>
> The BUN test is typically performed with the creatinine test. The healthcare provider then uses the BUN/creatinine ratio to evaluate the patient's condition.

What Is Being Measured?

- BUN level in blood

How Is the Test Performed?

- See "How to Collect Blood Specimen From a Vein" in Appendix A.

Rationale for the Test

- Screen for
  - Kidney function
  - Dehydration
- Assess
  - The treatment for kidney disease
  - Need for kidney dialysis

Nursing Implications

- Assess
  - If the patient has eaten meat or protein prior to the administration of the test
  - If the patient has taken Fungizone, Garamycin, Nebcin, Chloromycetin, nafcillin, Kantrex, tetracycline, or diuretics
  - The patient's age, since BUN levels increase with age

Understanding the Results

- Test results are available in 1 day. The laboratory determines normal values based on calibration of testing equipment with a control test. Test results are reported as high, normal, or low based on the laboratory's control test.
- Normal BUN range: 10 to 20 mg/dL
- Normal BUN/creatinine ratio: 10:1 to 20:1
- High BUN values may indicate
  - Kidney disease
  - Kidney stone
  - Addison disease
  - Kidney tumor
  - Burns
  - Heart failure
  - GI tract bleeding
  - Dehydration
  - High protein diet

- High BUN/creatinine ratio may indicate
  - Respiratory tract bleeding
  - GI tract bleeding
  - Shock
  - Kidney failure
  - Urinary tract blockage
  - Dehydration
- Low BUN values may indicate
  - Malnutrition
  - Liver damage
  - Overhydration
  - Low protein diet
- Low BUN/creatinine ratio may indicate
  - Rhabdomyolysis
  - Cirrhosis
  - Syndrome of inappropriate secretion of antidiuretic hormone (SIADH)
  - Muscle injury

NURSING ALERT

BUN level is higher than the creatinine level in dehydration. Both BUN and creatinine levels are high when there is blockage of urine flow.

Teach the Patient

- Explain
  - Why blood sample is taken.
  - That the patient should avoid eating meat or protein for 24 hours before the test is administered.
  - That the healthcare provider may ask the patient to stop taking Fungizone, Garamycin, Nebcin, Chloromycetin, nafcillin, Kantrex, tetracycline, or diuretics for 2 weeks prior to administration of the test.

6. Chemistry Screen

A chemistry screen test examines various components of the blood and is used to assess the patient's overall health. The various types of chemistry screens are called Chem 20, Chem 12, Chem 7, and so on, where the number represents the number of blood components examined in the test.

> ## NURSING ALERT
>
> A chemistry screen test is also called sequential multichannel analysis (SMA) or sequential multichannel analysis with computer (SMAC), followed by the number of components being examined. Other common names are comprehensive metabolic panel (CMP) or basic metabolic panel (BMP).

The following tests are included in a chemistry screen. Refer to each test for details.

- Albumin
- Alkaline phosphatase (ALP)
- Alanine aminotransferase (ALT)
- Aspartate aminotransferase (AST)
- Bilirubin
- Blood glucose
- Blood urea nitrogen (BUN)
- Calcium (Ca) in blood
- Carbon dioxide (CO_2)
- Chloride (Cl)
- Cholesterol and triglyceride tests
- Creatinine and creatinine clearance
- Lactic acid
- Phosphate in blood
- Potassium (K) in blood
- Sodium (Na) in blood
- Total serum protein
- Uric acid in blood

7. Cholesterol and Triglycerides Tests

Cholesterol is produced in the liver and is used for cell growth and hormone production. Cholesterol attaches to proteins in the blood forming lipoproteins. Excess cholesterol in the blood forms plaque on the side of blood vessels that can lead to cardiovascular disorders. The cholesterol and triglycerides tests profile lipoproteins to measure components of cholesterol. These components are:

- Total cholesterol: Total cholesterol is the total amount of LDL and HDL in the blood sample.
- Low-density lipoprotein (LDL): LDL transports lipids from the liver. High levels of LDL increase the risk of cardiovascular disorders.
- Very low-density lipoprotein (VLDL): VLDL distributes triglyceride that is produced in the liver. High levels of VLDL increase the risk of cardiovascular disorders.
- High-density lipoprotein (HDL): HDL binds with lipids in the blood returning lipids to the liver, where lipids are metabolized. High levels of HDL decrease the risk of cardiovascular disorders.
- Triglycerides: Triglycerides are stored lipids. High levels of both triglycerides and LDL increase the risk of cardiovascular disorders.

What Is Being Measured?

- Total cholesterol, low-density lipoprotein, very low-density lipoprotein, high-density lipoprotein, and triglycerides levels in blood.

How Is the Test Performed?

- See "How to Collect Blood Specimen From a Vein" in Appendix A.

Rationale for the Test

- Screen
  - For lipid disorder
- Assess
  - Treatment for lipid disorder

Nursing Implications

- Assess if the patient
  - Has eaten or drunk 12 hours before the test is administered
  - Has eaten a high fatty diet 24 hours before the test is administered
  - Has exercised before the test is administered
  - Has undergone a radioactive scan within a week before the test
  - Has an infection, hyperthyroidism, hypothyroidism, cirrhosis, hepatitis, diabetes, kidney disease
  - Has malnutrition
  - Abuse alcohol or medication
  - Is undergoing alcohol or medication withdrawal
  - Is pregnant
  - Has taken androgens, birth control pills, corticosteroids, estrogen, niacin, antibiotics, tranquilizers, or diuretics

Understanding the Results

- Test results are available in 1 day. The laboratory determines normal values based on calibration of testing equipment with a control test. Test results are reported as high, normal, or low based on the laboratory's control test.
- Normal total cholesterol range: Less than 240 mg/dL.
- Normal HDL range: Greater than 40 mg/dL.
- Normal total cholesterol: HDL ratio less than 5:1.
- Normal LDL range: Less than 160 mg/dL.
- Normal VLDL range: Less than 160 mg/dL.
- Normal triglycerides range: Less than 200 mg/dL.
- Lower HDL and higher LDL, VLDL, and triglycerides increase the risk of cardiovascular disorders including
  - Coronary artery disease
  - Acute coronary syndrome
  - Myocardial infarction

Teach the Patient

- Explain
  - Why blood sample is taken.
  - Not to eat or drink for 12 hours before the test.
  - Not to eat a fatty diet for 24 hours before the test.
  - Not to exercise before the test.
  - That the healthcare provider may request the patient to stop taking androgens, birth control pills, corticosteroids, estrogen, niacin, antibiotics, tranquilizers, or diuretics for 2 weeks prior to the test.

8. Cold Agglutinins

Agglutinins are antibodies that cause red blood cells to aggregate forming a clump called Rouleaux formation at low temperatures as an immune reaction to an infection. High levels of agglutinins can impede blood flow to the extremities when exposed to cold, resulting in tissue damage unless the extremity is warmed. High levels of agglutinins can cause hemolytic anemia. The cold agglutinins test measures the level of agglutinins in a blood sample.

What Is Being Measured?

Agglutinins level in the blood

How Is the Test Performed?

See Appendix A "How to Collect Blood Specimen."

Rationale for the Test

- Screen for
  - Hemolytic anemia
  - The underlying cause for pneumonia

Nursing Implications

- Assess if the patient has
  - Taken penicillin or cephalosporins

- Measles, malaria, congenital syphilis, pneumonia, chickenpox, anemia, infectious mononucleosis, cirrhosis, or multiple myeloma, since these diseases can produce a false positive test result

Understanding the Results

- Test results are available quickly. The laboratory determines normal values based on calibration of testing equipment with a control test. Test results are reported as high, normal, or low based on the laboratory's control test.
- Results are reported as a titer. A titer specifies how much of the sample of blood is diluted with saline before antibodies are no longer detected. The titer is reported as a ratio of parts of the blood sample and saline. The higher the second number of the ratio, the greater the number of antibodies in the blood sample.
- Normal cold agglutinins titer range: Less than 1 to 40 (1:40).
- High cold agglutinins titer may indicate
  - Pneumonia
  - Hepatitis C
  - Cirrhosis
  - Infectious mononucleosis
  - Rheumatoid arthritis
  - Malaria
  - Hemolytic anemia
  - Multiple myeloma
  - Lymphoma
  - Cytomegalovirus (CMV)
  - Scleroderma
  - Risk for thrombosis

Teach the Patient

- Explain
  - Why blood sample is taken.
  - That the healthcare provider may request that the patient stops taking penicillin or cephalosporins for 2 weeks prior to the test.

9. Complete Blood Count

The complete blood count (CBC) test measures several components of blood to assess the patient for various disorders; it is part of a routine blood screening. Components measured are

- Leukocyte count (WBC): Leukocytes normally increase when infection is present, but can also increase in the absence of infection if the patient has leukemia.
- Leukocyte cell type (WBC differential): There are five major types of leukocyte cells, each having a role in the immune process. These are neutrophils, lymphocytes, monocytes, eosinophils, and basophils. The quantity of each leukocyte cell type provides important information in diagnosing the patient's condition.
- Erythrocyte count (RBC): Erythrocyte cells carry oxygen and carbon dioxide.
- Erythrocyte indices
  - Mean corpuscular volume (MCV): This is the size of erythrocytes.
  - Mean corpuscular hemoglobin (MCH): This is the amount of hemoglobin in an erythrocyte cell.
  - Mean corpuscular hemoglobin concentration (MCHC): This is the concentration of hemoglobin in an erythrocyte cell.
  - Red cell distribution width (RDW): This shows the different sizes of erythrocyte cells.
- Hematocrit (HCT, packed cell volume): The hematocrit test measures the volume in percentage taken up by erythrocytes in the patient's blood.
- Hemoglobin (Hgb): The hemoglobin test measures the amount of hemoglobin in blood. Hemoglobin is the part of an erythrocyte that carries oxygen.
- Thrombocyte count (platelet): Platelets form blood clots.

> **NURSING ALERT**
>
> The healthcare provider may also order the erythrocyte sedimentation rate (ESR) test to detect inflammation and the reticulocyte count to identify the number of immature leukocytes.

What Is Being Measured?

- Leukocyte, erythrocyte, and thrombocyte levels in the blood

How Is the Test Performed?

- See Appendix A "How to Collect Blood Specimen."

Rationale for the Test

- Screen for
  - Anemia
  - Infection
  - Leukemia
  - Risk of bleeding
  - Asthma
  - Allergies
  - The cause of bruising
  - The cause of fatigue
  - Polycythemia
  - Blood loss

Nursing Implications

- Assess if the patient
  - Is taking antibiotics, steroids, Equanil, thiazide diuretics, Miltown, quinidine, Meprospan, or chemotherapy
  - Has high levels of triglycerides, since these can affect the hemoglobin test
  - Has an enlarged spleen, since this can reduce the platelet count
  - Is pregnant
  - Smokes
  - Is stressed
  - Has exercised before the test is administered

- Note
  - How long the tourniquet was tied when acquiring the blood sample.
  - If the blood sample clumps in the test tube, indicating that the sample is contaminated.

Understanding the Results

- Test results are available quickly. The laboratory determines normal values based on calibration of testing equipment with a control test. Test results are reported as high, normal, or low based on the laboratory's control test.
- Normal WBC count range
  - Men: 5,000 to 10,000 mcL^3
  - Nonpregnant women: 4,500 to 11,000 mcL^3
  - Pregnant women
    - First trimester: 6,600 to 14,100 mcL^3
    - Second trimester: 6,900 to 17,100 mcL^3
    - Third trimester: 5,900 to 14,700 mcL^3
    - Postpartum: 9,700 to 25,700 mcL^3
- Normal leukocyte cell type range
  - Neutrophils: 55% to 70%
  - Band neutrophils: 0% to 3%
  - Lymphocytes: 20% to 40%
  - Monocytes: 2% to 8%
  - Eosinophils: 1% to 4%
  - Basophils: 0.5% to 1%
- Normal RBC count range
  - Men: 4.7 to 6.1 million mcL
  - Women: 4.2 to 5.4 million mcL
  - Children: 4.0 to 5.5 million mcL
  - Newborn: 4.8 to 7.1 million mcL
- Normal hematocrit range
  - Men: 42% to 52%
  - Women: 37% to 47%

- Pregnant women
  - First trimester: 35% to 46%
  - Second trimester: 30% to 42%
  - Third trimester: 34% to 44%
  - Postpartum: 30% to 44%
- Children: 32% to 44%
- Newborn: 44% to 64%
- Normal hemoglobin range
  - Men: 14 to 18 g/dL
  - Women: 12 to 16 g/dL
  - Pregnant women
    - First trimester: 11.4 to 15 g/dL
    - Second trimester: 10 to 14.3 g/dL
    - Third trimester: 10.2 to 14.4 g/dL
    - Postpartum: 10.4 to 18 g/dL
  - Children: 9.5 to 15.5 g/dL
  - Newborn: 14 to 24 g/dL
- Normal erythrocyte indices range
  - MCV: 80 to 95 fL
  - MCH: 27 to 31 pg
  - MCHC: 32 to 36 g/dL
- Normal red cell distribution width range: 11% to 14.5%
- Normal thrombocyte count range
  - Adults and children: 150,000 to 400,000 mm^3
  - Babies: 200,000 to 475,000 mm^3
  - Newborn: 150,000 to 300,000 mm^3
- High WBC count might indicate
  - Inflammation
  - Infection
  - Leukemia
  - Tissue damage
  - Stress

- Malnutrition
- Burns
- Lupus
- Kidney failure
- Rheumatoid arthritis
- Tuberculosis
- Thyroid gland problems
- High RBC count might indicate
  - Lung disease
  - Alcoholism
  - Polycythemia vera
  - Smoking
  - Kidney disease
  - Dehydration
  - Burns
  - Sweating
  - Vomiting
  - Diarrhea
  - Spurious polycythemia
  - Carbon monoxide (CO) exposure
  - That the patient is using diuretics
- High thrombocyte count might indicate
  - That the patient is bleeding
  - Cancer
  - Bone marrow problems
  - Iron deficiency
- High MCV might indicate
  - Folate deficiency
  - Vitamin B_{12} deficiency
- Low WBC count might indicate
  - Alcoholism
  - Lupus

- Cushing syndrome
- AIDS
- Aplastic anemia
- Enlarged spleen
- Viral infection
- Malaria
- That the patient is undergoing chemotherapy
- Low RBC count might indicate
  - Anemia
  - Addison disease
  - Sickle cell disease
  - Inflammatory bowel disease
  - Cancer
  - Peptic ulcer
  - Lead poisoning
  - Removal of the spleen
  - Pernicious anemia
  - Heavy menstrual bleeding
- Low thrombocyte count might indicate
  - Risk for bleeding
  - Idiopathic thrombocytopenic purpura (ITP)
  - Pregnancy
  - Enlarged spleen
- Low mean corpuscular volume might indicate
  - Iron deficiency
  - Thalassemia deficiency

NURSING ALERT

Hematocrit and hemoglobin results indicate the same disorders as high and low erythrocyte (RBC) count. The mean corpuscular hemoglobin result indicates the same disorders as high and low mean corpuscular volume.

Teach the Patient

- Explain
  - Why the blood sample is taken.
  - That the patient should not exercise before the test is administered.
  - That the patient should tell the healthcare provider if he/she smokes.
  - That the healthcare provider may request that the patient stop taking antibiotics, steroids, Equanil, thiazide diuretics, Miltown, quinidine, or Meprospan for 2 weeks prior to the test.

10. C-peptide

Proinsulin is split into C-peptide and insulin. The level of C-peptide is considered equal to the amount of insulin, indicating the amount of insulin made by the pancreas. The C-peptide test measures the level of C-peptide in blood and is used to differentiate between types 1 and 2 diabetes.

NURSING ALERT

The healthcare provider will order a blood glucose test along with the C-peptide test. The healthcare provider may order a C-peptide stimulation test to differentiate between types 1 and 2 diabetes.

What Is Being Measured?

- C-peptide level in blood

How Is The Test Performed?

- See Appendix A "How to Collect Blood Specimen."

Rationale for the Test

- Differentiate between types 1 and 2 diabetes.
- Assess the result of removal of an insulinoma from the pancreas.
- Assess the underlying cause of hypoglycemia.

Nursing Implications

- Assess if the patient
  - Ate or drank 8 hours before the test is administered
  - Has taken insulin or oral type 2 diabetes medication, since this can affect the test results
  - Is taking alcohol, insulin, meglitinides or sulfonylureas, birth control pills, diuretics, or corticosteroids, since these medications can affect the test results
  - Has kidney failure
- Note if the patient is obese.

Understanding the Results

- Test results are available quickly. The laboratory determines normal values based on calibration of testing equipment with a control test. Test results are reported as high, normal, or low based on the laboratory's control test.
- The blood glucose test is performed along with the C-peptide test and the results of both tests are compared.
- Normal C-peptide range: 0.78 to 1.89 ng/mL
- High C-peptide and high blood glucose values may indicate
  - Type 2 diabetes
  - Cushing syndrome
  - Insulin resistance
- High C-peptide and low blood glucose values may indicate
  - Insulinoma/pancreatic insulin-producing tumor
  - That the patient is taking sulfonylureas
  - That the patient is taking meglitinides
- Metastasized insulinoma if the insulinoma was removed
- Low C-peptide and low blood glucose values may indicate
  - Addison disease
  - Liver disease
  - That the patient has taken insulin
  - Infection

- Low C-peptide and high blood glucose values may indicate
  - Type 1 diabetes
  - Pancreatectomy

NURSING ALERT

A patient with type 2 diabetes can develop low C-peptide level over time.

Teach the Patient

- Explain
  - Why blood sample is taken.
  - That the patient should not eat or drink 8 hours before the test is administered.
  - That the healthcare provider may ask the patient to stop taking alcohol, insulin, meglitinides or sulfonylureas, birth control pills, diuretics, or corticosteroids for 2 weeks prior to the test.

11. C-Reactive Protein

C-reactive protein (CRP) is protein produced by the liver a few hours after tissue injury, infection or other causes of the inflammation response. C-reactive protein attaches to damaged cells or microorganism enhancing phagocytosis in the destruction of the microorganism or damaged cell. The CRP test measures the CRP level in the blood. A high level indicates inflammation, but not the source of the inflammation. The healthcare provider will order other tests to identify the source of the inflammation.

NURSING ALERT

The healthcare provider may order a high-sensitivity CRP test (hs-CRP) to determine if inflammation has damaged the inner lining of arteries increasing the risk of a myocardial infarction. The healthcare provider may order the total cholesterol test and high-density lipoprotein (HDL) cholesterol test. These test results combined with the result from the CRP test help to determine the risk of cardiac problems.

What Is Being Measured?

- The CRP level in blood

How Is the Test Performed?

- See Appendix A "How to Collect Blood Specimen."

Rationale for the Test

- Screen for inflammation, arthritis, autoimmunity, irritable bowel syndrome (IBS), and smoking
- Assess
  - The treatment of inflammation
  - The treatment of diseases that cause inflammation
  - The response to cancer treatment

NURSING ALERT

The CRP level peaks 6 hours following surgery and decreases by the third day. Infection as a result of the surgery is suspected if the CRP level remains high after the third day. Elevated CRP level prior to surgery increases the risk of infection of the following surgery.

Nursing Implications

- Assess if the patient
- Has exercised immediately prior to administering the test
- Has taken nonsteroidal anti-inflammatory drugs (NSAIDs), birth control pills, aspirin, hormone replacement therapy, pravastatin, or corticosteroids
- Has an intrauterine device (IUD)
- Is pregnant
- Is obese

Understanding the Results

- Test results are available in 1 day. The laboratory determines normal values based on calibration of testing equipment with a control test. Test results are reported as high, normal, or low based on the laboratory's control test.

- Normal CRP range: 0 to 1 mg/mL
- High CRP values may indicate
  - Inflammation
  - Infection
  - Risk for a myocardial infarction

> **NURSING ALERT**
>
> The C-peptide level quickly raises, then returns to normal if treatment of infection or cancer is successful.

Teach the Patient

- Explain
  - Why blood sample is taken.
  - That the patient should not exercise before the test.
  - That the healthcare provider may ask the patient to stop taking NSAIDs, birth control pills, aspirin, hormone replacement therapy, pravastatin, or corticosteroids for 2 weeks.

12. Creatinine and Creatinine Clearance

Creatine phosphate provides energy to skeletal muscles. After 7 seconds of intense effort, creatine phosphate converts to creatine. Creatine is metabolized into creatinine and is carried in blood to the kidneys for filtering and excretion in urine. If kidneys are malfunctioning, creatinine levels in the blood increase and creatinine levels in urine decrease. There are three types of creatinine tests:

- Blood creatinine level test: This test measures the level of creatinine in blood.
- Creatinine clearance test: This test measures creatinine in a 24-hour urine sample and measures the level of creatinine in blood.
- Blood urea nitrogen/creatinine ratio (BUN/creatinine): This test compares the results of the blood urea test with the blood creatinine level test to assess for dehydration.

NURSING ALERT

Urea is a by-product of protein metabolism in the liver that is excreted in urine. Fetal kidney function is assessed by testing the level of creatinine in amniotic fluid. The healthcare provider may order the glomerular filtration rate test to determine kidney function.

NURSING ALERT

A normal blood creatinine level does not rule out kidney disease.

What Is Being Measured?

- Creatinine level in blood and urine

How Is the Test Performed?

- Avoid
  - Strenuous exercise for 2 days prior to the test
  - Ingesting protein for 1 day prior to the test
  - Drinking coffee and tea prior to the creatinine clearance test, since these increase urine production
- See "How to Collect Blood Specimen From a Vein" in Appendix A.

Rationale for the Test

- Screen for
  - Kidney function
  - Dehydration

Nursing Implications

- Assess if the patient
  - Has performed strenuous exercise for 2 days prior to the test
  - Has taken

- Diuretics, Proloprim, Trimpex, Aldomet, Tagamet, ascorbic acid, cephalosporins, or Mefoxin, since these can affect the results of the blood creatine level test.
- Dilantin, cephalosporins, Captopril, ascorbic acid, Garamycin, Tagamet, Proloprim, Trimpex, Cardioquin, Quinaglute, Quinine, Quinidex, amphotericin B, or procainamide, since these can affect the results of the creatinine clearance test.
- Tagamet or tetracycline, since these can affect the results of the BUN/creatine ratio test.
- Has ingested protein for 1 day prior to the test
- Drank coffee or tea before the creatinine clearance test

Understanding the Results

- The creatinine blood level test and creatinine clearance test results are available quickly. The laboratory determines normal values based on calibration of testing equipment with a control test. Test results are reported as high, normal, or low based on the laboratory's control test.
- Normal test results
  - Blood creatinine level
    - Men: 0.6 to 1.2 mg/dL
    - Women: 0.5 to 1.1 mg/dL
    - 13 to 19 years old: 0.5 to 1.0 mg/dL
    - 6 months to 12 years old: 0.3 to 0.7 mg/dL
    - Newborn: 0.3 to 1.2 mg/dL
  - Creatinine clearance
    - Men: 90 to 140 mL/min
    - Women: 87 to 107 mL/min
  - BUN/creatinine ratio
    - Over 11 months of age: 10:1 to 20:1
    - Under 12 months of age: 30:1 or less
- Higher levels may indicate
  - Blood creatinine level
    - Kidney disorder

- Shock
- Kidney stones
- Dehydration
- Shock
- Rhabdomyolysis
- Acromegaly
- Gigantism
- Polymyositis
- Muscular dystrophy
- Urinary tract blockage
- Cancer
- Creatinine clearance
  - Muscle injury
  - Pregnancy
  - Hypothyroidism
  - Burns
  - Strenuous exercise
  - Carbon monoxide poisoning
- BUN/creatinine ratio
  - Dehydration
  - Kidney stones
  - Shock
  - Acute kidney failure
- Lower levels may indicate
  - Blood creatinine levels
    - Protein-deficient diet
    - Decreased muscle mass
    - Pregnancy
    - Liver disease
  - Creatinine clearance
    - Cirrhosis

- Dehydration
- Infection
- Kidney disorder
- Urinary tract blockage
- Reduced blood to the kidneys
- BUN/creatinine ratio
  - Protein-deficient diet
  - Cirrhosis
  - Rhabdomyolysis
  - SIADH
  - Cancer
  - Pregnancy

Teach the Patient

- Explain
- Why blood sample is taken.
  - That the healthcare provider may ask the patient to refrain from taking the following medications prior to the individual test
    - Blood creatinine level test: Diuretics, Proloprim, Trimpex, Aldomet, Tagamet, ascorbic acid, cephalosporin, or Mefoxin
    - Creatinine clearance test: Dilantin, cephalosporins, Captopril, ascorbic acid, Garamycin, Tagamet, Proloprim, Trimpex, Cardioquin, Quinaglute, Quinine, Quinidex, amphotericin B, or procainamide
    - BUN/creatinine ratio test: Tagamet or tetracycline
- To avoid
  - Strenuous exercise for 2 days prior to the test
  - Ingesting protein for 1 day prior to the test
  - Drinking coffee and tea for the creatinine clearance test, since these increase urine production

13. D-xylose Absorption Test

D-xylose is a simple sugar that is absorbed by the intestines. The D-xylose absorption test measures the level of D-xylose in blood.

> ### NURSING ALERT
>
> D-xylose absorption can also be tested with a urine sample. A urine test is less accurate than the blood D-xylose absorption test for patients younger than 12 years of age. The healthcare provider may order an upper gastrointestinal (GI) series if the D-xylose test is positive.

What Is Being Measured?

- D-xylose level in blood

How Is the Test Performed?

- The patient drinks 8 oz of water that contains 25 g of D-xylose.
- A blood sample is taken after 2 hours and then again 5 hours after drinking the water.
- See Appendix A "How to Collect Blood Specimen."

Rationale for the Test

- Screen for malabsorption syndrome.

Nursing Implications

- The patient should avoid fruits, jams, pastries, and jellies 1 day before administration of the test.
- Adult patients should avoid eating or drinking, except water, 12 hours before the test.
- Patients younger than 9 years of age should avoid eating or drinking, except water, 4 hours before the test.
- Patients are not permitted to eat or drink until the last blood sample is taken.
- The patient should rest quietly until the last blood sample is taken.
- Assess if the patient is
  - Undergoing radiation treatment
  - Taking aspirin, antibiotics, indomethacin, or cardiac medication, since these medications can affect the test result

Understanding the Results

- Test results are available quickly. The laboratory determines normal values based on calibration of testing equipment with a control test. Test results are reported as high, normal, or low based on the laboratory's control test.
- Normal D-xylose range
  - Adult: 21 to 57 mg/dL
  - Younger than 13 years of age: Greater than 20 mg/dL
  - Younger than 6 months of age: Greater than 15 mg/dL
- High D-xylose levels may indicate
  - That the patient is undergoing radiation treatment
  - Hodgkin disease
  - Scleroderma
- Low D-xylose levels may indicate
  - Celiac disease
  - Hookworm
  - Malabsorption syndrome
  - Inflammation of the intestine
  - Crohn disease
  - Giardiasis
  - Whipple disease

Teach the Patient

- Explain
- Why the blood sample is taken.
- That the patient should avoid fruits, jams, pastries, and jellies 1 day before administering the test.
- That the adult patient should avoid eating or drinking, except water, 12 hours before the test and patients younger than 9 years of age for 4 hours.
- That the patient will not be permitted to eat or drink until after the last blood sample is taken.
- That the patient will be asked to rest quietly until the last blood sample is taken.

14. Ferritin

Ferritin is a protein found in bone marrow, liver, skeletal muscles, and the spleen that binds to iron. The ferritin test measures the level of ferritin in blood to determine the amount of iron in the body.

> **NURSING ALERT**
>
> Blood should contain a small amount of ferritin since most ferritin is bound to iron.

What Is Being Measured?

- Ferritin level in blood

How Is the Test Performed?

- See Appendix A "How to Collect Blood Specimen."

Rationale for the Test

- Screen for
  - Hemochromatosis (excess iron)
  - Iron deficiency anemia
  - Treatment of hemochromatosis and iron deficiency anemia
  - Inflammation

Nursing Implications

- Assess if the patient has
  - A diet high in red meat
  - Had a radioactive scan 3 days prior to the test
  - Taken birth control pills or antithyroid medication
  - Had a blood transfusion 4 months prior to the test
  - Inflammation, since inflammation increases ferritin levels
  - Had changes in the menstrual cycle recently
- Note the age of the patient since ferritin level increases with age.

Understanding the Results

- The ferritin test results are available quickly. The laboratory determines normal values based on calibration of testing equipment with a control test. Test results are reported as high, normal, or low based on the laboratory's control test.
- Normal ferritin test results
  - Men: 12 to 300 ng/mL
  - Women: 10 to 150 ng/mL
  - 6 months to 15 years: 7 to 142 ng/mL
  - 2 to 5 months: 50 to 200 ng/mL
  - 1 month: 200 to 600 ng/mL
  - Newborn: 25 to 200 ng/mL
- High ferritin level may indicate
  - Hemochromatosis
  - Thalassemia
  - Alcoholism
  - Iron deficiency anemia
  - Hepatitis
  - Cirrhosis
  - Hodgkin disease
  - Arthritis
  - Leukemia
  - Lupus
  - Excess dietary iron
- Low ferritin level may indicate
  - Iron deficiency
  - Excessive menstrual bleeding
  - Bleeding
  - Colon cancer
  - Ulcers
  - Colon polyps
  - Pregnancy
  - Insufficient dietary iron

Teach the Patient

- Explain why the sample is taken.

15. Folic Acid

Folic acid is a type of vitamin B that is necessary for cell development and maintenance. Women who are planning to become pregnant should increase the intake of folic acid to reduce the risk of spina bifida, and cleft lip and palate. The folic acid test measures the level of folic acid in blood.

> **NURSING ALERT**
>
> The healthcare provider may order a vitamin B_{12} blood test along with the folic acid blood test.

What Is Being Measured?

- Folic acid levels in the blood

How Is the Test Performed?

- The patient must refrain from eating and drinking other than water for 8 hours before the test.
- See Appendix A "How to Collect Blood Specimen."

Rationale for the Test

- Screen for
  - Malnutrition
  - Anemia
  - Malabsorption
  - Sufficient level of folic acid to reduce the risk of birth defects
  - Treatment of folic acid deficiency

Nursing Implications

- Assess if the patient has
  - Eaten or drunk, except water, for 8 hours before the test
  - Vitamin B_{12} anemia
  - Iron deficiency anemia
  - Taken Dyrenium, Proloprim, Dilantin, pentamidine, phenobarbital, Mysoline, or methotrexate, since these medications may affect the test result

Understanding the Results

- Folic acid test results are available quickly. The laboratory determines normal values based on calibration of testing equipment with a control test. Test results are reported as high, normal, or low based on the laboratory's control test.
- Normal folate range
  - In plasma
    - Adult: 2 to 20 ng/mL
    - Children: 5 to 21 ng/mL
  - In red blood cells
    - Adult: 140 to 628 ng/mL
    - Children: Greater than 160 ng/mL
- High folic acid may indicate
  - Increased dietary folic acid or supplements
  - Vitamin B_{12} deficiency
- Low folic acid may indicate
  - Alcohol abuse
  - Anorexia nervosa
  - Crohn disease
  - Cirrhosis
  - Celiac disease
  - Hemolytic anemia
  - Kidney disease
  - Cancer

Teach the Patient

- Explain
  - Why blood sample is taken.
  - That the patient must not eat or drink, except water, for 8 hours before the test.
  - That the healthcare provider may ask the patient to stop taking Dyrenium, Proloprim, Dilantin, pentamidine, phenobarbital Mysoline, or methotrexate for 2 weeks prior to the test.

16. Gastrin

Gastrin is a hormone produced by the G cells of the stomach lining when food enters the stomach. Gastrin stimulates the parietal cells in the stomach to secrete hydrochloric acid (HCl) that is used in digestion. Gastrin also stimulates the product of pepsin, which is a digestive enzyme. The gastrin test measures the level of gastrin in the blood.

> **NURSING ALERT**
>
> The healthcare provider may order an intravenous (IV) secretin test, where secretin, a digestive hormone, is injected into a vein and blood samples are taken immediately, then every 5 minutes for 15 minutes, and then at 30 minutes.

What Is Being Measured?

- Gastrin levels in blood

How Is the Test Performed?

- Refrain from drinking alcohol 1 day before the test is administered.
- Refrain from eating and drinking except for water 12 hours before the test.
- No smoking 4 hours before the test.
- Refrain from drinking water 1 hour before the test.
- Refrain from taking Rolaids, Prilosec, Pepcid, Zantac, or Tums 12 hours before the test.

- Rest 30 minutes before the test is administered.
- See Appendix A "How to Collect Blood Specimen."

Rationale for the Test

- Screen for
  - Zollinger-Ellison syndrome
  - Pernicious anemia
  - Pancreatic tumor
  - G-cell hyperplasia

Nursing Implications

- Assess if the patient has
  - Refrained from drinking alcohol 1 day before the test is administered
  - Refrained from eating and drinking except for water 12 hours before the test
  - Refrained from smoking 4 hours before the test
  - Refrained from drinking water 1 hour before the test
  - Refrained from resting 30 minutes before the test was administered
  - Taken calcium supplement or medication containing calcium
  - Taken tricyclic antidepressants, Urised, Lomotil, or Motofen
  - Taken Rolaids, Prilosec, Pepcid, Zantac, or Tums 12 hours before the test
  - Hypoglycemia
  - Cirrhosis, kidney failure, or rheumatoid arthritis
  - Undergone small bowel resection or peptic ulcer surgery

Understanding the Results

- Gastrin test results are available in 2 days. The laboratory determines normal values based on calibration of testing equipment with a control test. Test results are reported as high, normal, or low based on the laboratory's control test.
- Normal gastrin range
  - Adult: Less than 200 pg/mL
  - Children: Less than 125 pg/mL

- High gastrin level may indicate
  - Kidney failure
  - Pernicious anemia
  - Zollinger-Ellison syndrome
  - Hypercalcemia
  - Peptic ulcers
  - G-cell hyperplasia
  - Hyperparathyroidism
  - Stomach cancer
  - Sarcoidosis
  - Small bowel resection
- Low gastrin level may indicate
  - Hypothyroidism

Teach the Patient

- Explain
  - Why blood sample is taken.
  - That the healthcare provider may want the patient to stop taking tricyclic antidepressants, Urised, Lomotil, calcium supplements, or Motofen for 2 weeks before the test.
- Refrain from
  - Drinking alcohol 1 day before the test is administered
  - Eating and drinking except for water 12 hours before the test
  - Smoking 4 hours before the test
  - Drinking water 1 hour before the test
  - Taking Rolaids, Prilosec, Pepcid, Zantac, or Tums 12 hours before the test
- Rest 30 minutes before the test is administered.

17. Glycohemoglobin

Glucose binds to hemoglobin in red blood cells, which has a life span of 120 days. The glycohemoglobin (GHb), commonly known as the HgbAIC test, measures the level of glucose bound to hemoglobin. This differs from the blood glucose test, which measures the level of glucose in plasma. The health-care provider orders the GHb test to assess if treatment is controlling diabetes and if the patient is adhering to the treatment over a 120-day period.

> **NURSING ALERT**
>
> The GHb test can be administered at any time; however, the healthcare provider is likely to order the test four times a year. The GHb test is not a replacement for the blood glucose test and cannot dictate hypoglycemia.

What Is Being Measured?

- Glucose that adheres to hemoglobin

How Is the Test Performed?

- See Appendix A "How to Collect Blood Specimen."

Rationale for the Test

- Assess
  - Treatment for diabetes
  - If the patient is adhering to treatment for diabetes

Nursing Implications

- Assess if the patient has
  - Had a blood transfusion in the past 120 days
  - Hemolytic anemia, thalassemia, sickle cell anemia, polycystic ovary syndrome, pheochromocytoma, Cushing syndrome, or kidney disease
  - Had his/her spleen removed
  - Taken corticosteroids

Understanding the Results

- Normal GHb test results are available in 2 days. The laboratory determines normal values based on calibration of testing equipment with a control test. Test results are reported as high, normal, or low based on the laboratory's control test.

- Normal GHb level range
  - GHb A1c: 4.5% to 5.7%
  - Total GHb: 5.3% to 7.5%
- High GHb levels (8% or greater) may indicate
  - Poorly controlled diabetes
  - The patient is undergoing corticosteroid treatment
  - Pheochromocytoma
  - Polycystic ovary syndrome (PCOS)
  - Cushing syndrome

Teach the Patient

- Explain
  - Why the sample is taken.
  - Why the test is administered several times during the year.
  - That the GHb test is not an alternative to daily blood glucose tests.

18. Iron

Iron (Fe) is a mineral in food that is needed for cell growth. Once metabolized, iron binds to the transferrin protein, which transports iron to bone marrow and other tissues. The iron test measures the amount of iron that is bound to transferrin. There are three iron tests:

- Total iron-binding capacity (TIBC) test: This test measures the capacity of the blood to carry iron by determining the amount of iron needed to bind to all the available transferring protein.
- Serum iron test: This test measures the amount of circulating iron in the blood.
- Transferrin saturation test: This is the percentage of serum iron of TIBC.

NURSING ALERT

The healthcare provider may order the ferritin test, the siderocyte stain test, and a CBC along with the iron tests.

What Is Being Measured?

- Serum iron in blood

How Is the Test Performed?

- Avoid taking iron supplements 12 hours before the test is administered.
- Avoid taking vitamin B_{12} supplements 2 days before the test.
- Draw the blood in the morning to ensure the highest level of iron.
- See Appendix A "How to Collect Blood Specimen."

Rationale for the Test

- Screen for
  - Nutritional status of the patient
  - Iron deficiency anemia
  - Hemochromatosis
- Assess treatment of iron deficiency anemia.

Nursing Implications

- Assess if the patient
  - Has taken iron supplements 12 hours before the test is administered
  - Has taken vitamin B_{12} supplements 2 days before the test
  - Is sleep deprived
  - Is stressed
  - Has received a blood transfusion 4 months prior to the test
  - Is taking estrogen, birth control pills, Chloromycetin, aspirin, cortico-trophin, and St. John's wort
- Note if the sample was taken in the morning.

Understanding the Results

- The iron test results are available quickly. The laboratory determines normal values based on calibration of testing equipment with a control test. Test results are reported as high, normal, or low based on the laboratory's control test.

- Normal test results
  - Serum iron
    - Men: 80 to 180 mcg/dL
    - Women: 60 to 160 mcg/dL
    - Children: 50 to 120 mcg/dL
  - TIBC: 250 to 450 mcg/dL
  - Transferrin saturation
    - Men: 20% to 50%
    - Women: 15% to 50%
- High level may indicate
  - Hemochromatosis
  - Kidney disease
  - Cirrhosis
  - Lead poisoning
- Low level may indicate
  - Iron deficiency anemia
  - Iron deficient diet
  - Bleeding
  - Pregnancy
  - Rapid growth

Teach the Patient

- Explain
- Why the sample is taken.
- That the sample must be taken in the morning.
- That the healthcare provider may ask the patient to refrain from taking iron supplements, vitamin B_{12} supplements, estrogen, birth control pills, Chloromycetin, aspirin, corticotrophin, and St. John's wort prior to the test.

19. Lactic Acid

Muscle cells convert glucose into lactic acid and use lactic acid for energy when oxygen levels are low during strain of heart failure, exercise, shock, and sepsis. Lactic acid is not used for energy when there is a normal oxygen level in the blood. Lactic acid is metabolized by the liver. Liver disorders can result in lactic acidosis because of a high level of lactic acid in the blood. The lactic acid test measures the level of lactic acid in blood.

> **NURSING ALERT**
>
> The healthcare provider may order an arterial blood gas test to measure lactic acid in blood.

What Is Being Measured?

- Lactic acid level in blood

How Is the Test Performed?

- Avoid eating or drinking 10 hours before the test.
- Avoid exercising 12 hours before the test.
- Avoid clenching the fist during the test.
- See Appendix A "How to Collect Blood Specimen."

Rationale for the Test

- Screen for
  - Lactic acidosis
  - The underlying cause of acidosis
  - Tissue oxygenation

Nursing Implications

- Assess if the patient
- Has exercised 12 hours prior to the test
- Has eaten or drunk 10 hours before test
- Had clenched fist when the blood sample was drawn since clenched fist may increase lactic acid level
- Is taking alcohol, Glucophage, isoniazid, epinephrine, or Tylenol 12 hours prior to the test
- Has an infection

- Note the time the tourniquet has been in place when the blood sample is drawn, since the longer the tourniquet is in place, there is a risk of increased lactic acid level.

Understanding the Results

- The lactic acid test results are available in 1 day. The laboratory determines normal values based on calibration of testing equipment with a control test. Test results are reported as high, normal, or low based on the laboratory's control test.
- Normal lactic acid test results: 5 to 20 mg/dL
- High lactic acid level may indicate
  - Lactic acidosis
  - Heart failure
  - Pulmonary embolism
  - Anemia
  - Dehydration
  - Leukemia
  - Cirrhosis
  - Disruption of blood flow
  - Alcohol poisoning
  - The patient exercised prior to the test
  - The patient had taken Glucophage, or isoniazid prior to the test
  - Excess dietary iron

Teach the Patient

- Explain
  - Why the sample is taken.
  - That the healthcare provider may ask the patient to refrain from taking alcohol, Glucophage, isoniazid, epinephrine, or Tylenol 12 hours prior to the test.
- Avoid
  - Eating or drinking 10 hours before the test
  - Exercising 12 hours before the test
  - Clenching the fist during the test

20. Lead

Lead serves no benefit to the body. Lead can mimic the actions of calcium and interact with proteins.

Approximately 20% of lead is ingested. Inhaled lead is absorbed in the lower respiratory tract. Most lead is excreted in urine or feces. Repeated exposure to small amounts of lead causes a buildup of lead over time. The most common form of lead is inorganic lead that is not metabolized in the liver. Organic lead that is ingested is absorbed and metabolized in the liver. Lead that is absorbed and not excreted is found in blood, bones/teeth (94%), and liver, kidneys, lungs, brain, spleen, muscle, and heart. The half-life of lead in an adult is from 28 days to 35 days. Lead affects growth and development if lead-tainted water, paint chip, food, or dust is ingested or if lead is in contact with the skin. Pregnant women can pass lead to the fetus or to the newborn through breast milk. Children are more susceptible to lead poisoning because increased levels of lead in blood interfere with neural and brain development. Children who are in early development are at risk for permanent growth impairment if they ingest lead. The lead blood test measures the level of lead in the blood sample.

> **NURSING ALERT**
>
> The healthcare provider may order the urine aminolevulinic acid (ALA) test to determine the extent of lead poisoning (not for children). The lead mobilization urine test is performed during chelation therapy to assess if the therapy is removing lead in urine.

What Is Being Measured?

- Lead levels in the blood

How Is the Test Performed?

- See Appendix A "How to Collect Blood Specimen."

Rationale for the Test

- Assess
  - For lead poisoning
  - The treatment of lead poisoning

Nursing Implications

- Assess if the patient is taking herbal medicine.
- Test results of 10 mcg/dL or above from a finger or heel stick require blood to be drawn from a vein to confirm the results, since the blood sample might be contaminated from lead at the site of the stick.
- Consult your healthcare institution's policy to determine if a positive test result must be reported to the local health department. Lead levels above 10 mcg/dL on two occasions typically must be reported, so the source of the lead can be found. Tests are repeated within a few days or in a month following the initial test.
- Quick assessment using the United States Centers for Disease Control and Prevention (CDC) classes
  - Learning problems: Class 1 or 2
  - Slow growth: Class 2
  - Hearing problems: Class 2
  - Headache: Class 3
  - Neurologic problems: Class 3
  - Weight loss: Class 3
  - Anemia: Class 4
  - Seizures: Class 4
  - Brain damage: Class 5

Understanding the Results

- Test results are available in 1 week. The laboratory determines normal values based on calibration of testing equipment with a control test. Test results are reported as high, normal, or low based on the laboratory's control test.
- Normal range: 0 mcg/dL
- Abnormal Class 1: 1 to 9 mcg/dL
- Abnormal Class 2A: 10 to 14 mcg/dL
- Abnormal Class 2B: 15 to 19 mcg/dL
- Abnormal Class 3: 20 to 44 mcg/dL
- Abnormal Class 4: 45 to 69 mcg/dL
- Abnormal Class 5: Greater than 69 mcg/dL

NURSING ALERT

The lack of overt symptoms does not mean that the person is not experiencing lead poisoning. The Centers for Disease Control considers children with a threshold blood lead level (BLL) of 5 mcg/dL as living in an environment that exposes the child to lead hazards requiring institutional follow-up. Businesses whose employees work with lead must test lead levels in their employees and provide the employee with documentation if lead level in their blood is 40 mcg/dL or greater as required by the United States Occupational Safety and Health Administration (OSHA) regulation. Employees with a level higher than 45 mcg/dL should be seen by their healthcare providers.

Teach the Patient

- Explain
  - Why blood sample is taken.
  - That multiple samples may be taken.
  - Why the healthcare provider must report certain results to the local health department.

21. Lipase

Lipase is an enzyme in the pancreas. Level of lipase in the blood increases when the pancreatic duct is blocked or there is damage to the pancreas. The lipase test measures the level of lipase in the blood.

NURSING ALERT

The lipase test does not diagnose pancreatic disorder. A high level of lipase in the blood requires additional testing. The healthcare provider may order the amylase test at the same time as the lipase test.

What Is Being Measured?

- Lipase level in blood

How Is the Test Performed?

- Avoid eating or drinking, except water, 12 hours before the test is administered.
- See "How to Collect Blood Specimen From a Vein" in Appendix A.

Rationale for the Test

- Screen for
  - Pancreatic disease
  - Pancreatitis
  - Cystic fibrosis
- Assess treatment for
  - Pancreatitis
  - Cystic fibrosis

Nursing Implications

- Assess if the patient has
  - Eaten or drunk, except water, 12 hours before the test is administered.
  - High cholesterol, varicose veins, kidney disease, diabetes, or high blood pressure.
  - Taken narcotics, anticoagulants, or cholinergics.

Understanding the Results

- The lipase test results are available in 12 hours. The laboratory determines normal values based on calibration of testing equipment with a control test. Test results are reported as high, normal, or low based on the laboratory's control test.
- Normal lipase test result: Less than 200 U/L
- High lipase levels may indicate
  - Pancreatic cancer
  - Pancreatitis
  - Pancreatic disease
  - Cholecystitis
  - Gallstones

- Bowel obstruction
- Infarction
- Chronic kidney disease
- Inflammation
- Infection
- Drug abuse
- Peptic ulcer

Teach the Patient

- Explain
- Why blood sample is taken.
- That the patient must not eat or drink, except water, for 12 hours before the test is administered.
- That the healthcare provider may ask the patient to refrain from taking narcotics, anticoagulants, or cholinergics 2 weeks before the test is administered.

22. Partial Thromboplastin Time

When bleeding occurs, 12 blood clotting factors cause blood to coagulate to stop the bleeding in a process called hemostasis. Coagulation of blood is affected by a cascade of blood clotting factors where one factor activates other factors. A clotting factor may be absent or have a decreased or increased level changing the way blood clotting factors function. In addition, clotting inhibitors such as heparin and warfarin can reduce the effectiveness of clotting factors. Thromboplastin is a plasma protein from platelets and damaged endothelium cells of blood vessels that converts prothrombin to thrombin. The partial thromboplastin time (PTT) test measures the clotting time of blood in the intrinsic coagulation pathway and the common coagulation pathway. Assessed are clotting factors I, II, V, VIII, IX, XI, and XII. PTT is used to assess the therapeutic level of heparin. PTT is called partial since the test does not measure the tissue factor.

> **NURSING ALERT**
>
> Another blood clotting test is prothrombin time (PT). The heparin neutralization assay is performed to determine if substances other than heparin cause an increase in PTT.

What Is Being Measured?

- The time necessary for blood to clot

How Is the Test Performed?

- The test may be performed frequently for patients who experience a clotting or bleeding problem. The test is also performed before invasive procedures and before surgery.
- The test is performed frequently for patients taking heparin until the healthcare provider determines the proper dosage for the patient.
- See Appendix A "How to Collect Blood Specimen."

Rationale for the Test

- Assess
  - The blood's ability to clot prior to any invasive procedure
  - For hemophilia
  - For lupus anticoagulant syndrome or antiphospholipid antibody syndrome caused when the antibodies attack blood clotting factors
  - The effectiveness of the dose of heparin administered to the patient (PPT test)

Nursing Implications

- Assess
  - Prescription and nonprescription medications taken by the patient. Some medications such as aspirin and antihistamines affect the results of the test.
  - Herbal and natural remedies taken by the patient because these remedies can affect the test results.
- A patient with a high PTT value is at risk for bleeding and bruising. Pressure must be applied to the injection site longer than for a patient with a normal PTT value.

Understanding the Results

- The result is available quickly. The laboratory determines normal values based on calibration of testing equipment with a control test. Test results are reported as high, normal, or low based on the laboratory's control test.

- Generally normal range is
  - PTT: 30 to 40 seconds.
  - Proper heparin dose: The PTT is 1.5 to 2.5 seconds greater than the normal value.
- Longer times may indicate
  - Hemophilia.
  - vonWillebrand disease.
  - A blood clotting factor is low or absent.
  - Nephrotic syndrome.
  - Cirrhosis.
  - Antiphospholipid antibody syndrome.
  - Lupus anticoagulant syndrome.
  - Factor XII deficiency.
  - Disseminated intravascular coagulation (DIC).
  - The patient has been administered heparin.
  - Hypofibrinogenemia.

NURSING ALERT

Patients who have inherited bleeding disorders such as Hemophilia B may have normal PTT values. Patients who experience serious bleeding problems when taking heparin are likely to be administered protamine sulfate by slow infusion.

Teach the Patient

- Explain
  - Why blood sample is taken.
  - Why samples may be taken frequently until the healthcare provider determines the therapeutic dose of heparin for the patient.
  - That taking aspirin, antihistamines, and herbal and natural remedies may affect the test result.

23. Prothrombin Time (PT)/INR

Prothrombin time (PT) measures the extrinsic coagulation pathway and assesses clotting factors I, II, V, VII, and X by calculating the prothrombin ratio with the international normalized ratio (INR). The INR is used to standardize the results of the prothrombin time disregarding the testing method. The PT test is used to assess the therapeutic levels of warfarin (Coumadin) monthly because warfarin (Coumadin) has a narrow therapeutic range. The PT test is used to assess vitamin K. Vitamin K is required to make clotting factors such as prothrombin.

> ### NURSING ALERT
>
> PT/INR is performed at the same time each day to assess that the patient is receiving the proper dose of warfarin (Coumadin). A home PT test is available for patients who must frequently undergo the test. Patients who experience serious bleeding problems when taking warfarin (Coumadin) are likely to be administered vitamin K or a combination of prothrombin complex concentrate (PCC) and fresh frozen plasma as an emergency treatment to stop bleeding. There are new medications such as apixaban (Eliquis); dabigatran (Pradaxa); edoxban (Savaysa); and rivaroxaban (Xarelto) that perform similar to warfarin (Coumadin) but do not have a narrow therapeutic range and therefore do not require regular dose adjustments based on blood tests.

What Is Being Measured?

- The time necessary for blood to clot

How Is the Test Performed?

- The test may be performed frequently for patients who experience a clotting or bleeding problem. The test is also performed before invasive procedures and before surgery.
- The test is performed frequently for patients taking warfarin (Coumadin) until the healthcare provider determines the proper dosage for the patient.
- See Appendix A "How to Collect Blood Specimen."

Rationale for the Test

- Assess
  - The blood's ability to clot prior to any invasive procedure
  - For reason for abnormal bruising or bleeding.
  - For liver function along with liver function tests. The liver produces clotting factors.
  - The effectiveness of the dose of warfarin (Coumadin) administered to the patient.

Nursing Implications

- Assess
  - Prescription and nonprescription medications taken by the patient. Some medications such as aspirin and antihistamines affect the results of the test.
  - Herbal and natural remedies taken by the patient because these remedies can affect the test results.
  - Eating foods that have a high vitamin K content that include soybean products, broccoli, kale and turnip greens, and drinking high volumes of alcohol may lead longer PT/INR results.
  - A patient with a high PT/INR value is at risk for bleeding and bruising. Pressure must be applied to the injection site longer than for a patient with a normal PT/INR values.
- Severe diarrhea or vomiting resulting in fluid loss and dehydration may lead to longer PT/INR time related to poor absorption of nutrients, vitamins, and minerals leading to decreased vitamin K absorption.

Understanding the Results

- The result is available quickly. The laboratory determines normal values based on calibration of testing equipment with a control test. Test results are reported as high, normal, or low based on the laboratory's control test.
- Generally normal range is
  - PT: 11 to 13 seconds.
  - INR: 0.8 to 1.1 seconds.

- Proper warfarin (Coumadin) dose: The PT is 1.5 to 2.5 seconds greater than the normal value and INR is 2 to 3 times greater than the normal value.
- Longer times may indicate
  - Lack of or low level of one or more clotting factors (I, II, V, VII or X).
  - Vitamin K deficient
  - Liver disease or injury.
  - Disseminated intravascular coagulation (DIC).
  - Disseminated intravascular coagulation (DIC).
  - The patient has been administered warfarin (Coumadin).

> **NURSING ALERT**
>
> Patients who have an artificial heart valve may be treated with warfarin (Coumadin) and have a long PT/INR time.

Teach the Patient

- Explain
  - Why blood sample is taken.
  - Why samples may be taken frequently until the healthcare provider determines the therapeutic dose of warfarin (Coumadin) for the patient.
  - That taking aspirin, antihistamines, and herbal and natural remedies may affect the test result.

24. Reticulocyte Count

Reticulocyte is an immature red blood cell that is released by bone marrow and develops into a mature red blood cell in 2 days. The reticulocyte count test determines the amount of reticulocyte in a blood sample.

> **NURSING ALERT**
>
> The healthcare provider may order the reticulocyte index (RI).

What Is Being Measured?

- The percentage of reticulocyte in blood

How Is the Test Performed?

- See Appendix A "How to Collect Blood Specimen."

Rationale for the Test

- Screen for anemia.
- Assess the treatment of anemia.

Nursing Implications

- Assess if the patient
  - Is undergoing radiation therapy
  - Is pregnant
  - Has had a blood transfusion in the previous week
  - Has undergone a prostate biopsy in the past 8 weeks
  - Is taking Bactrim, Septra, corticotrophin, Imuran, levodopa, Chloromycetin, methotrexate, or Cosmegen

Understanding the Results

- The reticulocyte test results are available in 1 day. The laboratory determines normal values based on calibration of testing equipment with a control test. Test results are reported as high, normal, or low based on the laboratory's control test.
- Normal test results: 0.5% to 2.5%
- Higher levels may indicate
  - Hemolysis.
  - Anemia.
  - The patient is being treated for anemia.
  - The patient is in a high altitude location.
  - The patient has been hemorrhaging.

- Low levels may indicate
  - Aplastic anemia
  - Iron deficiency anemia
  - Folic acid deficiency
  - Vitamin B_{12} deficiency
  - Radiation exposure
  - Bone marrow cancer

Teach the Patient

- Explain
  - Why the sample is taken.
  - That the healthcare provider may ask the patient to avoid taking Bactrim, Septra, corticotrophin, Imuran, levodopa, Chloromycetin, methotrexate, and Cosmegen before the test.

25. Schilling Test

Vitamin B_{12} is the key to cell metabolism and energy production. Vitamin B_{12} attaches to the intrinsic factor produced by the parietal cells in the stomach. The intrinsic factor protects vitamin B_{12} from intestinal bacteria and enables absorption of vitamin B_{12} by the intestines. The Schilling test measures the absorption of vitamin B_{12}. There are two parts to the Schilling test:

- Part 1: The patient ingests vitamin B_{12} that is radioactively tagged. A 24-hour urine sample is examined for the presence of vitamin B_{12}. Up to 25% of the ingested vitamin B_{12} will normally be detected in the 24-hour urine sample. Little or no vitamin B_{12} detected is a sign of vitamin B_{12} malabsorption.
- Part 2: If part 1 is abnormal, then the healthcare provider may order part 2. The patient ingests radioactively tagged vitamin B_{12} and the intrinsic factor. A 24-hour urine sample is examined for the presence of vitamin B_{12}. Detection of vitamin B_{12} is a sign that the patient has pernicious anemia. Absence of vitamin B_{12} is a sign of an intestinal absorption problem.

NURSING ALERT

The healthcare provider may order a 48- or 72-hour urine sample if the patient has kidney disease. The healthcare provider may also order the methylmalonic acid (MMA) test and the homocysteine test.

> **NURSING ALERT**
>
> The Schilling test is not performed on a pregnant woman or a woman who is breast-feeding.

What Is Being Measured?

- The presence of vitamin B_{12} in a 24-hour urine sample

How Is the Test Performed?

- Part 1
  - Avoid eating or drinking, except water, for 12 hours before the test is administered.
  - Avoid taking vitamin B_{12} supplements for 3 days before the test is administered.
  - Avoid taking laxatives for 24 hours before the test is administered.
  - The patient swallows a small capsule containing radioactively tagged vitamin B_{12}.
  - The patient receives an intramuscular (IM) injection of nonradioactive vitamin B_{12} 2 hours after ingesting the capsule. This prevents the radioactively tagged vitamin B_{12} from binding with tissues.
- Part 2 (within 7 days of part 1)
  - Avoid eating or drinking except water for 12 hours before the test is administered.
  - Avoid taking vitamin B_{12} supplements for 3 days before the test is administered.
  - Avoid taking laxatives for 24 hours before the test is administered.
  - The patient swallows a small capsule containing radioactively tagged vitamin B_{12} and the intrinsic factor.
  - The patient receives an IM injection of nonradioactive vitamin B_{12} 2 hours after ingesting the capsule. This prevents the radioactively tagged vitamin B_{12} from binding with tissues.

> ### NURSING ALERT
>
> The amount of radioactivity in the radioactive vitamin B_{12} capsule is very low and poses no risk.

> ### NURSING ALERT
>
> The patient may have an allergic reaction to radioactive vitamin B_{12}, but this is rare.

Rationale for the Test

- Screen for
  - Absorption of vitamin B_{12}
  - Production of the intrinsic factor

Nursing Implications

- Assess if the patient
  - Is pregnant
  - Properly collected the 24-hour urine sample
  - Is taking Mycitracin, Dilantin, or colchicine
  - Has kidney disease
  - Used a laxative prior to administration of the test
  - Has had a radioactive scan 2 weeks prior to the test

Understanding the Results

- The Schilling test results are available quickly. The laboratory determines normal values based on calibration of testing equipment with a control test. Test results are reported as high, normal, or low based on the laboratory's control test.
- Normal test results: 8% to 10% of vitamin B_{12} is found in urine.

- Lower levels may indicate
  - Part 1
    - Pernicious anemia
    - Celiac disease
    - Hypothyroidism
    - Cirrhosis
    - Hepatitis
  - Part 2
    - Celiac disease
    - Hypothyroidism
    - Cirrhosis
    - Hepatitis

Teach the Patient

- Explain
  - Why sample is taken.
  - That the patient will not feel any discomfort when ingesting the capsule.
  - That the radioactivity in the radioactive vitamin B_{12} is low and not dangerous.
  - And demonstrate how to take a 24-hour urine sample.
  - That the healthcare provider may ask the patient to refrain from taking Mycitracin, Dilantin, or colchicines prior to the test.

26. Sedimentation Rate

An increase in fibrinogen in blood during the inflammatory process causes erythrocytes (RBC) to adhere to each other, forming a stack called rouleaux. The sedimentation rate (SR) test measures how many millimeters per hour erythrocytes settle to the bottom of a test tube. Rouleaux settles quicker than erythrocytes, therefore the increased sedimentation rate indicates that the patient has inflammation.

> **NURSING ALERT**
>
> The healthcare provider might order other tests in addition to the SR test to diagnose inflammation. The healthcare provider might order the CRP test to determine if the patient has inflammation.

> **NURSING ALERT**
>
> Not all inflammation increases the SR, therefore a normal SR does not rule out inflammation.

What Is Being Measured?

- The SR test measures how many millimeters per hour erythrocytes settle to the bottom of a test tube.

How Is the Test Performed?

- See Appendix A "How to Collect Blood Specimen."

Rationale for the Test

- Screen for inflammation.
- Assess treatment of inflammation.

Nursing Implications

- Assess if the patient
  - Is pregnant
  - Has her menstrual period
  - Has anemia
- Note the patient's age, since SR increases with age.

Understanding the Results

- The SR test results are available quickly. The laboratory determines normal values based on calibration of testing equipment with a control test. Test results are reported as high, normal, or low based on the laboratory's control test.

- Normal test results
  - Men: 0 to 15 mm/h
  - Women: 0 to 20 mm/h
  - Children: 0 to 10 mm/h
  - Newborn: 0 to 2 mm/h
- Higher levels may indicate
  - Inflammation
  - Rheumatoid arthritis
  - Systemic lupus erythematosus
  - Appendicitis
  - Pneumonia
  - Chronic kidney disease
  - Lymphoma
  - Pelvic inflammatory disease
  - Graves disease
  - Giant cell arteritis
  - Polymyalgia rheumatica
  - Toxemia of pregnancy
- Lower levels may indicate
  - Sickle cell disease
  - Hyperglycemia
  - Polycythemia

Teach the Patient

- Explain
  - Why sample is taken.
  - That additional tests are necessary to diagnose inflammation.
  - That normal results do not rule out inflammation.

27. Serum Osmolality

Serum osmolality is the number of particles of substances that are dissolved in blood serum (liquid portion of blood). These substances include glucose, chloride, sodium, proteins, and bicarbonate. Serum osmolality should be within a normal range—a balance between fluid and particles of substances.

Serum osmolality is controlled adjusting the fluid output of the kidneys, using the antidiuretic hormone (ADH) produced by the pituitary gland. ADH is a vasopressin that reduces fluid output from the kidneys. Therefore, when ADH is released into the blood stream, it increases fluid in the blood. A decrease in ADH production increases fluid output by the kidneys and decreases fluid in the blood.

A decrease in fluid results in an increase in serum osmolality—there is less fluid in the blood. This signals the pituitary gland to release ADH, which stimulates the kidneys to retain fluid, thereby increasing fluid in the blood and decreasing serum osmolality—fluid level in the blood is restored.

An increase in fluid results in a decrease in serum osmolality—there is more fluid in the blood. This signals the pituitary gland to stop releasing ADH, which causes the kidneys to increase the output of fluid, thereby decreasing fluid in the blood and increasing serum osmolality—fluid level in the blood is restored.

NURSING ALERT

The healthcare provider may test urine osmolality. The result of the urine test is compared with the serum osmolality to estimate kidney function.

What Is Being Measured?

- Serum osmolality of blood

How Is the Test Performed?

- See Appendix A "How to Collect Blood Specimen."

Rationale for the Test

- Screen
  - For dehydration.
  - For overhydration.
  - The quantity of poison ingested by the patient.

- For the underlying cause of a seizure.
- For the underlying cause of a coma.
- The function of the hypothalamus. The hypothalamus signals the pituitary gland to release ADH.
- The presence of syndrome of inappropriate antidiuretic hormone (SIADH) secretion.

Nursing Implications

- Assess if the patient
  - Has ingested alcohol, since this can affect the test results
  - Recently received a blood transfusion

Understanding the Results

- Test results are available in 4 hours.
- Normal range: 280 to 300 mOsm/kg of water.
- High values may indicate
  - Buildup of urea in the blood
  - Poisoning
  - High level of salt in the blood
  - Diabetes insipidus (DI)
  - High level of glucose in the blood
  - Dehydration
- Low values may indicate
  - Lung cancer
  - Overproduction of ADH
  - Overhydration
  - Low salt level in the blood

Teach the Patient

- Explain
  - Why blood sample is taken.
  - Not to ingest alcohol 12 hours before the test is administered.

28. Serum Protein Electrophoresis

Blood serum contains two groups of protein. These are albumin and globulin. Serum protein electrophoresis (SPE) separates albumin and globulin into five groups by placing the sample of blood serum on an agarose gel, and then exposing the gel to an electric current. These groups are

- Albumin
- Alpha-1 globulin
- Alpha-2 globulin
- Beta globulin
- Gamma globulin (antibodies)

NURSING ALERT

The healthcare provider may order urine protein electrophoresis. The healthcare provider may also order total serum protein test along with the SPE test.

NURSING ALERT

Serum protein electrophoresis is not used to diagnose liver disorders, kidney disorders, or rheumatoid arthritis although abnormal protein level may be associated with these disorders.

What Is Being Measured?

- Albumin and globulin in blood

How Is the Test Performed?

- See Appendix A "How to Collect Blood Specimen."

Rationale for the Test

- Screen for
  - The underlying cause of hypogammaglobulinemia (HGG)
  - Amyloidosis
  - Multiple myeloma
  - Macroglobulinemia

Nursing Implications

- Assess if the patient
  - Has hyperlipidemia
  - Is pregnant
  - Has taken birth control pills, chlorpromazine, corticosteroids, aspirin, sulfonamides, neomycin, or isoniazid
  - Is undergoing chemotherapy

Understanding the Results

- The SPE test results are available in 3 days. The laboratory determines normal values based on calibration of testing equipment with a control test. Test results are reported as high, normal, or low based on the laboratory's control test.
- Normal test results
  - Albumin: 58% to 74%
  - Alpha-1 globulin: 2% to 3.5%
  - Alpha-2 globulin: 5.4% to 10.6%
  - Beta globulin: 7% to 14%
  - Gamma globulin: 8% to 18%
- High level may indicate
  - Leukemia
  - Multiple myeloma
  - Lymphoma
  - Rheumatoid arthritis
  - Liver disease
  - Systemic lupus erythematosus
  - Pregnancy
  - Dehydration
  - Infection
  - Kidney disease
  - Heart disease
- Low level may indicate
  - Leukemia
  - Multiple myeloma

- Lymphoma
- Rheumatoid arthritis
- Liver disease
- Systemic lupus erythematosus
- Pregnancy
- Dehydration
- Infection
- Kidney disease
- Heart disease
- Hypothyroidism
- Burns
- Emphysema
- Celiac disease
- Crohn disease
- Malnutrition

Teach the Patient

- Explain
  - Why the sample is taken.
  - That the sample must be taken in the morning.
  - That the healthcare provider may ask the patient to refrain from taking birth control pills, chlorpromazine, corticosteroids, aspirin, sulfonamides, neomycin, or isoniazid prior to the test.

29. Total Serum Protein

The total serum protein test assesses the levels of albumin, globulin, and total protein in a blood sample. The result compares the ratio of albumin to globulin. Protein is not stored. It is continuously metabolized into amino acids, which are used to make enzymes, hormones, and new proteins.

- Albumin is a protein produced by the liver and resides in blood plasma that keeps blood from leaking from blood vessels by regulating colloidal osmotic pressure of blood. Albumin is also important for tissue growth and healing because it carries water, sodium, potassium, calcium, hormones, fatty acids; bilirubin, thyroxine and medicine to tissues.

- Globulin is a group of proteins made by the liver and the immune system that binds with hemoglobin and transports iron and metals in the blood to help fight infection. Globulin is composed of three different proteins: alpha, beta, and gamma. Alpha globulins inhibit an enzyme that digests protein and an enzyme that is involved in coagulation. As a result more protein is available to the body and blood can freely distribute globulins throughout the body. Beta globulin binds with iron and transports iron throughout the body and is involved in targeting foreign material so the foreign material can be destructed by the immune system. Both alpha and beta globulin increase when there is inflammation in the body. Gamma globulins are antibodies called immunoglobulins and consist of IgG antibodies to bacteria and viruses; IgE protects against parasites and triggers the histamine response to allergens; IgM is the first response to infection; IgD function is not understood; and IgA protects body surface and found in mucous membranes; blood, saliva, and tears.

A test for total serum protein reports separate values for total protein, albumin, and globulin. The amounts of albumin and globulin are also compared (albumin/globulin ratio).

What Is Being Measured?

- Total protein in the blood sample particularly albumin and globulin

How Is the Test Performed?

- See Appendix A "How to Collect Blood Specimen."

Rationale for the Test

- Screen for
  - Liver and kidney functions (albumin)
  - Malnutrition (albumin)
  - Cause of edema, ascites, and pulmonary edema (albumin)
  - Risk of infection (globulin)
  - Multiple myeloma (globulin)
  - Macroglobulinemia (globulin)

Nursing Implications

- Assess if the patient
  - Is taking androgens (male sex hormones), estrogen, corticosteroids, insulin, and growth hormone, which can affect the test results
  - Has a chronic illness that interferes with nutrition
  - Has any recent injuries or infections
  - Is pregnant
  - Has been on extended bed rest

Understanding the Results

- Test results are available in 12 hours. The laboratory determines normal values based on calibration of testing equipment with a control test. Test results are reported as high, normal, or low based on the laboratory's control test.
- The healthcare provider will likely order a serum protein electrophoresis if there are abnormal globulin levels.
- Generally the normal range is
  - Total protein: 5.5 to 9.0 g/dL
  - Albumin: 3.5 to 5.5 g/dL
  - Globulin: 2.0 to 3.5 g/dL
  - Albumin/globulin ratio: Greater than 1.0
- High albumin levels may indicate
  - Severe dehydration
- High globulin levels may indicate
  - Liver disease
  - Kidney disease
  - Hodgkin lymphoma
  - Leukemia
  - Hemolytic anemia
  - Macroglobulinemia
  - Rheumatoid arthritis
  - Lupus

- Sarcoidosis
- Autoimmune hepatitis
- Tuberculosis
- Low albumin levels may indicate
- Malnutrition
- Kidney disease
- Liver disease
- Uncontrolled diabetes
- Hodgkin lymphoma
- Severe burns
- Systemic lupus erythematosus (SLE)
- Rheumatoid arthritis
- Heart failure
- Hyperthyroidism
- Crohn disease
- Celiac disease
- A ratio less than 1 indicates abnormal function in the body.

NURSING ALERT

Liver damage reduces the protein level in blood, but this level may not be reduced for 2 weeks after the damage because protein stays in blood for up to 18 days.

Teach the Patient

- Explain
- Why the blood sample is taken.
- The function of albumin and globulin and the meaning of abnormal values.

30. Toxicology Tests (Tox Screen)

A toxin is a substance that disrupts the body's function and includes prescription medication, nonprescription medication, and illegal medication. Toxicology tests measure the levels of one or up to 30 different drugs toxins in a blood sample. A toxicology test typically identifies if the drug is present but not the level of the drug. Furthermore, the toxicology test does not identify specific medications. For example, a toxicology test may detect a high level of opioids. Further testing is required to determine the source of the opioid (i.e., Dilaudid, Demerol, Vicodin, methadone).

> **NURSING ALERT**
>
> The healthcare provider may order a urine toxicology test because traces of toxins can remain in urine longer than in blood. The healthcare provider may order a saliva toxicology test.

What Is Being Measured?

- Toxin level in the blood

How Is the Test Performed?

- See Appendix A "How to Collect Blood Specimen."

Rationale for the Test

- Screen for
  - The underlying cause of the patient's unusual behavior
  - The underlying cause why the patient is unconscious
  - Use of medication (toxin)

Nursing Implications

- Ask the patient to sign a consent form before administering the test unless the patient is incapacitated and unable to provide written consent.
- Ask the patient to list medications, vitamins, and herbal supplements that have been taken in the previous 4 days prior to the test.
- Assess if the patient has
  - Taken cough medicine in the previous 4 days
  - Eaten poppy seeds in the previous 4 days
- The chain of custody must be adhered to if the patient is suspected of drug abuse. Each person who handles the blood sample maintains the chain of

custody by signing the chain of custody document. The chain of custody document must be attached to the test result.

- Note on the specimen the time when the blood sample is taken.

Understanding the Results

- Test results are available quickly.
- Normal toxin range: 0 except for therapeutic levels of medication taken by the patient.
- Abnormal toxin range: Greater than 0 or higher than the therapeutic levels of medication taken by the patient.

NURSING ALERT

The healthcare provider may order a quantitative toxicology test to determine the level of toxin in the blood sample if the toxicology test is positive.

NURSING ALERT

A positive test result must be confirmed by two or more testing methods to rule out a false positive result.

Teach the Patient

- Explain
  - Why blood sample is taken.
  - That the patient must provide written consent otherwise the toxicology test cannot be administered unless the patient is incapacitated and unable to provide written consent.
  - That patient should identify any medication, vitamins, herbal supplements, cough medicine, and poppy seeds that have been taken in the previous 4 days.

31. Uric Acid in Blood

Some foods contain purine. Uric acid is produced when purine found in wine, beer, liver, anchovies, mackerel, and dried beans is metabolized. Purine is also created as a result of normal breakdown of cells. Uric acid is excreted by the kidneys through the urine and a small amount in stool. The uric acid test measures the level of uric acid in the blood.

> **NURSING ALERT**
>
> The healthcare provider may order a 24-hour uric acid urine test.

What Is Being Measured?

- Uric acid level in blood

How Is the Test Performed?

- See Appendix A "How to Collect Blood Specimen."

Rationale for the Test

- Screen for
  - Uric acid kidney stones
  - Gout
  - Adverse reaction of radiation therapy and chemotherapy
- Assess treatment of hyperuricemia.

Nursing Implications

- Assess
  - The patient for starvation, strenuous exercise, and a high-protein diet, since these can raise the level of uric acid
  - If the patient is taking aspirin, theophylline, diuretics, niacin, caffeine, vitamin C, ascorbic acid, epinephrine, levodopa, warfarin, diazoxide, cisplatin, cyclosporine nicotinic acid, phenothiazines, tacrolimus, methyldopa, or ethambutol, which can affect the test results
  - If the patient is pregnant, since uric acid level can increase during pregnancy that assists the healthcare provider in diagnosing preeclampsia
  - If the patient has eaten liver, red meats, game meat, herring, sardines, scallops, or beer

- Uric acid levels are higher in the morning and lower in the evening, therefore note the time when the test is administered.

Understanding the Results

- Test results are available in 2 days. The laboratory determines normal values based on calibration of testing equipment with a control test. Test results are reported as high, normal, or low based on the laboratory's control test.
- Normal uric acid range is
  - Men: 3.4 to 7.0 mg/dL
  - Women: 2.4 to 6.0 mg/dL
  - Children: 2.5 to 5.5 mg/dL
- High uric acid values may indicate
  - Kidney disease
  - Multiple myeloma
  - Lymphoma
  - Hemolytic anemia
  - Heart failure
  - Leukemia
  - Sickle cell anemia
  - Preeclampsia
  - Cirrhosis
  - Alcohol abuse
  - Hypoparathyroidism
  - Hypothyroidism
  - Starvation
  - Lead poisoning
  - Malnutrition
  - Psoriasis
  - Lesch-Nyhan syndrome
  - Obesity
  - High-purine diet

- Low uric acid values may indicate
  - Low-protein diet
  - SIADH
  - Wilson disease
  - Cancer
  - Liver disease
  - Taking Aloprim, Zyloprim, Benemid, and Probalan, sulfinpyrazone, 1,500 mg or more aspirin each day

Teach the Patient

- Explain
- Why blood sample is taken.
- That the patient should avoid eating liver, red meat, game meat, herring, sardines, scallops, and beer for 24 hours before the test is administered.
- That the healthcare provider may ask the patient to stop taking the following for 2 weeks: aspirin, theophylline, diuretics, niacin, caffeine, vitamin C, ascorbic acid, epinephrine, levodopa, warfarin, diazoxide, cisplatin, cyclosporine, nicotinic acid, phenothiazines, tacrolimus, methyldopa, or ethambutol.

NURSING ALERT

Uric acid crystals can form in joints leading to gout even when uric acid levels are normal. A high level of uric acid does not mean that the patient has gout. Gout is diagnosed by testing fluid from the affected join for uric acid crystals.

32. Vitamin B$_{12}$

Vitamin B$_{12}$ is a water-soluble vitamin that can be stored in the liver. Excess vitamin B$_{12}$ is excreted through urine. Vitamin B$_{12}$ is used to metabolize protein; assists in formation of red blood cells and maintains the central nervous system. The vitamin B$_{12}$ test measures the level of vitamin B$_{12}$ in a blood sample.

> **NURSING ALERT**
>
> The healthcare provider may order the folic acid test along with the vitamin B_{12} test. The healthcare provider may order a Schilling test to assess the patient's ability to absorb vitamin B_{12}.

What Is Being Measured?

- Vitamin B_{12} level in the blood

How Is the Test Performed?

- See Appendix A "How to Collect Blood Specimen."

Rationale for the Test

- Screen for
  - The underlying cause of anemia, peripheral neuropathy, and dementia
  - Vitamin B_{12} deficiency

Nursing Implications

- Assess if the patient
- Has eaten or drunk 12 hours before the test is administered
- Has taken vitamin C
- Is pregnant
- Is breast-feeding
- Has been diagnosed with pernicious anemia
- Has undergone dye testing less than a week prior to the test
- Has taken birth control pills, Prilosec, neomycin, Dilantin, Protonix, Glucophage, Prevacid, colchicines, para-aminosalicylic acid, rabeprazole, triamterene, or methotrexate

Understanding the Results

- Test results are available quickly. The laboratory determines normal values based on calibration of testing equipment with a control test. Test results are reported as high, normal, or low based on the laboratory's control test.

- Normal vitamin B_{12} range: 160 to 950 pg/mL
- High values of vitamin B_{12} may indicate
  - Hepatitis
  - Cirrhosis
  - Leukemia
- Low values of vitamin B_{12} may indicate
  - Folic acid deficiency anemia
  - Pernicious anemia
  - Hyperthyroidism
  - Fish tapeworm infection
  - Multiple myeloma

Teach the Patient

- Explain
- Why the blood sample is taken.
- Not to eat or drink 12 hours before the test.
- That the healthcare provider may request that the patient stop taking birth control pills, Prilosec, neomycin, Dilantin, Protonix, Glucophage, Prevacid, colchicines, para-aminosalicylic acid, rabeprazole, triamterene, vitamin C, or methotrexate for 2 weeks prior to the test.

Summary

Hematology clinical laboratory tests examine blood and its components to assess for signs of disease. A sample of blood can be collected from a vein, a finger, or from the heel, depending on the amount of the blood sample that is required for the test.

The clinical laboratory then measures the sample and compares the results to a range of values that the clinical laboratory has determined to be normal. For many hematology tests, the clinical laboratory sets the normal range daily. The results contain the measured value of the sample, the clinical laboratory's normal range, and an indicator if the sample is higher or lower than the range. A test result that is outside the normal range is assessed by the healthcare provider to determine if it is a significant sign of a disease.

The pancreas secretes insulin and glucagon based on the level of glucose in the blood. A high level of blood glucose signals the pancreas to secrete insulin, which assists glucose to cross cell membranes where glucose is used for energy.

A low level of blood glucose causes the pancreas to secrete glucagon. Glucagon is a hormone that signals the liver, muscles, and other organs to release stored glucose into the blood, resulting in an increase in blood glucose levels. The balance between insulin and glucagon secretions maintains a narrow range of blood glucose. However, diseases such as diabetes can cause an imbalance, resulting in high levels of blood glucose (hyperglycemia) or lower levels of blood glucose (hypoglycemia) that cannot be brought into range naturally. Glucose tests are used by healthcare providers to monitor a patient's blood glucose level to determine if the patient has a disease that affects insulin and/or glucagon. These tests are also used to monitor treatment of these diseases.

QUIZ

1. **What test is ordered to screen for malabsorption syndrome?**
   A. D-xylose absorption test
   B. Fasting blood glucose (FBG) test
   C. Two-hour postprandial blood sugar test
   D. Oral glucose tolerance test (OGTT)

2. **What should you do if the patient ate breakfast before fasting blood glucose (FBG) test?**
   A. Postpone the test for 1 month.
   B. Administer the test. Estimate the sugar content of the breakfast and subtract that amount from the test results.
   C. Reschedule the test after 2 weeks.
   D. Postpone the test for at least 8 hours.

3. **What test is used to differentiate between Type 1 and Type 2 diabetes?**
   A. C-peptide
   B. Two-hour postprandial blood sugar test
   C. Fasting blood glucose (FBG) test
   D. Random blood glucose test

4. **Why is C-reactive protein (CRP) test used to test for inflammation?**
   A. C-reactive protein is leaked from damaged cells shortly after cells are injured increasing the amount of C-reactive protein in blood.

B. A low level of C-reactive protein indicates that the liver is responding to reduce the inflammation process.

C. C-reactive protein attaches to damaged cells or microorganism enhancing phagocytosis in the destruction of the microorganism or damaged cell shortly after cells are injured.

D. C-reactive protein attaches to the liver causing an increase of white blood cells in blood to enhance phagocytosis in the destruction of the microorganism or damaged cell shortly after cells are injured.

5. **What might be suspected if the patient has increase leukocyte count but no signs of infection?**

   A. Polycythemia

   B. Risk of bleeding

   C. Anemia

   D. Leukemia

6. **A low level of folic acid may indicate**

   A. Malabsorption

   B. Malnutrition

   C. Treatment of folic acid deficiency

   D. All of the above

7. **A patient arrives for a gastrin level test and tells you he is feeling better since taken Prilosec this morning. What should you do?**

   A. Reschedule the test and tell the patient to refrain from taking Prilosec 12 hour before coming for the test.

   B. Continue with the test.

   C. Ask the patient to rest 30 minutes before the test.

   D. Refrain from drinking water 1 hour before the test is administered.

8. **Why would a practitioner order the total iron-binding capacity (TIBC) test?**

   A. To measure the amount of circulating iron in the blood.

   B. To measure the capacity of blood to carry iron.

   C. To assess the amount of vitamin B_{12} supplements taken by the patient.

   D. To determine if the patient has been taken St. John's wort.

9. **Why would a practitioner order an INR test?**

   A. To assess the volume of blood in the body.

   B. To assess the therapeutic level of heparin.

   C. The INR is used to standardize the results of the prothrombin time disregarding the testing method.

   D. To assess the dose of a vasopressin.

10. **Why is the Shilling test ordered?**
    A. To assess the absorption of vitamin B_{12}.
    B. Screen for pregnancy.
    C. To assess the vitamin B_6 level.
    D. To assess the vitamin folic acid level.

ANSWERS

1. A. D-xylose absorption test.
2. D. Postpone the test for at least 8 hours.
3. A. C-peptide.
4. C. C-reactive protein attaches to damaged cells or microorganism enhancing phagocytosis in the destruction of the microorganism or damaged cell shortly after cells are injured.
5. D. Leukemia.
6. D. All of the above.
7. A. Reschedule the test and tell the patient to refrain from taking Prilosec 12 hour before coming for the test.
8. B. To measure the capacity of blood to carry iron.
9. C. The INR is used to standardize the results of the prothrombin time disregarding the testing method.
10. A. To assess the absorption of vitamin B_{12}.

chapter 3

Electrolytes

Electrolytes are chemicals that help to generate an electrical impulse that contracts muscles, move fluids within the body, maintain stability of cells, and enables cells to generate an electrical charge. The concentration of electrolytes within the body is on constant change and the balance is maintained by the kidneys. Cells in the kidney monitor the amount of sodium, potassium, and fluid in the bloodstream. Hormones from the kidneys (renin), adrenal gland (aldosterone), and the pituitary gland (antidiuretic hormone) are used to adjust the electrolytes balance.

There are six key electrolytes that are monitored by clinical laboratory tests. These are calcium (Ca), magnesium (Mg), phosphate [contained in phosphorus (P)], potassium (K), sodium (Na), and chloride (Cl). All of these must be in balance to ensure proper physiology.

Electrolyte tests are referred to as an electrolyte panel, basic metabolic panel, or comprehensive metabolic panel. An electrolyte panel measures only electrolytes in a sample of blood. Basic metabolic and comprehensive metabolic panels measure electrolytes and other components.

In this chapter you will learn how each electrolyte is tested.

1. Calcium

Calcium (Ca) is required for growth of bone and teeth and for muscle contraction and blood clotting. Nearly all calcium in the body is stored in bone with a minimum amount in blood. Calcium has a homeostasis relationship with phosphate. As calcium increases in blood, phosphate decreases and when phosphate increases in blood, calcium decreases.

The parathyroid keeps calcium and phosphate balanced. When there is too much phosphate (too little calcium) in blood, the parathyroid releases the parathyroid hormone (PTH) that stimulates osteoclast, breaking down bone to increase calcium level in blood. PTH also activates vitamin D to increase absorption of calcium in the gastrointestinal (GI) tract. Vitamin D is necessary for calcium absorption. And the kidneys retain calcium. Too much calcium in the blood causes the thyroid gland to release calcitonin, which moves calcium from blood to bone.

There are two kinds of calcium blood tests that are performed as part of a routine blood screening. The nonionized calcium test measures calcium attached to albumin in the blood. This test is affected by the amount of albumin in the blood. The ionized calcium test measures calcium not attached to albumin in the blood and therefore is not affected by the amount of albumin in the blood.

NURSING ALERT

Calcium is also measured in urine.

What Is Being Measured?

- Calcium level in the blood

How Is the Test Performed?

- See "How to Collect Blood Specimen From a Vein" in Appendix A.

Rationale for the Test

- Screen for
  - Parathyroid gland function
  - Kidney function
  - Kidney stones
  - Pancreatitis
  - Bone disease
  - Underlying cause:
    - Muscle spasms, depression, confusion, tingling around the mouth and fingers, and muscle cramping and twitching are caused by low calcium level in blood.

- Of an abnormal electrocardiographic (ECG) result.
- Nausea, vomiting, bone pain, lack of appetite, weakness, abdominal pain, and constipation and increased urination are caused by a high calcium level in blood.

NURSING ALERT

Symptoms appear only when calcium levels are either very high or very low.

NURSING ALERT

The blood calcium test is not used to diagnose osteoporosis. The bone mineral density test is used for this purpose.

Nursing Implications

- Assess if the patient has
- Taken milk, antacid, calcium salt, or calcium supplements 8 hours before administering the test, since this will affect the test result
- Eaten or drunk 12 hours before the test is administered
- Taken Diamox, estrogen, albuterol, corticosteroids, vitamin D, lithium, laxatives, aspirin, theophylline, or birth control pills, since these medications can affect the test result
- Has had a blood transfusion recently

Understanding the Results

- Test results are available quickly. The laboratory determines normal values based on calibration of testing equipment with a control test. Test results are reported as high, normal, or low based on the laboratory's control test.
- Normal range
  - Nonionized calcium in adults: 9.0 to 10.5 mg/dL or 2.25 to 2.75 mmol/L
  - Nonionized calcium in children: 7.6 to 10.8 mg/dL or 1.9 to 2.7 mmol/L
  - Ionized calcium in adults: 4.65 to 5.28 mg/dL

- High-level values may indicate
  - Hyperparathyroidism
  - Cancer metastasized to the bone
  - Kidney disease
  - That the patient has been on bed rest for a long period
  - Tuberculosis
  - Sarcoidosis
  - Addison disease
  - Dehydration
  - Hyperthyroidism
  - Paget disease
  - Chronic liver problems
  - Ingesting too much calcium, vitamin D, or vitamin A
  - Decreased phosphate blood level
- Low-level values may indicate
  - Hypoparathyroidism
  - Malabsorption syndrome
  - Pancreatitis
  - Hypoalbuminemia
  - Low magnesium
  - Kidney disease
  - Increasing phosphate blood level

NURSING ALERT

Calcium values are high in children who are growing. Calcium values are low in older men and pregnant women. If calcium levels in blood are abnormal, the healthcare provider may order additional tests for the parathyroid hormone, vitamin D, alkaline phosphatase, acid phosphatase, and chloride, which can affect the calcium levels in blood.

Teach the Patient

- Explain
  - Why the blood sample is taken.

- That the patient should not eat or drink 12 hours before the test is administered.
- That the healthcare provider may ask the patient to stop taking Diamox, estrogen, albuterol, corticosteroids, vitamin D, lithium, laxatives, aspirin, theophylline, or birth control pills 2 weeks before the test is administered, since these can affect the test result.

2. Magnesium

Magnesium (Mg), found mostly in bones and inside cells, is an electrolyte and is used to transfer potassium and sodium in and out of cells and to activate nerves, muscles, and enzymes. The magnesium blood test measures the level of magnesium in a blood sample and is tested along with other electrolytes.

> **NURSING ALERT**
>
> Levels of calcium and magnesium have an inverse relationship.

What Is Being Measured?

- Magnesium level in the blood

How Is the Test Performed?

- See "How to Collect Blood Specimen From a Vein" in Appendix A.

Rationale for the Test

- Screen for
  - Underlying cause of
    - Muscle weakness, muscle twitches, and muscle irritability
    - Arrhythmia
    - The source of nausea, vomiting, low blood pressure, and dizziness
  - The effects of medication that cause changes in the level of magnesium
  - The therapeutic treatment of high or low levels of magnesium

Nursing Implications

- Assess if the patient
  - Has taken antacids, laxatives, Milk of Magnesia, diuretics, Epsom salts, or magnesium supplements 3 days before administering the test, since these medications and supplements can affect the test result
  - Has taken insulin or antibiotics or received intravenous (IV) fluids before the test is administered
  - Is in the second or third trimester of pregnancy, since magnesium levels are normally low at this stage

Understanding the Results

- Test results are available quickly. The laboratory determines normal values based on calibration of testing equipment with a control test. Test results are reported as high, normal, or low based on the laboratory's control test.
- Normal range
  - Adults: 1.3 to 2.1 mEq/L
  - Children: 1.4 to 1.7 mEq/L
  - Newborn: 1.4 to 2 mEq/L
- High values may indicate
  - Hyperparathyroidism
  - Addison disease
  - Hypothyroidism
  - Dehydration
  - Kidney failure
  - Overmedication with antacids and laxatives that contain magnesium
- Low values may indicate
  - Diabetic ketoacidosis
  - Pancreatitis
  - Hypercalcemia
  - Kidney disease
  - Alcohol abuse
  - Alcohol withdrawal

- Sprue
- Preeclampsia
- Hyperthyroidism
- Hypoparathyroidism
- Burns
- Starvation
- Insufficient ingestion of magnesium
- Diarrhea

Teach the Patient

- Explain
- Why the blood sample is taken.
- Not to take antacids, laxatives, Milk of Magnesia, diuretics, Epsom salts, or magnesium supplements 3 days before administering the test, since these medications can affect the test results

3. Phosphate

Phosphorus (P) is a mineral that contains a particle called phosphate, which is necessary for growth of bones and teeth and for contracting muscles. Most phosphate is in bone. Phosphate and calcium have an inverse relationship. The phosphate test measures the level of phosphate in blood.

> **NURSING ALERT**
>
> Phosphate is measured along with other electrolytes.

What Is Being Measured?

- Phosphate level in blood

How Is the Test Performed?

- See "How to Collect Blood Specimen From a Vein" in Appendix A.
- See "How to Collect Blood Specimen From a Heel Stick" in Appendix A.

Rationale for the Test

- Screen for
  - Bone disease
  - Kidney disease
  - Parathyroid glands function

Nursing Implications

- Assess if the patient has
  - Ingested alcohol, since this can affect the test results
  - Taken vitamin D supplements, antacids, insulin, epinephrine, acetazolamide, anabolic steroids, or phosphate-based enemas
  - Diabetes insipidus (DI)
  - Lymphoma
  - Type 2 diabetes

Understanding the Results

- Test results are available in 2 hours. The laboratory determines normal values based on calibration of testing equipment with a control test. Test results are reported as high, normal, or low based on the laboratory's control test.
- Normal range
  - Adults: 3.0 to 4.5 mg/dL or 0.97 to 1.45 mmol/L
  - Children: 4.5 to 6.5 mg/dL or 1.45 to 2.1 mmol/L
  - Children younger than 1 year of age: 4.3 to 9.3 mg/dL or 1.4 to 3 mmol/L
- Low values may indicate
  - Overuse of diuretics
  - Malnutrition
  - Hyperparathyroidism
  - Hypokalemia
  - After treatment diabetic ketoacidosis
  - Rickets
  - Excess vitamin D

- Hypothyroidism
- Alcoholism
- Severe burns
- High values may indicate
  - Kidney failure
  - Liver disease
  - Hypoparathyroidism
  - Increase intake of phosphate supplements
  - Before treatment diabetic ketoacidosis

Teach the Patient

- Explain
  - Why the blood sample is taken.
  - Not to ingest alcohol 12 hours before the test is administered.
  - That the healthcare provider may ask the patient to stop taking vitamin D supplements, antacids, epinephrine, acetazolamide, anabolic steroids, or phosphate-based enemas 2 weeks prior to the test.

4. Potassium

Potassium (K) is a mineral stored inside the cell that has multiple functions, including muscle contractions, neural transmission, and fluid balance. Potassium is excreted by the kidneys, regulated by aldosterone hormone, and released by the adrenal glands. Potassium and sodium have an inverse relationship. The potassium test measures the level of potassium in blood.

> ### NURSING ALERT
>
> Potassium is measured along with other electrolytes. The healthcare provider may order a urinalysis to determine the level of potassium that is being excreted by the kidneys.

What Is Being Measured?

- Potassium level in blood

How Is the Test Performed?

- See "How to Collect Blood Specimen" from Appendix A.

Rationale for the Test

- Screen for tumor lysis syndrome.
- Assess the
  - Effects of total parenteral nutrition (TPN) being administered to the patient
  - Adverse effect of diuretics, which can decrease potassium levels
  - Source of high blood pressure
  - Effect of kidney dialysis

Nursing Implications

- Assess if the patient has
- Taken potassium supplements
- Taken heparin, glucose, nonsteroidal anti-inflammatory drugs (NSAIDs), and antibiotics that contain potassium, natural licorice, corticosteroids, angiotensin-converting enzyme (ACE) inhibitors, or insulin
- Experienced severe vomiting
- Improperly used laxatives

Understanding the Results

- Test results are available quickly. The laboratory determines normal values based on calibration of testing equipment with a control test. Test results are reported as high, normal, or low based on the laboratory's control test.
- Normal range
  - Adults: 3.5 to 5.0 mEq/L
  - Children: 3.4 to 4.7 mEq/L
  - Children younger than 1 year of age: 3.9 to 5.3 mEq/L
- High values may indicate
  - Myocardial infarction
  - Ingestion of too many potassium supplements
  - Intake of ACE inhibitors

- Diabetic ketoacidosis
- Kidney damage
- Low values may indicate
  - Alcoholism
  - Cystic fibrosis
  - Diarrhea
  - Hyperaldosteronism
  - Use of diuretics
  - Bartter syndrome
  - Vomiting
  - Burns
  - Malnutrition
  - Dehydration

Teach the Patient

- Explain
  - Why the blood sample is taken.
  - That the healthcare provider may ask the patient to stop taking for 2 weeks heparin, glucose, NSAIDs, and antibiotics that contain potassium, natural licorice, corticosteroids, or ACE inhibitors.

5. Sodium

Sodium (Na) is a mineral stored outside the cell in blood and lymph fluid that has multiple functions, including muscle contractions, neural transmission, and fluid balance. Sodium is excreted by the kidneys, regulated by aldosterone hormone, and released by the adrenal glands. Sodium and potassium have an inverse relationship. The sodium test measures the level of sodium in blood.

NURSING ALERT

Sodium is measured along with other electrolytes. The healthcare provider may order a fractional excretion of sodium (FENa) urine test to determine the amount of sodium and creatinine in the urine.

What Is Being Measured?

- Sodium level in blood

How Is the Test Performed?

- See "How to Collect Blood Specimen From a Vein" in Appendix A.

Rationale for the Test

- Screen for
  - Adrenal gland diseases
  - Electrolyte balance
  - Water balance
  - Kidney disease

Nursing Implications

- Assess if the patient has
  - Elevated protein levels
  - Received IV fluid containing sodium
  - High triglyceride levels
  - Heparin, birth control pills, NSAIDs, antibiotics, tricyclic antidepressants (TCAs), corticosteroids, lithium, or estrogen

Understanding the Results

- Test results are available quickly. The laboratory determines normal values based on calibration of testing equipment with a control test. Test results are reported as high, normal, or low based on the laboratory's control test.
- Normal range: 136 to 145 mEq/L
- High values may indicate
  - Diabetic ketoacidosis
  - Cushing syndrome
  - Dehydration

- Kidney disease
- Diabetes insipidus
- High sodium intake
- Vomiting
- Diarrhea
- Hyperaldosteronism
- Low values may indicate
  - Psychogenic polydipsia (drinking too much water)
  - Heart failure
  - Vomiting
  - Diarrhea
  - Burns
  - Syndrome of inappropriate antidiuretic hormone (SIADH) secretion
  - Cirrhosis
  - Malnutrition
  - Kidney disease

Teach the Patient

- Explain
  - Why the blood sample is taken.
  - That the healthcare provider may ask the patient to stop taking heparin, birth control pills, NSAIDs, antibiotics, TCAs, corticosteroids, lithium, or estrogen for 2 weeks.

6. Chloride

Chloride (Cl) is an electrolyte found outside the cell and is involved in fluid balance. The chloride test measures the level of chloride in blood.

NURSING ALERT

The healthcare provider may order a chloride urine test or a skin sweat test. The healthcare provider will likely order the chloride test along with tests for other electrolytes.

What Is Being Measured?

- Chloride level in blood

How Is the Test Performed?

- See "How to Collect Blood Specimen From a Vein" in Appendix A.

Rationale for the Test

- Screen for the underlying cause of
  - Confusion, muscle spasm, muscle weakness, and difficulty breathing
  - Metabolic alkalosis
  - Kidney disorder
  - Adrenal gland disorder

Nursing Implications

- Assess if the patient
  - Is pregnant
  - Has taken Coumadin, aspirin, NSAIDs, corticosteroids, cholestyramine, diuretics, androgens, or estrogens
  - Is dehydrated or overhydrated

Understanding the Results

- The chloride test results are available quickly. The laboratory determines normal values based on calibration of testing equipment with a control test. Test results are reported as high, normal, or low based on the laboratory's control test.
- Normal test results
  - Adults: 98 to 106 mEq/L
  - Children: 90 to 110 mEq/L
  - Newborn: 96 to 106 mEq/L
  - Premature: 95 to 110 mEq/L
- Higher levels may indicate
  - Dehydration

- Anemia
- Kidney disease
- Hyperparathyroidism
- Ingestion of salt
- Lower levels may indicate
- Kidney failure
- Burns
- Cushing syndrome
- Heart failure
- Vomiting
- Diabetic ketoacidosis
- SIADH

Teach the Patient

- Explain
- Why the sample is taken.
- That the healthcare provider may ask the patient to refrain from taking Coumadin, aspirin, NSAIDs, corticosteroids, cholestyramine, diuretics, androgens, or estrogens prior to the test.

Summary

Electrical impulses within the body are conducted by electrically charged ions called electrolytes. The concentration of electrolytes must be within normal limits and are managed by the kidneys.

Diseases can cause one or more electrolytes to fall outside the normal range, resulting in signs and symptoms of the underlying disease. Healthcare providers order an electrolyte panel, a basic metabolic panel, or a comprehensive metabolic panel to measure a patient's electrolytes. These tests measure calcium, magnesium, phosphate, potassium, sodium, and chloride.

Knowing which electrolytes are outside the normal range enables the healthcare provider to compare the test results with other signs and symptoms to assist the healthcare provider in arriving at a medical diagnosis.

QUIZ

1. **What is the function of electrolytes?**

   A. Maintain blood flow across cell membranes

   B. Maintain voltage across cell membranes and carry electrical impulses within the body

   C. Balance leukocytes and erythrocytes

   D. Balance leukocytes and potassium

2. **A high level of calcium may indicate?**

   A. Addison disease

   B. Low magnesium

   C. Malabsorption syndrome

   D. Pancreatitis

3. **Why might a practitioner test for potassium levels?**

   A. The patient shows signs of arrhythmia

   B. The patient shows signs of muscle weakness

   C. The patient reports nausea and vomiting

   D. All of the above

4. **When the patient arrives in the morning for the metabolic panel, the patient states that she arrived home at three in the morning following a bachelorette party. How should you reply?**

   A. When did the party begin?

   B. When was the last time you drank alcohol?

   C. How much alcohol did you drink?

   D. Where was the party held?

5. **What should be asked of the patient if the patient has high level potassium?**

   A. Do you have a bacterial infection?

   B. Are you taking potassium supplements?

   C. Do you usually have a high level of potassium?

   D. Are you pregnant?

6. **Potassium has an inverse relationship with**

   A. Sodium

   B. Magnesium

   C. Phosphate

   D. Chloride

7. **What regulates sodium?**
   A. Bone marrow
   B. Aldosterone hormone
   C. Leukocytes level
   D. Erythrocytes level

8. **What might influence the level of calcium?**
   A. Corticosteroids
   B. Estrogen
   C. Albuterol
   D. All of the above

9. **What is a function of magnesium?**
   A. It is used to transfer potassium and sodium in and out of cells.
   B. It is used in deactivating nerves.
   C. It is used to relax the patient.
   D. It is used to balance the leukocytes and erythrocytes.

10. **Why would phosphate levels be normally higher in children?**
   A. Bones are actively growing.
   B. Children have more energy than adults.
   C. Children are more likely to be injured than adults.
   D. Children rarely eat a balanced diet.

ANSWERS

1. B. Maintain voltage across cell membranes and carry electrical impulses within the body.
2. A. Addison disease.
3. D. All of the above.
4. B. When was the last time you drank alcohol?
5. B. Are you taking potassium supplements?
6. A. Sodium.
7. B. Aldosterone hormone.
8. D. All of the above.
9. A. It is used to transfer potassium and sodium in and out of cells.
10. A. Bones are actively growing.

chapter 4

Arterial Blood Gases Test

KEY WORDS

Acidity range   Carboxyhemoglobin (COHb)
Arterial

Gas exchange in the alveoli and the network of capillaries in the walls of the lungs replaces carbon dioxide on hemoglobin in blood with oxygen. The arterial circulation system then distributes the oxygenated hemoglobin throughout the body. Disorders can lead to an ineffective gas exchange resulting in the pH of the patient's blood to fall outside the normal pH range of 7.35 to 7.45. The patient's blood may become acidosis or alkalosis.

Arterial blood gases test indicates how well the patient's lungs transfer oxygen and carbon dioxide to and from blood. Blood taken from an artery is analyzed to identify the concentration of oxygen, carbon dioxide, and bicarbonate in arterial blood. In addition, this test determines the pH value of the blood sample. The concentration of blood is altered through the body depending on the patient's condition. The body is able to compensate for these changes by adjusting the levels of acid and bicarbonate in the blood.

In this chapter you'll learn about arterial blood gases test and how these test results determine if the patient is experiencing metabolic disorders.

1.   Arterial Blood Gases

Blood contains oxygen and carbon dioxide. Measuring the partial pressure of these gases indicates how well lungs exchange oxygen and carbon dioxide. In addition, measuring the oxygen saturation of the blood indicates the amount of hemoglobin (Hgb) that is carrying oxygen, and measuring the oxygen content of blood indicates the amount of oxygen in the blood.

Blood must be within acidity range. Acidity is measured using the pH scale, which measures the hydrogen ions (H^+). The pH of blood must be between 7.35 and 7.45. If pH is less than 7.35, the blood is considered too acidic. If pH is greater than 7.45, the blood is too alkaline (basic). Bicarbonate (HCO_3^-) is a chemical in the blood that ensures that the blood remains within the acceptable pH range. If blood becomes too acidic, the amount of bicarbonate is increased by increasing the absorption of bicarbonate by the kidneys.

What Is Being Measured?

- Partial pressure of oxygen (Pao_2)
- Partial pressure of carbon dioxide ($Paco_2$)
- Oxygen saturation (O_2Sat)
- Oxygen content (O_2CT)
- Blood pH
- Bicarbonate (HCO_3^-)

How Is the Test Performed?

- See "How to Collect Blood Specimen From a Vein" in Appendix A.

Rationale for the Test

- Screen for
  - Gas exchange capabilities of the lungs
  - Effectiveness of treatment of lung disease
  - Blood acidity level
  - Effectiveness of treatment of an imbalance of blood acidity
  - Kidney function

Nursing Implications

- Assess whether the patient has been taking anticoagulants (aspirin, Coumadin, nonsteroidal anti-inflammatory drugs [NSAIDs]). Ask the patient if any over-the-counter (OTC) medications have been taken since some contain aspirin. The test can still be performed; however, coagulation time following the test may be longer than 10 minutes.
- Assess for allergies especially to anesthetics.
- Discontinue oxygen therapy 20 minutes before the test unless the patient is unable to breathe without oxygen therapy. This ensures that gas exchange measurement is based on room air without supplemental oxygen.

- Assess for following conditions that might affect the test and therefore may prevent the test from being performed:
  - Anemia
  - Polycythemia
  - Exposure to smoke (including second-hand smoke), paint removers, or carbon monoxide
  - Abnormally high or low body temperature

Understanding the Results

- Results are available quickly. The laboratory determines normal values based on calibration of testing equipment with a control test. Test results are reported as high, normal, or low based on the laboratory's control test.
- Generally normal ranges are
  - Partial pressure of oxygen (Pao_2): 75 to 100 mm Hg
  - Partial pressure of carbon dioxide ($Paco_2$): 34 to 45 mm Hg
  - Oxygen saturation (O_2Sat): 95% to 100% (means 95 to 100 mL per 100 mL of blood)
  - Oxygen content (O_2CT): 15% to 22% (means 15 to 22 mL per 100 mL of blood)
  - Blood pH: 7.35 to 7.45
  - Bicarbonate (HCO_3^-): 20 to 29 mEq/L or mmol/L
- High values can be a sign of
  - Chronic obstructive pulmonary disease (COPD)
  - Pulmonary edema
  - Cushing disease
  - Conn syndrome
  - Kidney failure
  - Sepsis
  - Dehydration
  - Drug overdose
  - Diabetes
  - The patient who is taking hydrocortisone, prednisone, or diuretics
- Low values can indicate
  - Liver disease (low bicarbonate)

- Aspirin overdose (low bicarbonate)
- Alcohol overdose (low bicarbonate)
- Severe malnutrition (low bicarbonate)
- Diarrhea (low bicarbonate)
- Dehydration (low bicarbonate)
- Hyperventilation (low bicarbonate)
- Kidney disease (low bicarbonate)
- Hyperthyroidism (low bicarbonate)
- Shock (low bicarbonate)
- Severe burns (low bicarbonate)

Teach the Patient

- Explain
- Why the blood sample is taken.
- The function of blood gases and the meaning of abnormal values.
- That pressure may be applied to the site for 10 minutes or more especially if the patient is taking anticoagulants.
- That oxygen therapy will be discontinued for 20 minutes before the test unless the patient is unable to breathe without oxygen therapy.

2. Total Carbon Dioxide

Carbon dioxide is a gaseous by-product of metabolism that is transported to the lungs where carbon dioxide is exhaled. Blood contains three forms of carbon dioxide. These are bicarbonate (HCO_3^-), carbonic acid (H_2CO_3), and dissolved carbon dioxide (CO_2). Most of the carbon dioxide is in the form of bicarbonate. Levels of these types of carbon dioxide are balanced by the lungs and kidneys. The total carbon dioxide test measures the level of all three types of carbon dioxide and is administered for the same amount of time as the arterial blood gas is administered.

NURSING ALERT

The total carbon dioxide test is part of the chemistry screen.

What Is Being Measured?

- Total carbon dioxide level in the blood

How Is the Test Performed?

- See "How to Collect Blood Specimen From a Vein" in Appendix A.

Rationale for the Test

- Assess
  - Lungs
  - Kidney function

Nursing Implications

- Assess if the patient
  - Has taken corticosteroids, antibiotics, antacids, diuretics, aspirin, sodium bicarbonate, or barbiturates
  - Has hyperthermia

Understanding the Results

- Test results are available quickly. The laboratory determines normal values based on calibration of testing equipment with a control test. Test results are reported as high, normal, or low based on the laboratory's control test.
- Normal range is
  - Adult: 23 to 29 mmol/L
  - Children: 20 to 28 mmol/L
  - Younger than 1 year old: 13 to 22 mmol/L
- High-level values may indicate
  - Vomiting
  - Pneumonia (respiratory acidosis)
  - COPD (respiratory acidosis)
  - Conn syndrome (metabolic acidosis)
  - Alcoholism (metabolic acidosis)
  - Cushing syndrome (metabolic acidosis)

- Low-level values may indicate
  - Hyperventilation (respiratory alkalosis)
  - Cirrhosis (respiratory alkalosis)
  - Liver failure (respiratory alkalosis)
  - Pneumonia (respiratory alkalosis)
  - Diabetes (metabolic alkalosis)
  - Aspirin overdose (metabolic alkalosis)
  - Diarrhea (metabolic alkalosis)
  - Heart failure (metabolic alkalosis)
  - Kidney failure (metabolic alkalosis)
  - Chronic starvation (metabolic alkalosis)
  - Ingestion of antifreeze (metabolic alkalosis)
  - Ingestion of methanol (metabolic alkalosis)

Teach the Patient

- Explain
- Why blood sample is taken.
- That the healthcare provider may ask the patient to stop taking for 2 weeks prior to the test corticosteroids, antibiotics, antacids, diuretics, aspirin, sodium bicarbonate, or barbiturates.

3. Carbon Monoxide

Carbon monoxide (CO) is a colorless, odorless gas that replaces oxygen attached to the hemoglobin (red blood cells), creating a compound called carboxyhemoglobin that decreases oxygenation of blood and can result in death. The carbon monoxide blood test measures the level of carboxyhemoglobin in blood.

What Is Being Measured?

- Carboxyhemoglobin level in the blood

How Is the Test Performed?

- See "How to Collect Blood Specimen From a Vein" in Appendix A.

Rationale for the Test

- Screen for
  - Exposure to breathing carbon monoxide
  - Underlying cause of headache, dizziness, vision problem, muscle weakness, confusion, extreme sleepiness, and nausea or vomiting which is caused by carbon monoxide

Nursing Implications

- Assess
  - If the patient has smoked before administering the test
  - If the patient has been exposed to carbon monoxide from automobiles and gas burning machine such as an old heating system
- Quick assessment
  - 20% to 30%
    - Nausea
    - Vomiting
    - Headache
    - Poor judgment
  - 30% to 40%
    - Vision problems
    - Dizziness
    - Confusion
    - Increasing heart rate (HR)
    - Increasing respiratory rate (RR)
    - Muscle weakness
  - 50% to 60%
    - Loss of consciousness
  - Greater than 60%
    - Seizures
    - Risk of death

Understanding the Results

- Test results are available right away. The laboratory determines normal values based on calibration of testing equipment with a control test.

Test results are reported as high, normal, or low based on the laboratory's control test.

- Normal range is
  - Nonsmoker: Less than 3% of total hemoglobin
  - Smoker: 2% to 10% of total hemoglobin
- High-level values may indicate carbon monoxide poisoning.

NURSING ALERT

Patients exposed to automobile traffic have normal carbon monoxide levels of 8% to 12%. A patient with 20% carbon monoxide level will show no symptoms of carbon monoxide poisoning. Women and children have fewer red blood cells than men and therefore have more severe symptoms at lower carbon monoxide levels. The healthcare provider will likely order arterial blood gases and complete blood count tests if carbon monoxide levels are high.

Teach the Patient

- Explain
  - Why the blood sample is taken.
  - That the patient must stop smoking before the test is administered.

Summary

The effective transfer of oxygen and carbon dioxide by the lungs is determined by the arterial blood gases tests. A sample of arterial blood is taken from the patient and is analyzed for the concentration of oxygen, carbon dioxide, bicarbonate, and pH value.

Based on the test results, the healthcare provider can assess gas exchange and the patient's metabolic status. If the blood sample is too acidic, the body compensates by removing carbon dioxide, which is an acid, and by retaining bicarbonate. If the blood sample is too alkaline, then the body retains carbon dioxide and removes bicarbonate. This is referred to as compensation where the body automatically makes adjustments to bring blood within an acceptable range.

QUIZ

1. **Why is hemoglobin important to arterial blood gases test?**

   A. Hemoglobin is used to measure the acidity of the blood that is used to calculate blood gases.

   B. Hemoglobin carries oxygen. A low level of hemoglobin may indicate a low blood oxygen level.

   C. Hemoglobin is used to measure the alkalinity of the blood that is used to calculate blood gases.

   D. Low hemoglobin indicates respiratory disease.

2. **Why should oxygen therapy be discontinued 20 minutes for the arterial blood gas test?**

   A. The test measures oxygen levels at room air.

   B. To determine if the patient has difficulty breathing.

   C. To make the patient more comfortable for the test.

   D. Supplemental oxygen will artificially decrease the results of the test.

3. **What is the potential risk if the patient is on aspirin therapy prior to drawing the arterial blood sample?**

   A. Inaccurate test results.

   B. The patient must take a baby aspirin following the test.

   C. Coagulation time may be longer than normal.

   D. The test should not be performed.

4. **What might a high level of carbon dioxide indicate?**

   A. Respiratory acidosis

   B. Metabolic acidosis

   C. Pneumonia

   D. All of the above

5. **How does carbon monoxide impede blood oxygenation?**

   A. Carbon monoxide can result in instant death.

   B. Carbon monoxide is a colorless, odorless gas.

   C. Carbon monoxide attaches to hemoglobin replacing oxygen.

   D. Carbon monoxide is irreversible.

6. **What can influence the test for carbon monoxide?**

   A. The patient smokes before taking the test.

   B. The patient refuses to take deep breaths before the test is administered.

   C. The patient takes shallow breaths before the test is administered.

   D. The patient vomits before the test.

7. **How long must pressure be applied to the blood sample site after the needle is removed from the patient who is not taking anticoagulation medication?**

    A. 3.5 minutes

    B. 1 minute

    C. 10 minutes

    D. 20 minutes

8. **Hyperventilation affects the arterial blood gas values and may result in which of the following?**

    A. Respiratory alkalosis

    B. Metabolic acidosis

    C. Metabolic alkalosis

    D. Respiratory acidosis

9. **Which of the following conditions would you expect to find in a patient who is diagnosed with alcoholism?**

    A. Respiratory alkalosis

    B. Metabolic alkalosis

    C. Metabolic acidosis

    D. Respiratory acidosis

10. **Bicarbonate is a form of**

    A. Carbon monoxide

    B. Oxygen

    C. Carbon dioxide

    D. Hemoglobin

ANSWERS

1. B. Hemoglobin carries oxygen. A low level of hemoglobin may indicate a low blood oxygen level.
2. A. The test measures oxygen levels at room air.
3. C. Coagulation time may be longer than normal.
4. D. All of the above.
5. C. Carbon monoxide attaches to hemoglobin replacing oxygen.
6. A. The patient smokes before taking the test.
7. C. 10 minutes.
8. A. Respiratory alkalosis.
9. C. Metabolic acidosis.
10. C. Carbon dioxide.

chapter 5

Liver Blood Tests

KEY WORDS

Conjugated bilirubin

Direct bilirubin

Gamma glutamyltransferase (GGT)

Gamma glutamyltranspeptidase

IgG anti-HAV

IgM anti-HAV

Indirect bilirubin

Lactulose

Serum glutamate oxaloacetatetrans-
aminase (SGOT)

Serum glutamate pyruvate transaminase (SGPT)

Total bilirubin

Unconjugated bilirubin

The liver detoxifies blood, produces clotting factors, and metabolizes medication and nutrients. The liver synthesizes albumin, which maintains blood volume and clotting factors, and synthesizes, stores, and metabolizes fatty acids and cholesterol. Fatty acids are used for energy by the body. The liver stores and metabolizes carbohydrates. Carbohydrates are converted into glucose for energy.

The liver forms and secretes bile. Bile contains acids that help the intestines absorb fats and vitamins A, D, E, and K, which are fat-soluble vitamins. In addition, the liver clears the body of medication and harmful chemicals, such as bilirubin, which is the result of the metabolism of aged red blood cells, and ammonia, which is the result of the metabolism of proteins. The liver transforms these chemicals into components that are easily excreted by the body in urine or stool.

The practitioner orders liver blood tests to assess if the liver is functioning normally. Liver blood tests measures liver enzymes in the blood. A liver enzyme is a catalyst that increases the speed of chemical reactions in liver cells. There is a high level of liver enzymes in the patient's blood if liver cells are destroyed by injury or disease.

In this chapter you will learn about blood tests that determine how well the liver is performing.

1. Hepatitis A Virus Test

A patient who is or has been infected with the hepatitis A virus (HAV) will have hepatitis A antibodies in his/her blood. A patient who received the HAV will also have these antibodies, indicating the effectiveness of the vaccine. There are two types of antibodies:

- IgM anti-HAV: Presence of this antibody indicates that the patient was recently infected. This antibody is detectable 2 weeks after being infected and remains in the blood for 3 to 12 months.
- IgG anti-HAV: Presence of this antibody indicates that the patient has at some point been infected. This antibody is detectable between 8 and 12 weeks following the infection and remains in the blood.

What Is Being Measured?

- The presence or absence of the IgM anti-HAV and IgG anti-HAV antibodies

How Is the Test Performed?

- See "How to Collect Blood Specimen From a Vein" in Appendix A.

Rationale for the Test

- Screen for
  - HAV infection
- Assess
  - The effectiveness of the hepatitis A vaccine
  - If the patient is protected against the hepatitis A vaccine
  - If the infection from hepatitis A is the source of abnormal liver function tests

Nursing Implications

- Assess
  - Whether the patient has been taking anticoagulants (aspirin, Coumadin, nonsteroidal anti-inflammatory drugs [NSAIDs]). Ask the patient if any over-the-counter medications have been taken since some contain aspirin. The test can still be performed; however, coagulation time following the test may be longer than 10 minutes.
  - If the vein is swollen after the test (phlebitis). If so, apply a warm compress several times a day.
- Consult the state's regulations to determine if cases of hepatitis A infection must be reported to the health department.

Understanding the Results

- Results are available in 5 to 7 days and reported as positive (the presence of the antibody) or negative (the antibody was not found in the blood sample).
- A negative test result does not mean that the patient is not infected with HAV. It can take 2 weeks or more before the antibodies are detectable. This is referred to as a false negative.
- A positive test result in the absence of the patient previously receiving the hepatitis A vaccine may be followed with liver function tests.

Teach the Patient

- Explain
  - Why the test is administered.
  - A negative test result does not mean that the patient is infection free. It takes 2 weeks or more to develop antibodies.
  - A positive test result indicates the presence of antibodies and not the presence of the HAV.

2. Hepatitis B Virus Tests

Hepatitis B is a virus that can cause an infection. There are several hepatitis B virus (HBV) tests used to determine if blood has signs of an HBV. There are three signs:

- HBV antibodies: HBV antibodies are produced as a part of the immune response to the presence of the HBV in the patient and may remain in the patient's blood long after the HBV is destroyed.
- HBV antigens: HBV antigens are markers created by the HBV when the HBV infects the patient.
- HBV DNA: HBV DNA is present when HBV infects the patient.

There are seven types of HBV tests:

- Hepatitis B surface antigen (HBsAg): This is the first test that detects HBV antigen even before symptoms are present. It is also used to detect if the patient will be an HBV carrier if the HBsAg level is elevated for more than 6 months.

- Hepatitis B surface antibody (HBsAb): This test detects HBV antibodies, which are elevated 4 weeks after HBsAg is no longer detectable, and is used to determine if the patient requires an HBV vaccination.

- Hepatitis B e-antigen (HBeAg): This test detects the HBeAg antigen, which is present if the patient is currently infected and is used to monitor HBV treatment.

- Hepatitis DNA test: This test determines the level of HBV DNA in the patient's blood and is used to monitor treatment of chronic HBV infection.

- Hepatitis B core antibody (HBcAb): This test detects the HBcAb antibody a month after the HBV infection and is used to screen transfused blood for hepatitis B.

- Hepatitis B core antibody IgM (HBcAbIgM): This test detects the HBcAbIgM antibody within 6 months of the patient becoming infected with HBV.

- Hepatitis B e-antibody (HBeAb): This test detects the HBeAb antibody, indicating that the patient has almost recovered from an acute HBV infection.

NURSING ALERT

The healthcare provider may also order tests for alanine aminotransferase (ALT), alkaline phosphatase (ALP), bilirubin, and aspartate aminotransferase (AST) to assess the patient's liver function.

What Is Being Measured?

- HBV antibody levels in blood
- HBV antigen levels in blood
- HBV DNA level in blood

How Is the Test Performed?

- See "How to Collect Blood Specimen From a Vein" in Appendix A.

Rationale for the Test

- Assess
  - For HBV infection
  - If transfused blood is or was infected with HBV
  - The effect of hepatitis B vaccination
  - The treatment of HBV

Nursing Implications

- A negative test result does not rule out HBV since signs of HBV can take weeks to develop.
- A patient who received an HBV vaccination may have HBsAb antibodies.
- A patient who received an HBV vaccination is protected against hepatitis D infection.

Understanding the Results

- HBV test results are available quickly.
- Normal HBV level is (negative): No presence of antigens, antibodies, or DNA.
- Abnormal HBV level is (positive): Antigens, antibodies, or DNA are present.

> **NURSING ALERT**
>
> Consult your local laws to determine if HBV infections must be reported to the health department.

Teach the Patient

- Explain why sample is taken.

3. Alanine Aminotransferase

Alanine aminotransferase (ALT), formerly called serum glutamate pyruvate transaminase (SGPT), is an enzyme mainly found in the liver, and is also in the heart, pancreas, muscles, and kidneys in small amounts. Damage to the liver caused by injury or disease results in the release of ALT in the blood. The ALT test measures the level of ALT in the blood as a way to detect liver disease. The ALT test is typically performed with the aspartate aminotransferase (AST) test to detect liver damage. Other tests that detect liver problems are the lactate dehydrogenase (LDH) test and the bilirubin test.

What Is Being Measured?

- The level of the ALT in the blood

How Is the Test Performed?

- See "How to Collect Blood Specimen From a Vein" in Appendix A.

Rationale for the Test

- Screen for liver disorder.
- Assess
  - The effects of medications that can cause liver damage
  - The underlying cause of jaundice

Nursing Implications

- Assess if the patient
  - Has performed strenuous exercise before the test is administered. Strenuous exercise can affect the test results.
  - Is pregnant. This can affect the test results.
  - Has taken Echinacea or valerian and other herbal and natural treatments. If so, the patient should refrain from taking these for several days before the test since they can affect the test results.
  - Is allergic to any medications.
  - Received any intramuscular (IM) injections, injured a muscle, cardiac catheterization, or surgery recently. These can release ALT from injured muscle and affect the results of the test.
- Identify prescription and nonprescription medications taken by the patient. Medications such as narcotics, barbiturates, antibiotics, chemotherapy, and statins affect the test results and should be stopped several days before taking the test.

Understanding the Results

- Test results are available in 12 hours. The laboratory determines normal values based on calibration of testing equipment with a control test. Test results are reported as high, normal, or low based on the laboratory's control test.
- Generally the normal range is 4 to 36 U/L or 0.07 to 0.62 microkat/L.
- Slightly high levels may indicate
  - Chronic diseases that affect the liver
  - Cirrhosis
  - Fat deposits in the liver
  - Medications such as narcotics, barbiturates, antibiotics, chemotherapy, and statins
- Moderately high levels may indicate
  - Excessive amounts of acetaminophen.
  - Alcohol abuse.
  - Mononucleosis.
  - Hepatitis.
  - Young child is growing quickly.
- Very high levels may indicate
  - Necrosis
  - Lead poisoning
  - Shock
  - Carbon tetrachloride exposure
  - Reaction to medication
  - Severe liver damage
  - Recent liver damage
  - Viral hepatitis
  - Rapid progression of acute lymphocytic leukemia (ALL) in a child

Teach the Patient

- Explain
  - Why blood sample is taken. ALT testing is part of routine blood screening.

- That the ALT enzyme can be abnormal for a number of reasons and therefore other tests are necessary to confirm an abnormal ALT test result.
- That the patient should make it known before the test is performed if the patient
  - Had strenuous exercise
  - Has taken narcotics, barbiturates, antibiotics, chemotherapy, and statins
  - Takes Echinacea or valerian and other herbal and natural treatments
  - Experienced anything that could cause a muscle injury such as IM injections, injured a muscle, cardiac catheterization, or surgery

4. Alkaline Phosphatase

Alkaline phosphatase (ALP) is an enzyme produced mainly in the liver and is also produced by bones, kidneys, intestines, and placenta. The ALP test measures the level of ALP in blood.

> **NURSING ALERT**
>
> An ALP isoenzymes test is likely to be ordered if the ALP level is high. The healthcare provider may order an ultrasound or CT scan. The gamma glutamyltransferase (GGT) test, 5-nucleotidase, or the gamma glutamyltranspeptidase test might be ordered if the ALP level is high to differentiate between bone ALP and liver ALP.

What Is Being Measured?

- ALP level in blood

How Is the Test Performed?

- See "How to Collect Blood Specimen From a Vein" in Appendix A.

Rationale for the Test

- Screen for
- Liver disease

- Side effects of medication on liver
- Rickets
- Osteomalacia
- Paget disease
- Bone tumor
- Assess
  - For treatment of Paget disease, rickets, and osteomalacia
  - The underlying cause of high calcium level in blood

Nursing Implications

- The ALP test is given as part of routine blood screening.
- There is no special preparation required for this test.
- If ALP is high, the healthcare provider may order a second test and ask the patient to refrain from eating or drinking 10 hours before the test. ALP increases after eating.
- Assess if the patient is taking antibiotics, birth control pills, oral diabetes medication, or is on aspirin therapy since these can affect the test results.
- Assess if the patient is pregnant and determine the gestational age of the fetus. The placenta produces ALP in the third trimester.
- Assess if the patient
  - Is postmenopausal. The patient will have a high level of ALP.
  - Is a child, since rapid bone growth increases ALP level?
  - Uses alcohol, since this affects the test result.

Understanding the Results

- Test results are available between 2 and 5 days. The laboratory determines normal values based on calibration of testing equipment with a control test.
- Test results are reported as high, normal, or low based on the laboratory's control test.
- Generally the normal range is
  - Adult: 30 to 126 U/L or 0.5 to 2.0 microkat/L
  - Children: 30 to 300 U/L or 0.5 to 5.0 microkat/L

- Very high level may indicate
  - Gallstones
  - Hepatitis
  - Obstructive jaundice
  - Cancer metastasized to the liver
  - Liver disease
- High level may indicate
  - Rickets
  - Paget disease
  - Osteomalacia
  - Cancer metastasized to the bone
  - Bone tumors
  - Hyperparathyroidism
  - Mononucleosis
  - Kidney cancer
  - Heart failure
  - Myocardial infarction
  - Sepsis
  - Bone healing
- Low level may indicate
  - Malnutrition
  - Scurvy
  - Celiac disease

NURSING ALERT

It is normal for a pregnant woman in the third trimester to have an increased ALP because the placenta makes ALP. It is normal for a child who is experiencing rapid bone growth to have an increased ALP.

Teach the Patient

Explain

- Why blood sample is taken.
- The function of ALP and the meaning of abnormal values.

- That the patient may be asked to take the ALP test a second time if the test result indicates a high level of ALP. For the second test, the patient will be asked to refrain from eating or drinking 10 hours before the test. ALP increases after eating.

5. Ammonia

Ammonia is formed when bacteria in the intestines breaks down protein. Ammonia is then converted into urea by the liver, which is excreted by the kidneys in urine. The ammonia test measures the ammonia level in the blood. If the liver is unable to convert ammonia to urea, ammonia levels in the blood increase, indicating that there may be a liver function problem.

What Is Being Measured?

- Ammonia level in blood

How Is the Test Performed?

- See "How to Collect Blood Specimen From a Vein" in Appendix A.

Rationale for the Test

- Screen for
  - Liver function
  - Reye syndrome
  - Hyperalimentation
  - Cirrhosis
  - Acute liver failure
- Assess for treatment of liver disease.

Nursing Implications

- High ammonia levels can result in symptoms of confusion, sleepiness, hand tremors, or coma.
- Assess if the patient
  - Has eaten or drunk other than water 8 hours before the test.

- Smoked for 8 hours before the test.
- Performed strenuous exercise before the test.
- Is constipated.
- Has eaten a high- or low-protein diet.
- Is taking furosemide, heparin, valproic acid, acetazolamide, neomycin, tetracycline, lactulose, Marplan, Nardil, diphenhydramine, or Parnate. The patient will be asked to refrain from taking these medications several days before the test.

Understanding the Results

- Test results are available in about 12 hours. The laboratory determines normal values based on calibration of testing equipment with a control test. Test results are reported as high, normal, or low based on the laboratory's control test.
- Generally the normal range is
  - Adult: 15 to 45 mcg/dL or 11 to 32 mcmol/L
  - Children: 40 to 80 mcg/dL or 28 to 57 mcmol/L
  - Newborn: 90 to 150 mcg/dL or 64 to 107 mcmol/L
- High level may indicate
  - Cirrhosis
  - Hepatitis
  - Reye syndrome
  - Heart failure
  - Bleeding from intestines or stomach
  - Hemolytic disease of the newborn (incompatible blood types of mother and fetus)
  - Kidney failure

NURSING ALERT

Lactulose is a laxative that reduces intestinal bacteria production of ammonia. Ammonia levels might be slightly elevated in a patient who has severe cirrhosis. Newborns normally have high levels of ammonia that is temporary.

Teach the Patient

- Explain
  - Why blood sample is taken.
  - The function of ammonia and the meaning of abnormal values.
  - That the patient must refrain from smoking, eating, or drinking, except water, for 8 hours before the test and avoid strenuous exercise before the test.
  - That the patient should consult the healthcare provider whether he/she should stop taking furosemide, heparin, valproic acid, acetazolamide, neomycin, tetracycline, lactulose, Marplan, Nardil, diphenhydramine, or Parnate several days before the test.

6. Aspartate Aminotransferase

Aspartate aminotransferase (AST), previously known as serum glutamate oxaloacetate transaminase (SGOT), is an enzyme in the liver, heart, pancreas, kidneys, red blood cells, and muscle tissues. When these tissues or cells are damaged, there is an increase of AST in the blood 6 to 10 hours after the damage and remains for 4 days. The AST test measures the level of AST in the blood.

> **NURSING ALERT**
>
> The healthcare provider orders tests to measure AST and ALT in a normal screen for liver damage and liver disease. The AST test is more effective in detecting liver damage caused by alcohol abuse than the ALT test. As the patient recovers from tissue damage, the AST level in the blood decreases.

What Is Being Measured?

- AST level in blood

How Is the Test Performed?

- See "How to Collect Blood Specimen From a Vein" in Appendix A.

Rationale for the Test

- Screen for
  - Liver damage
  - Hepatitis
  - Cirrhosis
- Assess
  - The treatment of liver disease
  - Underlying cause of jaundice
  - If medication is causing liver damage

Nursing Implications

- Assess if the patient
  - Performed strenuous exercise before administration of the test since this can affect the test result.
  - Is taking Echinacea, valerian, or other herbs since this can affect the test result. The patient may be required to stop taking these for several days before the test is administered.
  - Is pregnant.
  - Takes mega doses of vitamin A.
  - Has had surgery, cardiac catheterization, IM injections, or injury to muscle recently, since these can cause an increase in AST level in blood.
  - Has recently taken antibiotics, narcotics, statins, and barbiturates or is undergoing chemotherapy.

Understanding the Results

- Test results are available in about 12 hours. The laboratory determines normal values based on calibration of testing equipment with a control test. Test results are reported as high, normal, or low based on the laboratory's control test.
- Generally the normal range is 8 to 35 U/L or 0.14 to 0.58 microkat/L.
- Slightly high level may indicate
  - Fatty deposits in the liver
  - Alcohol abuse

- Excessive acetaminophen
- The patient has taken antibiotics, narcotics, statins, barbiturates, or is undergoing chemotherapy
- Moderately high level may indicate
  - Cirrhosis
  - Chronic disease that directly or indirectly affects the liver
  - Kidney damage
  - Lung damage
  - Duchenne muscular dystrophy
  - Mega dose of vitamin A
  - Myocardial infraction
  - Heart failure
  - Mononucleosis
  - Cancer
  - Myositis
  - Alcohol abuse
- Very high level may indicate
  - Viral hepatitis
  - Necrosis
  - Shock
  - Drug reaction
  - Burns
  - Pulmonary embolism
  - Trauma
  - Heatstroke
  - Poison

Teach the Patient

- Explain
  - Why blood sample is taken.
  - The function of AST and the meaning of abnormal values.
  - That the patient must refrain from taking Echinacea, valerian, or other herbs, vitamin A.

- That the patient must notify the healthcare provider if he/she is taking antibiotics, narcotics, statins, and barbiturates or is undergoing chemotherapy.

7. Bilirubin

The liver breaks down old red blood cells into bilirubin, which becomes the brownish yellow component of bile. Bilirubin is excreted through feces and gives feces its brown color. Indirect (unconjugated) bilirubin, which is insoluble in water, is carried by the blood to the liver, where indirect bilirubin is transformed into direct bilirubin, which is soluble in water. The bilirubin test measures the total and the direct bilirubin levels in the blood. Indirect bilirubin is measured by subtracting direct bilirubin level from the total bilirubin level.

> **NURSING ALERT**
>
> Bilirubin can also be measured in urine.

What Is Being Measured?

- Total bilirubin level in the blood
- Direct bilirubin level in the blood

How Is the Test Performed?

- See "How to Collect Blood Specimen From a Vein" in Appendix A.
- See "How to Collect Blood Specimen From a Heel Stick" in Appendix A.
- A transcutaneous bilirubin meter may be used to measure the bilirubin level in a newborn. This handheld meter is placed against the skin. The skin is not punctured. If the bilirubin level is high, then the heel stick test is used to collect a blood sample from the newborn.

Rationale for the Test

- Screen for
  - Liver function
  - Hepatitis

- Cirrhosis
- Block bile duct from gallstones or pancreatic tumor
- Hemolytic anemia
- Hemolytic disease
- Neonatal jaundice
- Liver damage caused by medication

Nursing Implications

- Assess if the patient
  - Has eaten or drunk 4 hours before the test.
  - Has taken aspirin or Coumadin.
  - Is pregnant.
  - Has taken caffeine. This can lower bilirubin levels.
  - Has fasted for a long period. This increases indirect bilirubin levels.
  - Has taken Dilantin, Valium, Indocin, birth control pills, or Dalmane, since these medications can increase bilirubin levels.
  - Has taken theophylline, phenobarbital, or ascorbic acid (vitamin C) since these can lower bilirubin levels.

Understanding the Results

- Test results are available in 2 hours. The laboratory determines normal values based on calibration of testing equipment with a control test. Test results are reported as high, normal, or low based on the laboratory's control test.
- Normal range is
  - Total bilirubin: 0.3 to 1.0 mg/dL or 5.1 to 17.0 mmol/L
  - Direct bilirubin: 0.1 to 0.3 mg/dL or 1.0 to 5.1 mmol/L
  - Indirect bilirubin: 0.2 to 0.7 mg/dL or 3.4 to 11.9 mmol/L
- Normal range for newborn
  - Younger than 24 hours
    - Full term: Less than 6.0 mg/dL or less than 103 mmol/L
    - Premature: Less than 8.0 mg/dL or less than 137 mmol/L

- Younger than 48 hours
  - Full term: Less than 10.0 mg/dL or less than 170 mmol/L
  - Premature: Less than 12.0 mg/dL or less than 205 mmol/L
- 3 to 5 days old
  - Full term: Less than 12.0 mg/dL or less than 205 mmol/L
  - Premature: Less than 15.0 mg/dL or less than 256 mmol/L
- 7 days or older
  - Full term: Less than 10.0 mg/dL or less than 170 mmol/L
  - Premature: Less than 15.0 mg/dL or less than 256 mmol/L
- High level may indicate
  - Cholecystitis
  - Infected gallbladder
  - Hepatitis
  - Cirrhosis
  - Mononucleosis
  - Blocked bile duct
  - Gallstones
  - Pancreatic cancer
  - Gilbert syndrome
  - Sickle cell disease
  - Transfusion reaction
  - That the patient has taken Dilantin, Valium, Indocin, birth control pills, Dalmane
- High level for newborn
  - 24 hours old or younger: More than 10 mg/dL or more than 170 mmol/L
  - 25 to 48 hours old: More than 15 mg/dL or more than 256 mmol/L
  - 49 to 72 hours old: More than 18 mg/dL or more than 205 mmol/L
  - Older than 72 hours: More than 20 mg/dL or more than 340 mmol/L
- Low level may indicate
  - That the patient has taken theophylline, phenobarbital, or ascorbic acid

> **NURSING ALERT**
>
> Newborns can experience physiologic jaundice between 1 and 3 days old because the newborn is unable to break down red blood cells. This usually resolves in a week. The healthcare provider may order phototherapy to prevent collateral problems from developing.

Teach the Patient

- Explain
  - Why blood sample is taken.
  - The function of bilirubin and the meaning of abnormal values.
  - That the patient must refrain from eating Echinacea, valerian, or other herbs.
  - That the patient should refrain from eating or drinking anything for 4 hours before the test is administered.
  - That the healthcare provider may want the patient to stop taking aspirin, Coumadin, Dilantin, Valium, Indocin, birth control pills, Dalmane, theophylline, phenobarbital, or ascorbic acid and caffeine several days before the test is administered.

Summary

The liver plays a critical role in maintaining various bodily functions. It is this organ that produces the clotting factor that stops bleeding. The liver also synthesizes albumin that is used to maintain blood volume.

The intestines are able to absorb fat and fat-soluble vitamins because the liver synthesizes and secretes bile. Bile contains acids that metabolize fat and fat-soluble vitamins into elements that are easily absorbed into the body.

The liver also provides an energy store for the body by storing carbohydrates and metabolizing carbohydrates into glucose and synthesizes, stores, and metabolizes fatty acids and cholesterol.

The liver can also be thought of as the garbage disposal because the liver metabolizes harmful biochemicals and medications into elements that can safely be excreted by the body in urine and stool.

QUIZ

1. **What does the presence of the IgG anti-HAV mean?**

   A. The patient was recently infected with hepatitis A virus.

   B. The patient at some point was infected with hepatitis A virus.

   C. The patient was recently infected with hepatitis B virus.

   D. The patient at some point was infected with hepatitis B virus.

2. **What would you say to the patient whose HAV test is negative?**

   A. You do not have Hepatitis A virus.

   B. You have never been exposed to Hepatitis A virus.

   C. You do not have any HAV antibodies; however, it takes 2 weeks or more to develop antibodies.

   D. You do not have Hepatitis A virus or Hepatitis B virus.

3. **If the ALT is high, then would you tell the patient that he has liver disease?**

   A. Yes. ALT is mainly found in the liver.

   B. No. ALT is also found in muscle. Assess if the patient performed strenuous exercise before the test was administered.

   C. Yes. No other tests need to be performed.

   D. No. ALT is used to assess damage to the pancreas.

4. **Why might a practitioner order the ALT test if the patient has taken excessive amounts of acetaminophen?**

   A. To assess liver damage as a result of accidental or intentionally overdosing with acetaminophen

   B. To assess the ammonia level in the patient's blood

   C. To assess the effect lactulose has interrupting the effects of acetaminophen

   D. To assess if the patient intentionally overdose with acetaminophen

5. **What is bilirubin?**

   A. The reddish coloring in the eyes

   B. The pigment formed by the breakdown of hemoglobin in the liver

   C. Brown spots that appear on hands

   D. The pigment formed by the breakdown of hemoglobin in the kidneys

6. **Why would a practitioner not be concerned about elevated ALP if the patient was pregnant?**

   A. Prenatal vitamins negatively affect the ALP test.

   B. Pregnancy interferes with the patient's liver function.

   C. The placenta also makes ALP.

   D. The practitioner would be concerned because elevated ALP jeopardizes the pregnancy.

7. **What forms ammonia in the body?**

   A. Bacteria in the intestine break down protein.

   B. The heme causes the liver to create ammonia.

   C. The heme causes the kidneys to create ammonia.

   D. Ammonia is the results of breakdown of hemoglobin.

8. **What might be the results of high ammonia levels?**

   A. The patient may become confused.

   B. The patient might experience hand tremors.

   C. The patient might experience increased sleepiness.

   D. All of the above.

9. **What might the practitioner prescribe if the patient has a high level of ammonia?**

   A. Echinacea

   B. Lactulose

   C. Nonsteroidal anti-inflammatory drugs

   D. Valerian

10. **What might a high ammonia level indicate?**

   A. The patient exercised before the ammonia test.

   B. The liver is unable to convert ammonia to urea.

   C. The liver is unable to convert heme to hemoglobin.

   D. All of the above.

ANSWERS

1. B. The patient at some point was infected with hepatitis A virus.
2. C. You do not have any HAV antibodies; however, it takes 2 weeks or more to develop antibodies.
3. B. No. ALT is also found in muscle. Assess if the patient performed strenuous exercise before the test was administered.
4. A. To assess liver damage as a result of accidental or intentionally overdosing with acetaminophen.
5. B. The pigment formed by the breakdown of hemoglobin in the liver.
6. C. The placenta also makes ALP.
7. A. Bacteria in the intestine break down protein.
8. D. All of the above.
9. B. Lactulose.
10. B. The liver is unable to convert ammonia to urea.

chapter 6

Cardiac Enzymes and Cardiac Markers Tests

LEARNING OBJECTIVES

1. Brain Natriuretic Peptide (BNP)
2. Cardiac Enzyme Studies
3. Homocysteine
4. Renin Assay

KEY WORDS

Aldosterone

Angiotensin

Creatine phosphokinase

N-terminal pro-brain natriuretic peptide

Protein troponin

Renin-angiotensin system

Cardiac cells contain enzymes and other substances. Cardiac cells rupture when there is damage to cardiac muscle. As a result, substances once inside the cardiac cells are released into the bloodstream. A practitioner who suspects that a patient has had an acute coronary syndrome or cardiac ischemia will likely order the cardiac enzymes test and the cardiac markers test. The cardiac enzymes test determines the level of cardiac enzymes in the patient's bloodstream. The cardiac markers test measures other substances in addition to cardiac enzymes that are produced if the heart is damaged or under stress.

Cardiac markers are substances that are released into the patient's bloodstream when the patient's heart is damaged or the heart is under stress.

Troponin I and troponin T are proteins contained in heart muscle and are released whenever there is damage to the patient's heart.

Creatine kinase (CK) is an enzyme found in muscles and other organs. Creatine kinase-MB (CK-MB) is an isoenzyme found in cardiac muscle.

Myoglobin is a protein found in muscle cells.

Brain natriuretic peptide (BNP) is a hormone released by the heart in response to changes in pressure inside the heart.

It can take between 2 and 24 hours for cardiac muscle enzymes to reach a detectable level in blood. Therefore, the practitioner typically uses an electrocardiogram (ECG) to diagnose the acute phase of a myocardial infarction. The cardiac enzymes and cardiac markers tests are used to confirm a previous acute myocardial infarction or cardiac stress.

Several cardiac enzymes and cardiac markers tests are commonly used by a practitioner to confirm a diagnosis of myocardial infarction. You will learn about these tests in this chapter.

1. Brain Natriuretic Peptide

The heart produces the hormone brain natriuretic peptide (BNP). Low level of BNP is normally found in blood. However, BNP level increases when the heart works harder for long periods such as in heart failure. The BNP test measures the level of BNP in the blood.

> **NURSING ALERT**
>
> The healthcare provider may order the N-terminal pro-brain natriuretic peptide (NT-proBNP) test that measures the NT-proBNP hormone. This test provides similar diagnostic results as the BNP test.

What Is Being Measured?

- BNP level in blood

How Is the Test Performed?

- See "How to Collect Blood Specimen From a Vein" in Appendix A.

Rationale for the Test

- Screen for heart failure.
- Assess the treatment of heart failure.

Nursing Implications

- Assess if the patient
  - Has eaten or drunk anything except water for 12 hours before the test is administered.
  - Is taking diuretics or cardiac glycosides, which affect the test results.
  - Has myocardial infarction, kidney disease and is on dialysis, and chronic obstructive pulmonary disease (COPD).
  - Is taking Echinacea, valerian, or other herbs, since these herbs can affect the test results. The patient may be required to stop taking these herbs for several days before the test is administered.

Understanding the Results

- Test results are available quickly. The laboratory determines normal values based on calibration of testing equipment with a control test. Test results are reported as high, normal, or low based on the laboratory's control test.

- Generally the normal range: 0 to 99 pg/mL or 0 to 99 ng/L
- Slightly high level (100–300 pg/mL or 100–300 ng/L) may indicate
  - Minimum heart failure
- Moderately high level (300 pg/mL or 300 ng/L) may indicate
  - Mild heart failure
- High level (600 pg/mL or 600 ng/L) may indicate
  - Moderate heart failure
- Very high level (900 pg/mL or 900 ng/L) may indicate
  - Severe heart failure

NURSING ALERT

An abnormal level of BNP indicates increased pressure inside the heart and may indicate heart failure if the patient is on kidney dialysis.

Teach the Patient

- Explain
  - Why the blood sample is taken.
  - The function of BNP and the meaning of abnormal values.
  - That the patient must refrain from taking Echinacea, valerian, or other herbs.
  - That the patient should refrain from eating or drinking anything except water for 12 hours before the test is administered.

2. Cardiac Enzyme Studies

The cells of heart muscles and other tissues contain the enzyme creatine phosphokinase (CK, CPK) and the protein troponin (TnT, TnI). Creatine phosphokinase and troponin enter the blood when heart muscle and other tissues are damaged. If levels of creatine phosphokinase and troponin are elevated, the healthcare provider orders an ECG to differentiate between heart muscle damage and other tissue damage. Troponin and CPK-MB are mostly found in cardiac muscle.

NURSING ALERT

Blood samples are taken every 12 hours for 2 days following a suspected myocardial infarction. It takes 6 hours for troponin levels to rise after a myocardial infarction. The healthcare provider may order a myoglobin test along with the cardiac enzymes test to help diagnose a myocardial infarction.

What Is Being Measured?

- Creatine phosphokinase and troponin levels in blood

How Is the Test Performed?

- See "How to Collect Blood Specimen From a Vein" in Appendix A.

Rationale for the Test

- Screen for
  - A myocardial infarction
  - Heart muscle injury following bypass surgery
  - Unstable angina
- Assess the results of percutaneous coronary intervention (PCI) or thrombolytic medication to restore blood flow through the coronary artery.

Nursing Implications

- Assess if the patient
  - Has Reye syndrome, muscular dystrophy, myocarditis, autoimmune diseases, or cardiac disease
  - Has undergone cardioversion or defibrillation
  - Has recently received an intramuscular (IM) injection
  - Has had recent surgery
  - Has undergone strenuous exercise before the test is administered
  - Is taking statins
  - Abuses alcohol
  - Has kidney failure

Understanding the Results

- Test results are available in 1 hour. The laboratory determines normal values based on calibration of testing equipment with a control test. Test results are reported as high, normal, or low based on the laboratory's control test.
- Normal troponin range is
  - TnI: Less than 0.3 mcg/L
  - TnT: Less than 0.1 mcg/L
- Normal total creatine phosphokinase range is
  - Men: 55 to 170 IU/L
  - Women: 30 to 135 IU/L
- Normal CPK-MB range: Less than 3.0 ng/mL
- High troponin values may indicate
  - Cardiac muscle injury. Troponin level increases in 4 hours and reaches the highest level in 24 hours after the cardiac muscle injury. Troponin level returns to normal in 10 days following the cardiac muscle injury.
- High total creatine phosphokinase values may indicate
  - Cardiac muscle injury or tissue injury. Total creatine phosphokinase increases in 4 hours and reaches the highest level in 24 hours after the cardiac muscle injury. Total creatine phosphokinase level returns to normal levels in 3 days following the cardiac muscle injury.
- High CPK-MB values may indicate
  - Cardiac muscle injury. CPK-MB increases within 2 hours and reaches the highest level within 24 hours after the cardiac muscle injury. CPK-MB level returns to normal in 3 days following the cardiac muscle injury. If levels are high after 3 days, then additional cardiac muscle is being damaged and the myocardial infarction is continuing.

Teach the Patient

- Explain
  - Why the blood sample is taken.
  - That the patient should not exercise before the test is administered.
  - That the patient should not receive an IM injection before the test is administered.

- That the healthcare provider may request that the patient stops taking statins for 2 weeks prior to the test.

3. Homocysteine

Homocysteine is an amino acid found in blood. Homocysteine levels increase along with increases in levels of cholesterol that can lead to a risk of stroke, deep venous thrombosis (DVT), myocardial infarction, and pulmonary embolism. The homocysteine test measures the level of homocysteine in blood. The healthcare provider may order the homocysteine test for a patient who has a family history of heart disease, but has not exhibited other risk factors.

> **NURSING ALERT**
>
> The healthcare provider may order a urine homocysteine test.

What Is Being Measured?

- Homocysteine level in blood

How Is the Test Performed?

- Avoid eating and drinking anything except water for 12 hours before the test is administered.
- See "How to Collect Blood Specimen From a Vein" in Appendix A.

Rationale for the Test

- Assess risk for stroke and myocardial infarction.

Nursing Implications

- Assess if the patient
- Has eaten or drunk anything except water for 12 hours before the test
- Is currently hypertensive
- Smokes
- Has psoriasis, leukemia, kidney disease, or homocystinuria

- Is experiencing menopause
- Is deficient of vitamin B_{12}, vitamin B_6, and folic acid
- Drinks three or more cups of coffee daily
- Is taking birth control pills, theophylline, tamoxifen, antibiotics, or anticonvulsants
- Has a family history of elevated homocysteine
- Is a diabetic

Understanding the Results

- The homocysteine test results are available in 24 hours. The laboratory determines normal values based on calibration of testing equipment with a control test. Test results are reported as high, normal, or low based on the laboratory's control test.
- Normal homocysteine test results: 4 to 14 mcmol/L
- High homocysteine level may indicate
  - Homocystinuria
  - Hypothyroidism
  - Kidney disease
  - Alzheimer disease
  - Inflammatory bowel disease
  - Diet deficient in vitamin B_{12}, vitamin B_6, or folic acid
- Low homocysteine level may indicate
  - Diabetes

NURSING ALERT

Homocysteine level naturally increases with age.

Teach the Patient

- Explain
- Why the sample is taken.
- That the patient cannot eat or drink anything except water for 12 hours before the test.

- That the healthcare provider may ask the patient to refrain from taking birth control pills, theophylline, tamoxifen, antibiotics, or anticonvulsants 2 weeks prior to the test.

4. Renin Assay

Blood pressure is regulated by the renin-angiotensin system (RAS). Low blood pressure causes the secretion of the renin enzyme by the kidneys, which increases angiotensin production that constricts blood vessels, resulting in an increase in blood pressure. Angiotensin causes the adrenal cortex to replace aldosterone, causing the kidneys to retain water and sodium, resulting in an increase in fluid volume and blood pressure. The renin assay test measures the level of renin in blood.

NURSING ALERT

The healthcare provider may also order the aldosterone test. The renin stimulation test may be ordered if the renin level is low.

What Is Being Measured?

- Renin level in blood

How Is the Test Performed?

- Avoid
  - Eating natural black licorice for 2 weeks before the test
  - Ingesting caffeine 24 hours before the test
  - Eating or drinking 8 hours before the test
  - Taking β-blockers, corticosteroids, angiotensin-converting enzyme (ACE) inhibitors, estrogen, aspirin, or diuretics 4 weeks before the test
- Maintain a low-sodium diet for 3 days before the test.
- The patient must
  - Relax for 2 hours before the first blood sample is taken
  - Ambulate for 2 hours after the first blood sample is taken and before the second blood sample is taken

- The patient should be upright when the sample is taken.
- See "How to Collect Blood Specimen From a Vein" Appendix A.

Rationale for the Test

- Assess the underlying cause of hypertension.

Nursing Implications

- Assess if the patient
  - Has eaten natural black licorice 2 weeks before the test
  - Has ingested caffeine 24 hours before the test
  - Has eaten or drunk 8 hours before the test
  - Maintained a low-sodium diet 3 days before the test
  - Has taken β-blockers, corticosteroids, ACE inhibitors, estrogen, aspirin, or diuretics 4 weeks before the test
  - Has relaxed 2 hours before the first blood sample is taken
  - Has ambulated for 2 hours after the first blood sample is taken and before the second blood sample is taken
  - Is pregnant
  - Was upright when the sample was taken

Understanding the Results

- The renin assay test results are available quickly. The laboratory determines normal values based on calibration of testing equipment with a control test. Test results are reported as high, normal, or low based on the laboratory's control test.
- Normal renin assay test results (patient in upright position)
  - Age 20 to 39 years (normal sodium diet): 0.1 to 4.3 ng/mL/h
  - Age 20 to 39 years (low-sodium diet): 2.9 to 24 ng/mL/h
  - Age 40 and older (normal sodium diet): 0.1 to 3.0 ng/mL/h
  - Age 40 and older (low-sodium diet): 2.9 to 10.8 ng/mL/h
- High renin assay test results may indicate
  - Malignant high blood pressure
  - Kidney disease

- Blocked artery
- Cirrhosis
- Addison disease
- Hemorrhage
- Low renin assay test results may indicate
- Conn syndrome

Teach the Patient

- Explain
- Why the sample is taken.
- That two samples are taken—one after resting for 2 hours and another after ambulating for 2 hours.
- That the healthcare provider may ask the patient to refrain from taking β-blockers, corticosteroids, ACE inhibitors, estrogen, aspirin, or diuretics 4 weeks prior to the test.
- Avoid
- Eating natural black licorice for 2 weeks before the test
- Ingesting caffeine 24 hours before the test
- Maintain a low-sodium diet for 3 days before the test.
- Avoid eating or drinking 8 hours before the test.

Summary

Healthcare providers use cardiac enzymes and cardiac markers tests to detect if a patient has experienced a myocardial infarction. Cardiac enzymes and cardiac markers tests determine the level of cardiac enzymes in the patient's blood.

Cardiac enzymes are normally contained inside cardiac muscle. In a myocardial infarction, some cardiac muscles rupture, releasing cardiac enzymes into the bloodstream. It can take between 2 and 24 hours for cardiac muscle enzymes to reach a detectable level. It is during this time when the cardiac enzymes can be detected by the cardiac enzymes and cardiac markers tests.

Healthcare providers use an ECG to diagnose the acute phase of a myocardial infarction and the cardiac enzymes and cardiac markers tests to confirm the diagnosis.

QUIZ

1. **Why would the practitioner order a BNP test?**

   A. BNP increases when the heart works harder for long periods.

   B. BNP decreases if the patient has a myocardial infarction.

   C. BNP indicates if the patient has taken Echinacea.

   D. BNP indicates if the patient will develop chronic obstructive pulmonary disease.

2. **Why would the practitioner order an ECG if creatine phosphokinase and troponin are elevated?**

   A. To differentiate between right ventricle and left ventricle failure

   B. To differentiate between right and left heart failure

   C. To differentiate between heart muscle damage and other tissue damage

   D. To determine if the patient ate within 12 hours of the test

3. **Cardiac muscle is the only source of Troponin.**

   A. True

   B. False

4. **Why are blood samples taken every 12 hours for 2 days following a suspected myocardial infarction?**

   A. The patient may have multiple myocardial infarctions during that period.

   B. It takes 6 hours for troponin levels to rise after a myocardial infarction.

   C. It takes 2 days for troponin levels to rise after a myocardial infarction.

   D. To confirm the test results.

5. **If a practitioner believes that the patient had a myocardial infarction 4 days ago, would the practitioner order a CPK-MB?**

   A. No. CPK-MB level returns to normal in 3 days.

   B. No. Total creatine phosphokinase levels is a better test.

   C. Yes.CPK-MB level indicates cardiac muscle injury.

   D. Yes. CPK-MB level returns to normal in 10 days.

6. **What causes increase in secretion of the renin enzyme?**

   A. High blood pressure

   B. Low blood pressure

   C. Increase water intake

   D. Arterial sclerosis

7. **Why would strenuous exercise before the cardiac enzyme study influence the test results?**

    A. Enzymes being studied are contained in other muscle cells that might be injured during exercising.
    B. The patient should be relaxed before taking the test.
    C. Exercise may cause the patient to have a myocardial infarction.
    D. Muscle pain caused by exercising might be misunderstood as cardiac pain.

8. **What would you tell the patient scheduled for the BNP test who is taking Echinacea and valerian?**

    A. Stop taking Echinacea and valerian for a week before the test.
    B. Reduce the amount of Echinacea and valerian for 2 days before the test.
    C. You cannot take the test.
    D. Tell the practitioner that you are taking Echinacea and valerian so the practitioner can adjust the test results accordingly.

9. **What other test might the practitioner order along with the cardiac enzymes test?**

    A. Aspartate aminotransferase test
    B. Alanine aminotransferase test
    C. IgG anti-HAV test
    D. Myoglobin test

10. **What would negatively affect the cardiac enzyme studies?**

    A. Intramuscular injection
    B. Recent surgery
    C. Statins
    D. All of the above

ANSWERS

1. A. BNP increases when the heart works harder for long periods.
2. C. To differentiate between heart muscle damage and other tissue damage.
3. B. False.
4. B. It takes 6 hours for troponin levels to rise after a myocardial infarction.
5. A. No. CPK-MB level returns to normal in 3 days.
6. B. Low blood pressure.
7. A. Enzymes being studied are contained in other muscle cells that might be injured during exercising.
8. A. Stop taking Echinacea and valerian for a week before the test.
9. D. Myoglobin test.
10. D. All of the above.

chapter 7

Serologic Tests

LEARNING OBJECTIVES

1. Antibody (Coombs) Tests
2. Antinuclear Antibodies (ANA)
3. Blood Culture
4. CD4+ Count
5. *Helicobacter pylori* Tests
6. Herpes Simplex Virus Tests (HSV)
7. Human Immunodeficiency Virus (HIV) Tests
8. Immunoglobulins
9. Lyme Disease Test
10. Mononucleosis Tests
11. Rheumatoid Factor (RF)
12. Rubella Test
13. Syphilis Tests
14. Viral Load Measurement

175

KEY WORDS

Agglutination test	IgD
Antibodies	IgE
Autoimmune	IgG
Blood transfusion reaction	IgM
Branched DNA (bDNA)	Indirect fluorescent antibody (IFA)
Congenital rubella syndrome (CRS)	Macroglobulinemia
Enzyme-linked immunosorbent assay (ELISA)	Monospot test
	Nephelometry test
Epstein-Barr virus (EBV)	Nucleic acid sequence–based amplification (NASBA)
Heterophil antibodies	
HIV RNA	Polymerase chain reaction (PCR)
Home blood test kits	Rapid test kits
HSV (herpes simplex virus)	Reverse-transcriptase polymerase chain reaction (RT-PCR)
HSV-1	
HSV-2	Saliva test
Human immunodeficiency virus	T-helper cells
IgA	Western blot

The patient's immune system reacts to bacteria, viruses, and foreign substances that are recognized as alien to the body referred to as an antigen. The reaction creates antibodies. An antibody is a protein called an immunoglobulin that is triggered in the presence of the antigen in the blood. The antibody chemically combines with the substance and metabolizes the substance into components that can be excreted safely by the body.

Serologic tests examine the patient's blood for antibodies. The provider orders serologic tests for a number of reasons. Serology tests can be ordered to diagnose an infection or to determine if the patient has developed immunity to a specific antigen. The practitioner may also order a serology test to determine the patient's blood type and to assess if he/she has an autoimmune disorder. An autoimmune disorder occurs when the patient's immune system identifies its own cells as foreign, resulting in the immune system creating antibodies to its own cells leading to the destruction of those cells.

In this chapter you will learn about common serologic tests.

1. Antibody Tests

Antibodies are proteins made by the immune system that bind to bacteria, viruses, and other microorganisms to destroy the microorganism. Antibodies can also bind to red blood cells and can destroy them. Antibody tests determine if antibodies are attacking red blood cells.

Antibodies are created as a result of

- Blood transfusion reaction: The transfused blood has different antigens on the surface of its red blood cells than the patient's red blood cells. This causes the immune system to produce antibodies that attack the transfused red blood cells.

- Rhesus factor sensitization: The Rh antigen is in the fetus's blood (Rh positive), but not in the pregnant woman's blood (Rh negative). During delivery, the fetus's blood mixes with the mother's blood causing the mother's immune system to create antibodies against the fetus's red blood cells. The mother becomes Rh sensitive. The antibodies can attack the fetus's red blood cells in future pregnancies if the fetus is Rh positive. Women with Rh-negative blood are given the Rh immune globulin (RhoGAM) that typically stops Rh sensitivity.

  - Rh antibody titer: The test is performed in early pregnancy to determine the mother's blood type and to determine if she is Rh negative.

- Autoimmune hemolytic anemia: The patient's immune system creates antibodies against his/her red blood cells.

  - Direct Coombs test: Identifies antibodies attached to the patient's red blood cells. This test is performed

    - On a newborn whose mother is Rh negative to determine if the antibodies crossed the placenta into the newborn's blood

    - On a patient who received a blood transfusion to determine if there is a transfusion reaction

    - On a patient to determine if an autoimmune response is occurring

  - Indirect Coombs test: Identifies antibodies that have not but could attach to the patient's red blood cells if he/she blood is mixed. This test is performed

    - On the blood transfusion recipient or donor before the transfusion to identify if antibodies exist in their blood.

What Is Being Measured?

- Antibodies that might attack the patient's red blood cells

How Is the Test Performed?

- See "How to Collect Blood Specimen From Vein" in Appendix A.

Rationale for the Test

- Assess
  - Blood transfusion reaction or potential reaction
  - Rh factor sensitization
  - Autoimmune hemolytic anemia

Nursing Implications

- Assess reason(s) the patient should refrain from taking the test
  - History of blood transfusions
  - Recently administered contrast material IV or dextran injections
  - Was pregnant 3 months ago
  - Has taken cephalosporins, tetracyclines, tuberculosis (TB) medication, sulfa medication, or insulin

Understanding the Results

- Negative test results
  - No antibodies found in the patient's blood (direct Coombs test).
  - The patient's blood is compatible with transfusion donor's blood (indirect Coombs test).
  - Rh-negative mother is not Rh sensitized (indirect Coombs test). The mother is administered the RhoGAM vaccine.
- Positive test results
  - The patient's blood contains antibodies for his/her red blood cells (direct Coombs test).
  - The patient's blood is incompatible with transfusion donor's blood (indirect Coombs test). The blood is not transfused.

- Rh-negative mother is Rh sensitized (indirect Coombs test). The health-care provider monitors the pregnancy closely to prevent problems with the fetus if the fetus is Rh positive.

Teach the Patient

- Explain
  - That no special preparation is needed for the test.
  - Why the test is ordered.
  - Rh sensitivity and the administration of RhoGAM vaccine if the patient is Rh negative.

2. Antinuclear Antibodies

In autoimmune diseases, the body produces antibodies that attach and destroy its own cells. The antinuclear antibody (ANA) test measures the pattern and amount of these antibodies.

What Is Being Measured?

- ANA

How Is the Test Performed?

- See "How to Collect Blood Specimen From a Vein" in Appendix A.

Rationale for the Test

- Screen for
  - Rheumatoid arthritis (RA)
  - Systemic lupus erythematosus (SLE)
  - Polymyositis
  - Scleroderma

Nursing Implications

- No special patient preparation is necessary for the test.

- Ask the patient for a list of prescription and nonprescription medications he/she has taken. Consult the laboratory to determine if these medications might affect the test results. Medication for high blood pressure, heart disease, and TB can cause the results to be high.

Understanding the Results

- Results are available in 1 week. The laboratory determines normal values based on calibration of testing equipment with a control test. Test results are reported as high, normal, or low based on the laboratory's control test.
- Results are reported as a titer. A titer specifies how much of the sample of blood is diluted with saline before antibodies are no longer detected. The titer is reported as a ratio of parts of the blood sample and saline. The higher the second number of the ratio, the greater the number of antibodies in the blood sample.
- Generally normal range is
  - 1:40 or less than 40
- Abnormally high values are not used to diagnose a condition. However, they can be a sign of
  - RA
  - SLE
  - Scleroderma
  - Polymyositis
  - Raynaud syndrome
  - Addison disease
  - Hashimoto thyroiditis
  - Hemolytic anemia
  - Vitamin B_{12} deficiency
  - Hepatitis
  - Idiopathic thrombocytopenia

> ### NURSING ALERT
>
> An elevated result can be caused by medication for high blood pressure, heart disease, and TB and a viral infection. Older adults also show an elevated result caused by aging. A patient who has a family history of autoimmune disease may have an elevated result.

Teach the Patient

- No special preparation is needed for the test.
- Explain
  - Why the test is ordered.
  - That the test result is a sign and not a definitive diagnosis. Additional assessment must be made before a diagnosis is reached.
  - The conditions that can cause an elevated test result other than disease.

3. Blood Culture

Blood can be infected by bacteria or fungi. A blood culture identifies the bacteria or fungi by allowing the microorganism to grow in a controlled environment and then examining the microorganism under a microscope.

> **NURSING ALERT**
>
> The healthcare provider typically orders a sensitivity test along with the blood culture. The sensitivity test identifies medication that kills the microorganism.

What Is Being Measured?

- Bacteria or fungi in the blood

How Is the Test Performed?

- A blood sample is obtained from three different veins and at two different times to assure that bacteria on the skin does not contaminate the blood sample.
- See "How to Collect Blood Specimen From a Vein" in Appendix A.

> **NURSING ALERT**
>
> Patients who have catheters in their vein will have the blood sample taken from the catheter.

Rationale for the Test

- Assess
  - The existence of bacteria or fungi in blood
  - For endocarditis
  - Medication that will kill the microorganism
  - The cause of unexplained fever
  - The effect of treatment of a microorganism infection

Nursing Implications

- Kidney, lung, and throat infections can lead to bacterial infection of the blood.
- Assess if the patient has recently been administered antibiotics, since this can affect the test results.

Understanding the Results

- Test results for bacterial infection are normally available in 3 days but can take longer than 10 days. Test results for a fungal infection can take up to 30 days.
- Normal is negative: No bacteria or fungi found in the blood sample.
- Normal false-negative: Improper processing or improper sampling results in bacteria or fungi not found in the blood sample but the patient's blood is infected.
- Abnormal is positive: Bacteria or fungi found in the blood sample.
- Abnormal false-positive: Contaminated sample or improper processing results in bacteria or fungi found in the blood sample but not in the patient's blood.

Teach the Patient

- Explain
  - Why blood sample is taken.
  - Multiple samples may be taken from different sites and at different times.
  - That the results of the sensitivity test will tell the healthcare provider about the medication that will kill the microorganism.

4. CD4+ Count

Three types of leukocytes (WBC) important in fighting infection are T-lymphocytes, T-cells, and T-helper cells. The CD4+ count test measures the level of these leukocytes to assess the patient's immune system. Patients who have a low CD4+ count are at risk for opportunistic infections.

> **NURSING ALERT**
>
> The CD4+ count test is used to assess the immune system of patients who have HIV. The result of the CD4+ count test and the viral load test determines when antiretroviral treatment of HIV is to be started. The healthcare provider may also order the CD4+ percentage test that determines the percentage of CD4+ cells in the total number of lymphocytes and the CD8 count test, which determines the level of T-suppressor cells.

What Is Being Measured?

- The CD4+ cells level in blood

How Is the Test Performed?

- See "How to Collect Blood Specimen From a Vein" in Appendix A.

Rationale for the Test

- Assess
  - The patient's immune system
  - The progress of HIV
  - The treatment of HIV
- Assist in the diagnosis of AIDS.
- Develop a baseline of CD4+ count. The healthcare provider compares CD4+ values over time to identify changes in levels.

Nursing Implications

- Note the time when the CD4+ blood sample is taken since CD4+ cells are normally lower in the morning.

- Be sure that the blood sample is refrigerated.
- Assess if the patient has influenza, pneumonia, or herpes simplex since these diseases can affect the test results.
- Assess if the patient has taken corticosteroids or is undergoing chemotherapy.

Understanding the Results

- Test results are available in 3 days.
- Normal CD4+ cell count range is
  - Not infected with HIV: 600 to 1,200 cells/μL
  - Low risk for opportunistic infection: Greater than 350 cells/μL
- Low CD4+ cell count may indicate
  - 200 to 350 cells/μL
    - Weak immune system
    - Risk for opportunistic infection
    - Start antiretroviral treatment
  - Under 200 cells/μL
    - High risk for opportunistic infection
    - AIDS
    - Start antiretroviral treatment

Teach the Patient

- Explain
  - Why blood sample is taken.
  - That the healthcare provider may request that the patient stops taking corticosteroids for 2 weeks prior to the test.

5. Helicobacter pylori Tests

Helicobacter pylori is a bacterium that infects the stomach and duodenum and may result in a peptic ulcer. Many patients have *H pylori* but few develop peptic ulcer disease. There are four tests used to detect *H pylori*

- *Helicobacter pylori* blood antibody test: This test determines if the blood sample has *H pylori* antibodies.

- Urea breath test: This test determines the presence of *H pylori* in the stomach.
- *Helicobacter pylori* stool antigen test: This test determines the presence of *H pylori* antigens in feces.
- Stomach biopsy: This is the endoscopic removal of the lining of the stomach and small intestine, which is examined for the presence of *H pylori*.

NURSING ALERT

All tests may produce a false-negative result if the H pylori count is low and undetectable. The stomach biopsy may produce a false-negative result if the sample is not infected. The blood test for H pylori antibodies may give a false-positive result since antibodies are present years after the H pylori infection is resolved.

What Is Being Measured?

- *H pylori* antibody levels in blood

How Is the Test Performed?

- See "How to Collect Blood Specimen From a Vein" in Appendix A.

Rationale for the Test

- Assess for the presence of *H pylori*.
- Assess if the treatment for *H pylori* is successful.

Nursing Implications

- Assess if the patient
  - Is pregnant or breast-feeding. The urea breath test is not performed.
  - Has taken antibiotics. This can reduce the *H pylori* count.
  - Has taken Prilosec, Carafate, Pepcid, AcipHex, Zantac, or Pepto-Bismol, since these can affect the test results.

Understanding the Results

- Blood test results are available in 1 day.
  - Normal results: No *H pylori* antibodies

- Abnormal blood test results: Presence of *H pylori* antibodies
- Urea breath test results are available in 3 hours.
  - Normal results: No tagged hydrocarbon
  - Abnormal blood test results: Tagged hydrocarbon present
- Stool antigen test results are available in 3 hours.
  - Normal results: No *H pylori* antigens
  - Abnormal blood test results: Presence of *H pylori* antigens
- Stomach biopsy test result is available between 2 and 10 days.
  - Normal results: No *H pylori*
  - Abnormal blood test results: Presence of *H pylori*

Teach the Patient

- Explain
- Why blood sample is taken.
- How to take a stool collection at home, if necessary.
- That there is no long-term effect of swallowing a capsule or water containing radioactive material in the urea breath test.
- That the healthcare provider may want the patient to refrain from taking Prilosec, Carafate, Pepcid, AcipHex, Zantac, or Pepto-Bismol 12 hours before the test.

6. Herpes Simplex Virus Tests

Herpes simplex virus (HSV) causes painful blisterlike sores on the skin and mucous membranes of the mouth, vagina, urethra, rectum, nose, and throat. There are two types of HSV. These are

- Herpes simplex virus type 1 (HSV-1): Commonly called a fever blister or cold sore that appears on the lips and is spread by direct contact or indirectly through sharing eating utensils
- Herpes simplex virus type 2 (HSV-2): Commonly called genital herpes that appears on the penis or vagina and is spread by direct contact

There are four common tests of HSV

- HSV antibody test: This test identifies HSV antibodies in the blood but cannot differentiate between HSV-1 and HSV-2 and can produce a false-negative result, since the immune system takes several days to develop sufficient antibodies to be detected by the HSV antibody test.

- Polymerase chain reaction (PCR) test: This test differentiates between HSV-1 and HSV-2 in cell scraping.
- Herpes virus antigen detection test: This test detects antigens on cells scraped from the HSV sore using a microscope.
- Herpes viral culture: This test cultures cells or fluid from a HSV sore to determine if the sore is from HSV-2.

> ### NURSING ALERT
>
> HSV-1 can infect the genitals. HSV-2 can infect the newborn if the mother has HSV-2. It can also infect the mouth. There is no cure for HSV; however, it can go into remission. Fatigue, stress, or sunlight can cause HSV sore to recur. Varicella zoster is a type of herpes virus that is better known as shingles and chickenpox.

What Is Being Measured?

- HSV
  - Antibodies in blood
  - Antibodies in cell scraping
  - Antigens in cell scraping
  - Antigens in culture

How Is the Test Performed?

- See "How to Collect Blood Specimen From a Vein" in Appendix A.
- The POC kit tests for HSV-2 antibodies in blood in 10 minutes.

Rationale for the Test

- Assess for HSV.
- Identify the types of HSV.

Nursing Implications

- Assess if the patient
  - Has had sexual contact before the test results are known

- Urinated 2 hours before the test (sore is on the urethra)
- Douched 24 hours before the test (sore is on the cervices)
- Has taken ganciclovir, acyclovir, valacyclovir, or famciclovir
- If a culture was taken from a crusted sore

Understanding the Results

- Rapid HSV culture test results take 3 days.
- The HSV culture test results take 14 days.
- The HSV antigen test results take 1 day.
- The polymerase chain reaction (PCR) test results take 3 days.
- The antibody blood tests take 2 days.
- Normal HSV test results (negative): No HSV, no HSV antigen, no HSV DNA, no HSV antibodies.
- Abnormal HSV test results (positive): HSV, HSV antigen, HSV DNA, HSV antibodies present.

NURSING ALERT

A negative test does not rule out an HSV infection. Additional testing is necessary if symptoms appear.

Teach the Patient

- Explain
- Why blood sample is taken.
- That the patient should not douche 24 hours before the test if the sore is on the crevices.
- That the patient should not urinate 2 hours before the test if the sore is on the urethra.
- That the patient should not have sexual contact before the test results are known.
- That the healthcare provider may request that the patient may avoid taking ganciclovir, acyclovir, valacyclovir, or famciclovir for 2 weeks prior to the test.

7. Human Immunodeficiency Virus Tests

The human immunodeficiency virus (HIV) infects the CD4+ white blood cells that are the body's defense against infection. There are two types of HIV. HIV-1 is common in nearly all AIDS cases. HIV-2 is associated with West Africa. HIV causes AIDS, which is incurable. There is a period when the HIV infection is not detectable in a patient. This is called the seroconversion period and also known as the window period. The patient can spread HIV during this period. The seroconversion period can be up to 2 weeks and as long as 6 months. After the seroconversion period, the HIV test is able to detect HIV antibodies or the HIV RNA in the patient's blood.

There are several HIV tests:

- Enzyme-linked immunosorbent assay (ELISA): The first test administered to screen a patient. This looks for HIV antibodies in the blood. If the test result is negative, then other tests are not performed. If the test result is positive, another ELISA test is performed. Other tests are performed if there are two positive ELISA tests because the ELISA test can produce a false positive.

- Western blot: This tests for HIV antibodies and is more difficult to perform than the ELISA test.

- Polymerase chain reaction (PCR): This looks for HIV RNA in the blood. PCR is used to identify a very recent infection and is administered to screen blood and organs before using them for donations and when HIV antibody tests are inconclusive. The PCR test is not performed often because of expense.

- Indirect fluorescent antibody (IFA): This tests for HIV antibodies and is performed secondary to two positive ELISA tests.

- Saliva test: This tests the presence of HIV in saliva. Results must be confirmed by the Western blot test.

- Rapid test kits: These test results are available in a half hour. Results must be confirmed by the Western blot test.

- Home blood test kits: Available without prescription. Samples are sent through the mail to the laboratory. Results are provided over the phone using an anonymous code.

NURSING ALERT

Detecting HIV in a newborn is difficult because the newborn's blood still has HIV antibodies from either HIV positive parent for 18 months.

Testing is performed when the patient

- Exhibits symptoms of HIV.
- Has HIV risk factors.
- Is donating blood or organs.
- Is pregnant. An infected mother can be treated, decreasing the likelihood that HIV will be passed to the fetus.

What Is Being Measured?

- HIV antibodies in blood
- HIV RNA in blood

How Is the Test Performed?

- The patient must consent to HIV testing.
- Tests are performed at 6 weeks, 3 months, and 6 months after the patient is exposed to HIV.
- The PCR test is performed days or a few weeks following exposure to HIV.
- There are no special preparations for this test.
- See "How to Collect Blood Specimen From a Vein" in Appendix A.

Rationale for the Test

- Assess if the patient has been infected with HIV.

Nursing Implications

- If the patient is diagnosed with HIV, then the healthcare provider will order regularly CD4+ count and viral load measurement tests. The CD4+ count determines the impact HIV has on the immune system. The viral load measurement test determines the amount of HIV in the blood.
- Consult with the healthcare institution's policy on reporting positive test results.
- Assess
  - For use of corticosteroids since this can affect the test results.
  - If the patient has an autoimmune disease, syphilis, or leukemia. These diseases can affect the test results.
  - If the patient consumes alcohol. This can affect the test results.

- Arrange for counselors to be available to assist the patient with the emotional, financial, and social repercussions of being HIV positive should there be positive test results.

Understanding the Results

- ELISA test results are available in 2 to 4 days. Results of other tests are available within 2 weeks.
- Normal (negative) is
  - No HIV antibodies detected.
  - The test is repeated for 6 months if the test is negative. The immune system can take up to 6 months to produce detectable HIV antibodies.
- Uncertain (indeterminate) is
  - Results are not clear if the patient is infected with HIV because another factor is possibly interfering with the results.
  - The PCR test is typically ordered.
  - After 6 months, the patient is said to be stable indeterminate and not infected with HIV.
- Abnormal (positive) is
  - HIV antibodies are found in the patient's blood.
- If the ELISA test is positive, the same blood sample is tested again. If the second ELISA test is positive, then the Western blot or IFA test is performed.
- A patient is considered HIV positive if the Western blot, IFA, or PCR tests are positive, confirming two positive ELISA test results.

Teach the Patient

- Explain
  - That HIV testing cannot be performed without the patient's consent.
  - Why blood sample is taken. HIV testing is part of routine blood screening.
  - That HIV testing does not determine if the person has AIDS.
  - That a negative test results will require retesting at 6 weeks, 3 months, and 6 months after the patient is exposed to HIV because of the seroconversion period.
  - That it is difficult to detect HIV in a newborn for 18 months because the newborn has antibodies from the mother.

- That a positive ELISA test result does not mean that the patient is HIV positive. Additional testing is necessary to confirm this result.
- That counselors will be available to assist the patient with the emotional, financial, and social repercussions of being HIV positive.
- The benefits of early detection and treatment.
- That treatment can be given to an infected mother, decreasing the likelihood that HIV will be passed on to the fetus.

8. Immunoglobulins

Immunoglobulins are antibodies made by the immune system in response to microorganisms that enter the body, an allergen, and abnormal cells such as cancer cells. An antibody is specific to an antigen. The immunoglobulin test measures the level of an immunoglobulin in the patient's blood. A low level of a specific immunoglobulin increases the risk of repeated infections from antigen. There are five major types of immunoglobulins:

- IgA: This is found in tears and saliva and protects the ears, eyes, breathing passages, digestive tract, and vagina that are exposed to outside antigens. Body produces 10% of this type of immunoglobulin.
- IgD: This is found in abdominal and chest tissues. Body produces less than 5% of this type of immunoglobulin.
- IgE: This is found on mucous membranes, lungs, and skin and defends against allergens. A high level of IgE immunoglobulins is common in patients who are hypoallergenic. Body produces less than 5% of this type of immunoglobulin.
- IgG: This is found in all body fluids and defends the body against viruses and bacteria. This immunoglobulin crosses the placenta. Body produces 80% of this type of immunoglobulin.
- IgM: This is found in blood and lymph fluid and is the first response to infection. Body produces 5% of this type of immunoglobulin, which form when an infection occurs for the first time.

NURSING ALERT

The immunoglobulin test is commonly administered as a follow-up to an abnormal result from the total blood protein test or from the blood protein electrophoresis test.

What Is Being Measured?

- IgA immunoglobulins
- IgD immunoglobulins
- IgE immunoglobulins
- IgG immunoglobulins
- IgM immunoglobulins

How Is the Test Performed?

- See "How to Collect Blood Specimen From a Vein" in Appendix A.

Rationale for the Test

- Assess
  - Levels of immunoglobulins to determine the strengths of the patient's immune system
  - The patient's immunization
  - The effectiveness of treatment of infection and bone marrow cancer
- Screen for
  - Allergies
  - Autoimmune diseases
  - Multiple myeloma and macroglobulinemia cancers

Nursing Implications

- Assess if there is reason for the patient not to take the test:
- Has taken hydralazine (Apresoline), phenylbutazone, birth control pills, anticonvulsants (phenytoin), methotrexate, aminophenazone, asparaginase, and corticosteroids
- Received a blood transfusion within 6 months before the test
- Used alcohol or illegal medication
- Received boosters of a vaccination or new vaccinations within 6 months before the test
- Received a radioactive scan within 3 days before the test
- Has undergone radiation and chemotherapy treatments

Understanding the Results

- Results are available in 2 days. The laboratory determines normal values based on calibration of testing equipment with a control test. Test results are reported as high, normal, or low based on the laboratory's control test.
- Generally normal ranges are
  - IgA: 85 to 385 mg/dL
  - IgD: Less than 8 mg/dL or 5 to 30 mcg/L
  - IgE: 10 to 1,421 mcg/L
  - IgG: 565 to 1,765 mg/dL
  - IgM: 55 to 375 mg/dL
- Abnormally high values are not used to diagnose a condition. However, they can be a sign of
  - IgA
    - SLE
    - RA
    - Multiple myeloma
    - Cirrhosis
    - Chronic hepatitis
  - IgD
    - Multiple myeloma
  - IgE
    - Asthma
    - Allergic reaction
    - Parasitic infection
    - Atopic dermatitis
    - Multiple myeloma
  - IgG
    - Chronic infection
    - Multiple sclerosis (MS)
    - Multiple myeloma
    - Chronic hepatitis

- IgM
  - Nephrotic syndrome
  - RA
  - Macroglobulinemia
  - Mononucleosis
  - Viral hepatitis
  - Parasite infection
  - Infection that started in a newborn before delivery
- Abnormally low values are not used to diagnose a condition. However, they can be a sign of
  - IgA
    - Enteropathy
    - Leukemia
    - Nephrotic syndrome
    - Ataxia/telangiectasia
  - IgD
    - Not significant
  - IgE
    - Ataxia/telangiectasia
  - IgG
    - Leukemia
    - Nephrotic syndrome
    - Macroglobulinemia
  - IgM
    - Multiple myeloma
    - Leukemia

Teach the Patient

- No special preparation is needed for the test.
- Explain why the test is ordered. An immunoglobulin test can help the healthcare provider diagnose the infection.

9. Lyme Disease Test

The *Borrelia burgdorferi* bacterium is carried by ticks and transmitted by a tick bite. The Lyme disease test detects *B burgdorferi* bacteria antibodies in blood. The healthcare provider will order at least two of three Lyme disease tests.

- IFA
- ELISA: quickest and most sensitive test for Lyme disease
- Western blot test: confirms positive IFA and ELISA test results

NURSING ALERT

The healthcare provider orders the Lyme disease test if the patient has symptoms of Lyme disease or is known to have been exposed to ticks.

NURSING ALERT

The Lyme disease test can produce a false-negative result if performed within 2 months of the tick bite because the patient's immune system may take 2 months to produce a detectable amount of B burgdorferi bacteria antibodies. Likewise, test can produce a false-positive result because B burgdorferi bacteria antibodies remain in the patient's blood years after the B burgdorferi bacteria was killed.

What Is Being Measured?

- *Borrelia burgdorferi* bacteria antibodies level in blood

How Is the Test Performed?

- See "How to Collect Blood Specimen From a Vein" in Appendix A.

Rationale for the Test

- Assess
  - For Lyme disease

Nursing Implications

- Assess if the patient
  - Has a viral or bacterial infection
  - Has high lipid level
  - Has ever been diagnosed with Lyme disease
  - Has ever been exposed to ticks

Understanding the Results

- The Lyme disease test results are available in 2 weeks. The laboratory determines normal values based on calibration of testing equipment with a control test. Test results are reported as high, normal, or low based on the laboratory's control test.
- Results are reported as a titer. A titer specifies how much of the sample of blood is diluted with saline before antibodies are no longer detected. The titer is reported as a ratio of parts of the blood sample and saline. The higher the second number of the ratio, the greater number of antibodies in the blood sample.
- Normal Lyme disease test results (negative)
  - IFA: Less than 1:256
  - ELISA: No *B burgdorferi* bacteria antibodies found
  - Western blot test: No *B burgdorferi* bacteria antibodies found
- Abnormal Lyme disease (positive).
  - IFA: Greater than 1:256
  - ELISA: *B burgdorferi* bacteria antibodies found
  - Western blot test: *B burgdorferi* bacteria antibodies found

Teach the Patient

- Explain
  - Why blood sample is taken.
  - That a negative test result does not rule out Lyme disease since the immune system can take 2 months to develop detectable antibodies.
  - That a positive test result must be confirmed by another Lyme disease test, which is usually the Western blot test.

- That a positive test result does not mean that the patient has Lyme disease since detectable antibodies remain in the blood for years after a *B burgdorferi* bacteria infection. The patient might have been infected in the past but is not currently infected.

10. Mononucleosis Tests

The Epstein-Barr virus (EBV) causes mononucleosis. The mononucleosis tests identify antibodies for the EBV in the blood sample. There are two kinds of mononucleosis tests

- Monospot test: This test identifies heterophil antibodies that form between 2 and 9 weeks after the patient becomes infected.
- EBV antibody test: This test is ordered when the patient shows symptoms of mononucleosis and the monospot test is negative.

What Is Being Measured?

- Antibodies for the EBV in blood

How Is the Test Performed?

- See "How to Collect Blood Specimen From a Vein" in Appendix A.
- See "How to Collect Blood Specimen From a Finger Stick" in Appendix A.

Rationale for the Test

- Assess for infectious mononucleosis

Nursing Implications

- A false-negative result can occur if the test is administered within 2 weeks of the patient being infected.
- Assess if the patient has lymphoma, hepatitis, rubella, cytomegalovirus, or lupus.

Understanding the Results

- Monospot test results are available in 1 hour.
  - Normal (negative) heterophil antibody range is 0.

- High (positive) heterophil antibody levels greater than 0 may indicate
  - Mononucleosis
  - RA
  - Leukemia
  - Hepatitis
  - Lymphoma
- EBV antibody test results are available in 3 days.
  - Results are reported as a titer. A titer specifies how much of the sample of blood is diluted with saline before antibodies are no longer detected. The titer is reported as a ratio of parts of the blood sample and saline. The higher the second number of the ratio, the greater the number of antibodies in the blood sample.
  - Normal (negative) EBV antibody titer range is below 1 to 40 (1:40).
  - High (positive) EBV antibody titer may indicate
    - Mononucleosis

> **NURSING ALERT**
>
> The presence of IgG antibody indicates that the patient was exposed to the EBV in the past. Most adults have the IgG antibody.

Teach the Patient

- Explain
  - Why blood sample is taken.
  - That a false-negative result can occur if the test is administered within 2 weeks of the patient being infected.

11. Rheumatoid Factor

The rheumatoid factor (RF) is an autoantibody that destroys the patient's own tissues, resulting in stiffness, joint pain, and inflammation. The RF test measures the amount of the RF in the blood sample and is used to differentiate RA from other forms of arthritis. The two types of RF tests are the agglutination test and the nephelometry test.

> **NURSING ALERT**
>
> A patient may have a high level of RF but no symptoms of RA. However, the patient is likely to develop RA in the future. A patient may have a normal level of RF and symptoms of RA will likely require a second RF test.

> **NURSING ALERT**
>
> The RF is one of other signs and symptoms used to diagnose RA.

What Is Being Measured?

- Measures the RF in blood

How Is the Test Performed?

- See "How to Collect Blood Specimen From a Vein" in Appendix A.

Rationale for the Test

- Screen for RA.

Nursing Implications

- Assess the patient's age. Patients older than 65 years of age normally have a higher RF level.

Understanding the Results

- The RF test results are available quickly.
- Results are reported as a titer. A titer specifies how much of the sample of blood is diluted with saline before antibodies are no longer detected. The titer is reported as a ratio of parts of the blood sample and saline. The higher the second number of the ratio, the greater the number of antibodies in the blood sample.
- Normal test results: 1:20 to 1:40 or less.
- Higher levels may indicate
  - RA

- SLE
- Vasculitis
- Scleroderma
- Cirrhosis
- Hepatitis
- Leukemia
- Endocarditis
- Mononucleosis
- Malaria
- TB
- Syphilis

Teach the Patient

- Explain
- Why the sample is taken.
- That the healthcare provider may ask for a second RF test if the first test is normal and the patient shows signs of RA.

12. Rubella Test

Rubella (German measles) is a virus that causes congenital rubella syndrome (CRS) if a pregnant woman is infected with the rubella virus and transmits the virus to the fetus in the first trimester. CRS consists of birth defects and possibly a miscarriage or stillbirth. The rubella test detects rubella virus antibodies in the blood. There are two rubella virus antibodies that are detected:

- IgG antibody: The patient has immunity against the rubella virus. The rubella virus antibody developed from a previous rubella virus infection or from the rubella virus vaccination.
- IgM antibody: The patient currently has or recently had a rubella virus infection.

What Is Being Measured?

- Rubella virus antibodies in blood

How Is the Test Performed?

- See "How to Collect Blood Specimen From a Vein" in Appendix A.

Rationale for the Test

- Assess if the patient
  - Is immune to the rubella virus
  - Currently or recently has had a rubella virus infection

Nursing Implications

- A woman who wants to become pregnant must receive the rubella test to determine if she is immune to the rubella virus.
- A woman who is not immune to the rubella virus can receive the rubella vaccination but must wait 1 month after receiving the vaccination before becoming pregnant.
- A pregnant woman who is not immune to the rubella virus cannot receive the rubella vaccination during the pregnancy and must avoid anyone who is at risk of being infected with the virus.

Understanding the Results

- The rubella test results are available quickly.
- Results are reported as a titer. A titer specifies how much of the sample of blood is diluted with saline before antibodies are no longer detected. The titer is reported as a ratio of parts of the blood sample and saline. The higher the second number of the ratio, the greater the number of antibodies in the blood sample.
- Normal test results (positive): 1:10 to 1:20.
- Lower levels (negative) may indicate risk for rubella virus infection.

Teach the Patient

- Explain
  - Why blood sample is taken.
  - That if the patient is pregnant, she should avoid others who might be at risk of rubella virus infection unless she is immune to the virus.

- That the patient should have the rubella test before becoming pregnant. The healthcare provider will likely order the rubella vaccination if she is not immune. She must wait 1 month after the vaccination before becoming pregnant.

13. Syphilis Tests

Treponema pallidum is the bacterium that causes syphilis. The syphilis tests identify *T pallidum* antibodies in a blood sample. There are seven types of syphilis tests:

- Veneral disease research laboratory (VDRL): This test identifies anticardiolipin antibodies that are produced by the patient who has syphilis. Diseases including syphilis cause the production of anticardiolipin antibodies; therefore, this test is used for screening of syphilis and not diagnosing syphilis.
- Rapid plasma reagin (RPR): This test is similar to VDRL except antibodies can be detected without the aid of a microscope.
- ELISA: This test identifies *T pallidum* antibodies and is used for screening of syphilis. Additional test is necessary to diagnose syphilis.
- Fluorescent treponemal antibody absorption (FTA-ABS): This test identifies *T pallidum* antibodies after the fourth week of the initial infection and is used to confirm other positive test results.
- *Treponema pallidum* particle agglutination assay (TPPA): This test is similar to the FTA-ABS except it is not used to test spinal fluid.
- Darkfield microscopy: This test identifies the *T pallidum* bacterium under a darkfield microscope and is used to diagnose the early stage of syphilis.
- Microhemagglutination assay (MHA-TP): This test is similar to TPPA.

> **NURSING ALERT**
>
> Many syphilis tests can use either blood sample or a sample of spinal fluid.

> **NURSING ALERT**
>
> A positive VDRL test or RPR test does not mean that the patient has syphilis. Other conditions can cause a positive test result. FTA-ABS, MHA-TP, and TPPA tests remain positive even after the patient is successfully treated for syphilis. VDRL and RPR tests are negative when treatment for syphilis is successful. A negative result does not rule out syphilis, since detectable antibodies can take 4 weeks following the initial infection to develop.

What Is Being Measured?

- *Treponema pallidum* antibodies in blood or spinal fluid
- Anticardiolipin antibodies in blood or spinal fluid
- *Treponema pallidum* bacterium in blood or spinal fluid

How Is the Test Performed?

- See "How to Collect Blood Specimen From a Vein" in Appendix A.
- The healthcare provider will insert a needle into the spinal canal and remove a sample of spinal fluid.

Rationale for the Test

- Assess
  - For syphilis infection
  - Treatment for syphilis infection

Nursing Implications

- Assess if the patient has
  - Had a blood transfusion recently
  - Liver disease, yaws, lupus, or HIV
  - Taken antibiotics
- Consult the healthcare facility's policy for reporting diagnosed cases of syphilis to the local health department.

Understanding the Results

- The syphilis test results are available in 10 days.
- Normal test results (nonreactive/negative): No antibodies found. No *T pallidum* bacterium seen under the microscope.
- Abnormal test results (reactive/positive): Antibody reagin found. *Treponema pallidum* bacterium seen under the microscope.
- Inconclusive test results (equivocal): Unclear if antibody reagin found. Unclear if *T pallidum* bacterium is seen under the microscope.

Teach the Patient

- Explain
  - Why the sample is taken.
  - That the sex partner must also be tested.
  - That the patient should refrain from sex until test shows that the patient and the sex partner are no longer infected.
  - That a diagnosis of syphilis may have to be reported to the health department.
  - That a negative test may not rule out syphilis since detectable antibodies can take 4 weeks following the initial infection to develop.

14. Viral Load Measurement

The HIV in a patient's blood is determined by the presence of HIV RNA. The amount of HIV RNA indicates if the infection is decreasing, stabilized, or increasing. The viral load measurement test determines the amount of HIV RNA in the patient's blood. A viral load measurement test is administered when the patient is diagnosed with HIV and becomes the baseline. Results of subsequent viral load measurement tests are compared to the baseline to determine the infection's progress.

There are three types of viral load measurement tests:

- Branched DNA (bDNA) test
- Nucleic acid sequence–based amplification (NASBA) test
- Reverse-transcriptase polymerase chain reaction (RT-PCR) test

> ## NURSING ALERT
>
> Although the viral load measurement test is more accurate, the healthcare provider may also order the CD4+ count test, which assesses the progress of the HIV infection. The viral load measurement test is not used to diagnose HIV.

> ## NURSING ALERT
>
> A patient diagnosed with HIV who has a negative viral load measurement test result can infect another person.

What Is Being Measured?

- HIV RNA in blood

How Is the Test Performed?

- Baseline every 4 months if the patient is not receiving highly active antiretroviral therapy (HAART).
- Baseline 8 weeks after the start of HAART, and then every 4 months if the patient is receiving HAART.
- See "How to Collect Blood Specimen From a Vein" in Appendix A.

Rationale for the Test

- Assess treatment of HIV infection.
- Assess progress of HIV infection.

Nursing Implications

- Assess if the patient has
  - Another infection
  - Received immunizations recently

Understanding the Results

- The viral load measurement test results take 2 weeks.
- Normal viral load measurement test result is (negative): No HIV RNA is found in blood.

- Abnormal viral load measurement test result: HIV RNA is found and is reported as copies per milliliter where a copy is an HIV RNA.
- The viral load measurement test result is compared to the baseline test result and to previous test results to determine the trend of the infection.

Teach the Patient

- Explain
  - Why the sample is taken.
  - That a negative test result does not mean that the patient is cured. The patient can still spread the infection.

Summary

When a foreign protein enters the body, the body's immune system is alerted and becomes defensive by creating antibodies that seek out the foreign protein. Once found, the antibody kills the foreign protein by metabolizing it into components that can be safely excreted by the body.

Once the antibody is produced, it remains in the body for a long time, providing protection against the related foreign protein. The patient is considered immune to that foreign protein. In this chapter, you learned that healthcare providers order serology tests to examine antibodies in the patient's blood serum.

The presence of an antibody can mean that the patient is currently infected with foreign protein or has been exposed to the foreign protein in the past either through an invasion by a microorganism or from a vaccination. The serology test is used to determine the status of a patient's immunization and can be used to determine if he/she has an autoimmune disorder.

QUIZ

1. **Why would a practitioner order the immunoglobulin test?**
   A. To measure antibodies made by the patient's immune system
   B. To determine if the patient has an infection
   C. To determine if the patient has leukemia
   D. To assess if the patient has internal bleeding

2. **What is IgE?**

   A. An immunoglobulin that forms when an infection occurs for the first time
   B. An immunoglobulin that crosses the placenta
   C. An immunoglobulin found on mucous membranes
   D. An immunoglobulin found in tears

3. **When is the immunoglobulin test typically ordered?**

   A. To diagnose pneumonia
   B. As a follow-up to an abnormal result from the total blood protein test or from the blood protein electrophoresis test
   C. To rollout pneumonia
   D. To measure erythrocytes levels

4. **What might a high level of IgM indicate?**

   A. RA
   B. Viral hepatitis
   C. Mononucleosis
   D. All of the above

5. **Why is the ANA test ordered?**

   A. Screen for autoimmune diseases
   B. Screen for infection
   C. Screen for pregnancy
   D. Screen for HIV

6. **Why would a practitioner order the CD4+ count test?**

   A. T-lymphocytes
   B. T-cells
   C. T-helper cells
   D. All of the above

7. **What is the seroconversion period?**

   A. The period when the HIV-2 infection is detectable in a patient
   B. The period when the HIV infection is detectable in a patient
   C. The period when the HIV infection is not detectable in a patient
   D. The period when the HIV-1 infection is detectable in a patient

8. **What should occur after a positive saliva test?**

   A. Results must be confirmed by the ANA test.
   B. Results must be confirmed by the Western blot test.
   C. Results must be confirmed by the immunoglobulins test.
   D. Results must be confirmed by the IgM test.

9. **Why are T-lymphocytes, T-cells, and T-helper cells important?**

   A. These are factors that spread HCV.
   B. These are factors that cause rheumatoid arthritis.
   C. These are factors that spread HAV.
   D. These are three types of leukocytes important in fighting infection.

10. **What would you tell the patient whose ELISA test is positive?**

   A. You have a confirmed diagnosis of HIV.
   B. You have a confirmed diagnosis of AIDS.
   C. The test result does not mean that you are HIV positive. Further testing is necessary.
   D. You do not have HIV.

ANSWERS

1. A. To measure antibodies made by the patient's immune system.
2. C. An immunoglobulin found on mucous membranes.
3. B. As a follow-up to an abnormal result from the total blood protein test or from the blood protein electrophoresis test.
4. A. RA.
5. A. Screen for autoimmune diseases.
6. D. All of the above.
7. C. The period when the HIV infection is not detectable in a patient.
8. B. Results must be confirmed by the Western blot test.
9. D. These are three types of leukocytes important in fighting infection.
10. C. The test result does not mean that you are HIV positive. Further testing is necessary.

chapter **8**

Endocrine Tests

KEY WORDS

Addison disease
Adrenal gland tumor
Adrenal glands
Aldactone
α-Fetoprotein (AFP)
Corticotropin-releasing hormone
  (CRH)
Cushing disease
Diabetes
Estradiol
Estriol
Estrone

Human chorionic gonadotropin (hCG)
Hyperaldosteronism
Hyperthyroidism
Hypoglycemic
Hypothyroidism
Inferior petrosal sinus
Insulin-like growth factor 1 (IGF-1)
Pituitary gland
Renin
Sheehan syndrome
Thyroxine (T4)
Triiodothyronine (T3)

The endocrine system is an organization of glands that create, store, and release hormones to regulate metabolism, moods, growth, and other functions of the body. Glands increase or decrease hormone production based on the level of hormones in the blood. Hormones act as chemical messengers that signal other glands and organs to react in a specific manner.

Disorders can disrupt hormone creation, storage, and release by glands resulting in an under- or overproduction of one or more hormones. As a result, functions of the body can become deregulated leading to disruption of normal bodily activities. Endocrine tests are ordered by the practitioner to assess the patient's endocrine system specifically looking for disorders that may explain signs and symptoms reported by the patient.

You will learn about endocrine tests in this chapter.

1. Adrenocorticotropic Hormone and Cortisol

The hypothalamus releases corticotropin-releasing hormone (CRH), which causes the pituitary gland to release the adrenocorticotropic hormone (ACTH). ACTH causes the adrenal gland to release cortisol. Cortisol increases blood pressure and glucose and reduces the immune response. The ACTH test measures the level of ACTH in the blood. ACTH levels fall when cortisol levels rise and ACTH levels rise when cortisol levels fall.

NURSING ALERT

The healthcare provider may request that a sample be taken from the inferior petrosal sinus near the pituitary gland to determine if the pituitary gland is producing ACTH or if ACTH is being produced elsewhere in the patient's body.

What Is Being Measured?

- The level of ACTH in the patient's blood
- The level of cortisol in the patient's blood

How Is the Test Performed?

- A blood specimen is taken either in the morning if the healthcare provider wants a peak level or in the evening if a trough level is required. ACTH is highest between 6 AM and 8 AM and lowest between 6 PM and 11 PM.
- See "How to Collect Blood Specimen From a Vein" in Appendix A.
- The sample must be placed in a special test tube, placed on ice and immediately processed.
- Note on the test tube the day and time when the sample was taken.

Rationale for the Test

- Assess
  - The pituitary gland function
  - The adrenal gland function

Nursing Implications

- Assess the patient for conditions that might affect the test results
  - Intoxication
  - Pregnancy
  - Menstruation
  - Emotional or physical stress or severe injury
  - Undergoing a radioactive tracer medical test the previous week before the ACTH test

- Taking corticosteroids acts like cortisol
- Taking amphetamines, insulin, and lithium carbonate, which causes the release of cortisol
- Assess whether or not the patient
  - Ate or drank 12 hours before the test
  - Has exercised within the previous 12 hours
- The patient may experience bruising if either the ACTH or cortisol levels are elevated.

Understanding the Results

- The result is available in 6 days. The laboratory determines normal values based on calibration of testing equipment with a control test. Test results are reported as high, normal, or low based on the laboratory's control test.
- Generally normal ranges for ACTH levels are
  - 6 AM to 8 AM: Less than 80 pg/mL or less than 18 pmol/L
  - 6 PM to 11 PM: Less than 50 pg/mL or less than 11 pmol/L
- Generally normal ranges for cortisol levels are
  - 6 AM to 8 AM: 5 to 23 mcg/dL or 138 to 635 nmol/L
  - 6 PM to 11 PM: 3 to 13 mcg/dL or 83 to 359 nmol/L
- High levels may indicate
  - Physical or emotional stress
  - Addison disease
  - Cushing disease
  - Adrenal gland tumor
  - Pituitary gland tumor
- Low levels might indicate
  - Head injury
  - Stroke
  - Pituitary gland damaged from radiation or surgery
  - Pituitary gland tumor
  - Adrenal gland tumor—Cushing syndrome (increased release of cortisol)

- Comparing levels of ACTH and cortisol can give a sign for the following diseases/conditions
  - High ACTH high cortisol: ACTH made outside the pituitary gland; Cushing disease
  - Low ACTH high cortisol: Adrenal tumor (Cushing syndrome)
  - High ACTH low cortisol: Addison disease
  - Low ACTH low cortisol: Hypopituitarism

NURSING ALERT

Levels of ACTH vary by the minute, making test results difficult to interpret.

Teach the Patient

- Don't exercise 12 hours before the test.
- Avoid stressful situations 12 hours before the test.
- Explain
  - That there might be bruising if the ACTH and cortisol levels are high.
  - That the test cannot be taken if the patient is pregnant, menstruating, or intoxicated or if he/she has taken corticosteroids, amphetamines, insulin, and lithium carbonate. If the patient is taking these medications, then he/she must stop taking them for 2 days before the test.
  - When and why blood samples are taken.
  - That the healthcare provider may ask the patient not to eat or drink 12 hours before the test. The patient may be permitted to eat low-carbohydrate foods for 2 days before the test.

2. Overnight Dexamethasone Suppression Test

The pituitary gland releases ACTH whenever there is a low level of cortisol in the blood. ACTH signals the adrenal glands to release cortisol. An adrenal gland tumor causes the release of cortisol in the absence of ACTH.

Dexamethasone is medication similar to cortisol in that dexamethasone signals the pituitary gland that there is a high level of cortisol in the blood, causing the pituitary gland to suppress the release of ACTH.

The overnight dexamethasone suppression test examines the patient's cortisol level after dexamethasone has been administered. The cortisol level should be lower because there is no ACTH in the blood to signal the adrenal glands to release cortisol. If cortisol levels remain high, then this is a sign of Cushing syndrome as a result of an adrenal gland tumor, which is producing cortisol.

What Is Being Measured?

- The level of ACTH in the patient's blood
- The level of cortisol in the patient's blood

How Is the Test Performed?

- Dexamethasone is administered at 11 PM the night before the test.
- Administer dexamethasone with antacid or milk to reduce the risk of heartburn or stomach upset.
- Patient is not permitted to eat or drink anything 12 hours before the specimen is drawn.
- A blood specimen is taken at 8 AM.
- See "How to Collect Blood Specimen From a Vein" in Appendix A.

Rationale for the Test

- Assess
  - The adrenal gland function
  - For Cushing syndrome

Nursing Implications

- Assess the patient for conditions that might affect the test results by preventing a decrease in cortisol levels
  - Severe obesity
  - Pregnancy
  - Dehydration
  - Uncontrolled diabetes
  - Severe weight loss

- Acute alcohol withdrawal
- Severe injury
- Stress
- Taking birth control pills, phenytoin (Dilantin), monoamine oxidase inhibitors (MAOIs), lithium, morphine, aspirin, barbiturates, methadone, diuretics, or Aldactone

- Assess the patient's metabolism. Some patients metabolize dexamethasone quickly, resulting in a lower than expected blood level when the blood specimen is taken. In this case, the healthcare provider will increase the dose of dexamethasone. The patient may be given up to 8 doses of dexamethasone over 2 days.

- The patient should refrain from taking birth control pills, phenytoin (Dilantin), MAOIs, lithium, morphine, aspirin, barbiturates, methadone, diuretics or Aldactone for 48 hours before the blood specimen is drawn.

- A patient with high ACTH and cortisol levels may experience bruising.

Understanding the Results

- The result is available in 3 days. The laboratory determines normal values based on calibration of testing equipment with a control test. Test results are reported as high, normal, or low based on the laboratory's control test.
- Generally normal ranges for cortisol levels
  - Less than 5 mcg/dL or less than 150 nmol/L
- High levels may indicate
  - Cushing syndrome
  - Hyperthyroidism
  - Uncontrolled diabetes
  - Heart failure
  - Myocardial infarction
  - Poor diet
  - Fever
  - Alcoholism
  - Depression
  - Anorexia nervosa
  - Lung cancer

> **NURSING ALERT**
>
> Further testing is indicated if there is a high cortisol level. Also, a normal result does not rule out Cushing syndrome. The healthcare provider may prefer conducting a 24-hour urine free cortisol test, since this is not influenced by the timing of the blood specimen.

Teach the Patient

- Don't exercise 12 hours before the test.
- Avoid stressful situations 12 hours before the test.
- Explain
  - That there might be bruising if the ACTH and cortisol levels are high.
  - That the test cannot be administered if the patient has taken birth control pills, phenytoin (Dilantin), MAOIs, lithium, morphine, aspirin, barbiturates, methadone, diuretics, or Aldactone. If the patient is taking these medications, he/she must stop taking them for 2 days before the test.
  - When and why the blood sample is taken.
- Don't eat or drink 12 hours before the test.

3. Aldosterone in Blood

Kidneys release renin. Renin is a hormone that signals the adrenal glands to release aldosterone to control blood pressure and fluids and electrolyte balance by retaining fluid and sodium. The aldosterone test determines the level of aldosterone in the blood. This test is typically performed with the renin activity test.

What Is Being Measured?

- Aldosterone level in blood

How Is the Test Performed?

- See "How to Collect Blood Specimen From a Vein" in Appendix A.

NURSING ALERT

The healthcare provider may choose to use a 24-hour urine test in place of measuring aldosterone levels in the blood if the patient is unable to change position.

Rationale for the Test

- Assess
  - For an adrenal gland tumor
  - The cause of high blood pressure
  - The cause of a low potassium level in the blood
  - For an overactive adrenal gland

Nursing Implications

- The aldosterone test is administered as a part of routine blood screening.
- There is no special preparation required for this test.
- If the test result is abnormal, the healthcare provider may order subsequent aldosterone tests. For subsequent aldosterone tests, the patient should
  - Refrain from eating natural black licorice 2 weeks prior to the test.
  - Eat 3 g/d of sodium for 2 weeks prior to the test.
  - Avoid a low-salt diet, since this increases aldosterone levels.
  - Avoid a high-salt diet, since this decreases aldosterone levels. Do not eat olives, soy sauces, pretzels, potato chips, canned soups, bacon, and vegetables.
  - Might be asked to stand, sit, or lie when the test is administered, since the patient's position may affect the test results. Standing or sitting for 2 hours before the test increases the aldosterone level.
- Assess
  - Prescription and nonprescription medication that the patient takes. Diuretics, estrogen, corticosteroids, progesterone, opiates, nonsteroidal anti-inflammatory drugs (NSAIDs), heparin, and Aldactone affect the test and should be stopped 2 weeks before the test.

- If the patient is in the third trimester of pregnancy, since aldosterone level can be high at this stage of pregnancy.
- If the patient is under emotional stress or experiences strenuous exercise prior to the test. This can affect the test results.
- The patient's age, since aldosterone level decreases with age.

> **NURSING ALERT**
>
> A patient who has muscle cramps, muscle weakness, tingling in the hands, or high blood pressure may have a high level of aldosterone.

Understanding the Results

- Test results are available between 2 and 5 days. The laboratory determines normal values based on calibration of testing equipment with a control test. Test results are reported as high, normal, or low based on the laboratory's control test.
- The healthcare provider will likely order subsequent aldosterone tests if there is an abnormal result.
- Generally the normal range is
  - Lying down: 3 to 10 ng/dL or 0.08 to 0.3 nmol/L
  - Standing or sitting: 5 to 30 ng/dL or 0.14 to 0.8 nmol/L
  - Child 1 year and older: 5 to 80 ng/dL or 0.14 to 2.13 nmol/L
  - Child younger than 1 year: 1 to 160 ng/dL or 0.03 to 2.26 nmol/L
- High level may indicate
  - Primary hyperaldosteronism directly affects the adrenal glands—renin activity test is low.
    - Adrenal hyperplasia
    - Conn syndrome/adrenal gland tumor
  - Secondary hyperaldosteronism does not directly affect the adrenal glands—renin activity test is high.
    - Cirrhosis
    - Heart failure
    - Kidney disease
    - Preeclampsia

- Low level may indicate
  - Addison disease

> **NURSING ALERT**
>
> The healthcare provider may order a potassium blood test if there is abnormal adrenal growth or if overactive adrenal glands are suspected as the cause of an abnormal aldosterone test result.

Teach the Patient

- Explain
  - Why blood sample is taken.
  - The function of aldosterone and the meaning of abnormal values.
  - That the patient may be asked to stand, sit, or lie during the test.
  - That the healthcare provider may ask the patient to stop taking diuretics, estrogen, corticosteroids, progesterone, opiates, NSAIDs, heparin, or Aldactone 2 weeks prior to the test, since these medications affect the test results.
- Ask the patient to refrain from
  - Eating natural black licorice 2 weeks prior to the test.
  - Keeping a low- or high-salt diet.

4. Cortisol in Blood

Cortisol, produced by the adrenal glands, is a hormone that causes an increase in blood pressure and glucose while decreasing the immune response. Cortisol levels reach the highest at 7 AM and the lowest 3 hours after sleep based on the diurnal rhythm. However, the diurnal rhythm reverses if the patient works at night and sleeps during the day.

The pituitary gland releases ACTH whenever there is a low level of cortisol in the blood. ACTH signals the adrenal glands to release cortisol.

> **NURSING ALERT**
>
> The healthcare provider may also order the dexamethasone suppression test, adrenocorticotropic hormone test, or a 24-hour urine test.

What Is Being Measured?

- Cortisol level in the blood

How Is the Test Performed?

- A blood sample is taken in the morning to measure peak level.
- See "How to Collect Blood Specimen From a Vein" in Appendix A.

Rationale for the Test

- Assess the function of the
  - Pituitary gland
  - Adrenal glands

Nursing Implications

- Ask the patient to lie down for 30 minutes before administering the test to reduce stress levels.
- Assess if the patient
  - Has had strenuous physical activity 24 hours before the test is administered
  - Is pregnant, since this test can increase cortisol levels
  - Is hypoglycemic
  - Has had a radioactive scan a week before the test
  - Has taken amphetamines, estrogen, birth control pills, or corticosteroids, since these medications affect the test results
  - Has eaten or drunk before the test, since this can affect the test results

Understanding the Results

- Test results are available quickly. The laboratory determines normal values based on calibration of testing equipment with a control test. Test results are reported as high, normal, or low based on the laboratory's control test.
- Normal range
  - Adults (morning): 5 to 23 mcg/dL or 138 to 635 nmol/L

- Adults (afternoon): 3 to 13 mcg/dL or 83 to 359 nmol/L
- Children (morning): 3 to 21 mcg/dL or 83 to 580 nmol/L
- Children (afternoon): 3 to 10 mcg/dL or 83 to 276 nmol/L
- Newborn: 1 to 24 mcg/dL or 27 to 663 nmol/L
- High level values may indicate
  - Adrenal gland tumor
  - Overactive adrenal gland
  - Cushing syndrome
  - Cushing disease
  - Adenoma
  - Depression
  - Severe liver disease
  - Obesity
  - Hyperthyroidism
  - Severe kidney disease
  - Surgery
  - Sepsis
- Low level values may indicate
  - Addison disease
  - Shock
  - Sheehan syndrome
  - Autoimmune disease

Teach the Patient

- Explain
  - Why blood sample is taken.
  - That the healthcare provider may ask the patient to stop taking amphetamines, estrogen, birth control pills, or corticosteroids 2 weeks prior to the test, since these medications affect the test results.
  - That the healthcare provider may ask the patient not to eat or drink 12 hours before the test.

5. Estrogens

Estrogen is a hormone produced in the ovaries, placenta, muscle tissue, adipose tissue, adrenal glands, and testicles in men. There are three types of estrogen hormones:

- Estradiol: This is an estrogen found in non-pregnant women that varies with the menstrual cycle.
- Estriol: This is an estrogen that is produced by the placenta and is measured in pregnant women who are in at least the ninth week of pregnancy.
- Estrone: This is an estrogen measured in women who have finished menopause and in both men and women suggestive of having testicular cancer, ovarian cancer, or an adrenal gland tumor.

NURSING ALERT

Estrogen levels can also be measured in urine. The healthcare provider may order a triple test or quad marker screen to assess for fetal birth defects. The maternal serum triple test measures levels of estrogen, α-fetoprotein (AFP), and human chorionic gonadotropin (hCG). The quad marker screen measures the same as the triple test and also tests inhibin A hormone.

What Is Being Measured?

- Estrogen levels in blood

How Is the Test Performed?

- See "How to Collect Blood Specimen From a Vein" in Appendix A.

Rationale for the Test

- Assess
  - The effect of fertility therapy
  - For abnormal sexual characteristics in men
  - For estrogen-producing tumors
  - For fetal birth defects

Nursing Implications

- Assess
  - The stage of the patient's menstrual cycle
  - If the patient is pregnant
  - If the patient has completed menopause
  - If the patient is undergoing hormone replacement therapy
  - Type of birth control that is used by the patient
  - If the patient has undergone a radioactive scan in the week prior to administering the test
  - If the patient has taken prednisone, Clomid, or Serophene, since these medications might affect the test result

Understanding the Results

- Estrogen test results are available in 1 day. The laboratory determines normal values based on calibration of testing equipment with a control test. Test results are reported as high, normal, or low based on the laboratory's control test.
- Normal estradiol range
  - Before menopause: 30 to 400 pg/mL
  - After menopause: 0 to 30 pg/mL
  - Men: 10 to 50 pg/mL
  - Children: 0 to 15 pg/mL
- Normal estriol range in pregnant women
  - First trimester: Less than 38 ng/mL
  - Second trimester: 38 to 140 ng/mL
  - Third trimester: 31 to 460 ng/mL
- High estrogen values may indicate
  - Cirrhosis
  - Multiple fetuses
  - Early puberty
  - Infertility treatment is working
  - Ovarian cancer
  - Testicular cancer
  - Adrenal gland tumor

- Low estrogen values may indicate
  - Turner syndrome
  - Anorexia nervosa
  - Dysfunctional pituitary gland
  - Dysfunctional placenta
  - Fetal disorder

Teach the Patient

- Explain
  - Why blood sample is taken.
  - That the healthcare provider may ask the patient to stop taking predni-sone, Clomid, or Serophene for 2 weeks prior to the test.

6. Growth Hormone

The human growth hormone (HGH), secreted by the pituitary gland, stimu-lates cell growth and reproduction and insulin-like growth factor 1 (IGF-1). The GH test measures the level of GH in blood.

> **NURSING ALERT**
>
> The healthcare provider may order the IGF-1 test, the GH suppression test (glucose loading test), and the GH stimulation test (insulin tolerance test) along with the GH test.

What Is Being Measured?

- GH level in blood

How Is the Test Performed?

- Avoid eating and drinking for 10 hours before the test.
- Avoid exercising 10 hours before the test.
- Rest for 30 minutes before the test.
- See "How to Collect Blood Specimen From a Vein" in Appendix A.

Rationale for the Test

- Assess for
  - Abnormal growth
  - Treatment of abnormal growth
  - A pituitary gland tumor

Nursing Implications

- Assess if the patient
  - Has eaten or drunk 10 hours before the test
  - Has exercised 10 hours before the test
  - Rested for 30 minutes before the test
  - Is taking St. John's wort, insulin, estrogen, amphetamines, birth control pills, or corticosteroids, since these medications can affect the test result
  - Is hypoglycemic
  - Is obese

Understanding the Results

- Normal GH test results are available quickly. The laboratory determines normal values based on calibration of testing equipment with a control test. Test results are reported as high, normal, or low based on the laboratory's control test.
- Normal GH level range
  - Men: Less than 5 ng/mL
  - Women: Less than 10 ng/mL
  - Children: 0 to 10 ng/mL
  - Newborn: 10 to 40 ng/mL
- High GH levels may indicate
  - Acromegaly
  - Gigantism
  - Pituitary gland tumor
  - Starvation
  - Diabetes
  - Kidney disease

- Low growth hormone levels may indicate
  - Dwarfism
  - Hypopituitarism
  - Sarcoidosis

Teach the Patient

- Explain
- Why sample is taken.
- That the patient must avoid eating and drinking for 10 hours before the test.
- That the patient must avoid exercising for 10 hours before the test.
- That the patient must rest for 30 minutes before the test.
- That the healthcare provider may want the patient to refrain from taking St. John's wort, insulin, estrogen, amphetamines, birth control pills, or corticosteroids 2 weeks before the test.

7. Luteinizing Hormone

Luteinizing hormone (LH) is produced by the pituitary gland that stimulates production of testosterone and ovulation and regulates the menstrual cycle.

> **NURSING ALERT**
>
> Home ovulation testing kits detect LH levels in urine.

What Is Being Measured?

- LH level in blood

How Is the Test Performed?

- The healthcare provider may order several samples taken on 1 day or samples taken over several days.
- See "How to Collect Blood Specimen From a Vein" in Appendix A.

Rationale for the Test

- Assess for
  - Underlying cause of infertility
  - Infertility treatment
  - Underlying cause of irregular menstrual period or amenorrhea
  - Menopause
  - Precocious puberty and delayed puberty
  - Erectile dysfunction

Nursing Implications

- Assess
  - First day of the patient's last menstrual period
  - If the patient experiences light or heavy bleeding on the first day of the menstrual period
  - If the patient has hyperthyroidism
  - If the patient has undergone a radioactive tracer test 1 week prior to the test
  - If the patient is taking phenothiazine, cimetidine, clomiphene, spironolactone, digitalis, naloxone, anticonvulsants, levodopa, or birth control pills a month before the test is administered
  - If the patient has liver disease

NURSING ALERT

Age, menstrual cycle, and stage of sexual development affect the test results.

Understanding the Results

- The LH test results are available quickly. The laboratory determines normal values based on calibration of testing equipment with a control test. Test results are reported as high, normal, or low based on the laboratory's control test.
- Normal LH test results
  - Menstruating
    - Follicular phase: 1 to 18 IU/L

- - Midcycle phase: 8.7 to 80 IU/L
  - Luteal phase: 0.5 to 18 IU/L
  - Postmenopause: 12 to 55 IU/L
- Men: 1 to 9 IU/L
- Before puberty: 0 to 1 IU/L
- Male puberty: 0.4 to 7 IU/L
- Female puberty: 0.4 to 12 IU/L
- High LH level may indicate
  - Women
    - Polycystic ovary syndrome
    - Early puberty
    - No ovaries
  - Men
    - Klinefelter syndrome
    - No testicles
    - Malfunctioning testicles
- Low LH level may indicate
  - Malfunctioning pituitary gland
  - Malfunctioning hypothalamus
  - Anorexia nervosa
  - Underweight
  - That the patient is stressed

Teach the Patient

- Explain
- Why the sample is taken.
- That the healthcare provider may order several samples taken on 1 day or samples taken over several days.
- That the healthcare provider may ask the patient to refrain from taking phenothiazine, cimetidine, clomiphene, spironolactone, digitalis, naloxone, anticonvulsants, levodopa, or birth control pills a month before the test is administered.

8. Parathyroid Hormone

The parathyroid glands release parathyroid hormone (PTH) when calcium level in the blood is low, causing the kidneys to retain calcium and bone to release calcium into the blood. PTH converts vitamin D to an active form, resulting in an increase in absorption of calcium by the intestine. Calcium and phosphorus have an inverse relationship. When calcium level in blood is high, phosphorus level in blood is low. Therefore, PTH also controls the phosphorus level in the blood. The PTH test measures the level of PTH in the blood.

> **NURSING ALERT**
>
> The healthcare provider may also order tests for calcium and phosphorus levels in the blood and creatinine tests to assess kidney function.

What Is Being Measured?

- PTH level in blood

How Is the Test Performed?

- Avoid eating or drinking anything except water 10 hours before the test.
- Take the blood sample shortly after the patient awakens.
- See "How to Collect Blood Specimen From a Vein" in Appendix A.

Rationale for the Test

- Assess for hyperparathyroidism.
- Assess the underlying cause of abnormal calcium level in blood.

Nursing Implications

- Assess if the patient
  - Works days or nights to determine the patient's sleep habits
  - Has high cholesterol levels
  - Has high triglyceride levels
  - Is pregnant

- Is breast-feeding
- Has eaten or drunk anything except water 10 hours before the test
- Has taken calcium supplements or is on a high-calcium diet
- Has taken phosphorus supplements or is on a high-phosphorus diet
- Has undergone a radioactive tracer test in 1 week prior to the test
- Has taken Tagamet, Betachron ER, or Inderal, since these medications lower test results
- Has taken diuretics, lithium, rifampin, furosemide, thiazide, or an anticonvulsant, since these medications increase the test results

Understanding the Results

- The PTH test results are available in 2 days. The laboratory determines normal values based on calibration of testing equipment with a control test. Test results are reported as high, normal, or low based on the laboratory's control test.
- Normal PTH test results: 10 to 65 pg/mL
- High PTH test results may indicate
  - Hyperplasia
  - Parathyroid tumor
  - Low calcium level in blood
  - Kidney disease
  - Pancreatic cancer
  - Lung cancer
  - Ovarian cancer
  - Absorption disorder of the intestines
  - Vitamin D deficiency
- Low PTH test results may indicate
  - Lymphoma
  - Low magnesium level in blood
  - Excess calcium intake
  - Malfunctioning parathyroid gland
  - Multiple myeloma
  - Sarcoidosis

Teach the Patient

- Explain
  - Why the sample is taken.
  - To avoid eating or drinking anything except water 10 hours before the test.
  - That the sample will be taken shortly after the patient awakens.
  - That the healthcare provider may ask the patient to refrain from taking Tagamet, Betachron ER, Inderal, diuretics, lithium, rifampin, furosemide, thiazide, or anticonvulsant medication 2 weeks prior to the test.

9. Thyroid Hormone Tests

The hypothalamus gland releases thyrotropin-releasing hormone (TRH), which stimulates the anterior pituitary gland to release thyroid-stimulating hormone (TSH). TSH causes the thyroid gland to release thyroxine (T4) and triiodothyronine (T3), both of which regulate metabolism. T4 and T3 are produced only if there is sufficient iodine in the thyroid gland. T4 and T3 are transported in blood either freely or bound to globulin. Free T4 and T3 affect metabolism. The thyroid gland also releases calcitonin when the patient has hypercalcemia. Calcitonin regulates calcium levels in blood by moving calcium from the blood to bone. The thyroid hormone tests measure the level of T4 and T3 in the blood. There are four thyroid hormone tests:

- Total T4 test: This test measures the amount of T4 hormone that is bound to globulin and the amount of unbound T4 hormone, called free thyroxine in the blood.
- Free thyroxine (FT4) test: This test measures the amount of unbound T4 hormone.
- Free thyroxine index (FTI) test: This test compares the amount of bound thyroxine to total thyroxine and thereby indirectly measures unbound thyroxine.
- T3 test: This test measures T3 hormone that is bound to globulin and the amount of unbound T3 hormone, called free triiodothyronine (FT3).

What Is Being Measured?

- T4 level in blood
- T3 level in blood

How Is the Test Performed?

- See "How to Collect Blood Specimen From a Vein" in Appendix A.
- See "How to Collect Blood Specimen From a Heel Stick" in Appendix A.

Rationale for the Test

- Assess
  - The underlying cause for an abnormal TSH test
  - For hyperthyroidism
  - For treatment of hyperthyroidism
  - For hypothyroidism
  - For treatment of hypothyroidism

Nursing Implications

- Assess if the patient
  - Is taking Dilantin, Tegretol, Coumadin, aspirin, heparin, propranolol, lithium, amiodarone, estrogen, birth control pills, corticosteroids, or progesterone
  - Is pregnant
  - Has had an iodine dye X-ray 4 weeks before the test

Understanding the Results

- Thyroid hormone test results are available in 3 days. The laboratory determines normal values based on calibration of testing equipment with a control test. Test results are reported as high, normal, or low based on the laboratory's control test.
- Normal test results
  - Total T4
    - Adults: 5 to 14 mcg/dL
    - Children: 5.6 to 16.6 mcg/dL
    - Newborn: 9.8 to 22.6 mcg/dL
  - Total T3
    - Adults: 80 to 230 ng/dL

- Children: 83 to 280 ng/dL
- Newborn: 32 to 250 ng/dL
- FT4: 0.8 to 2.4 ng/dL
- FTI
  - Adults: 4.2 to 13
  - Children: 5 to 12.8
  - Newborn: 7.5 to 17.5
  - FT3: 0.2 to 0.6 ng/dL
- High levels may indicate
  - Hyperthyroidism
  - Graves disease
  - Goiter
  - Thyroiditis
  - Overdose of T4 replacement therapy
- Low levels may indicate
  - Hypothyroidism
  - Thyroid radiation treatment
  - Thyroid surgery
  - Pituitary gland disorder
  - Thyroiditis

Teach the Patient

- Explain
- Why the sample is taken.
- That the healthcare provider may ask the patient to refrain from taking Dilantin, Tegretol, Coumadin, aspirin, heparin, propranolol, lithium, amiodarone, estrogen, birth control pills, corticosteroids, or progesterone before the test.

10. Thyroid-Stimulating Hormone

The hypothalamus gland releases TRH, which stimulates the anterior pituitary gland to release TSH. TSH causes the thyroid gland to release T4 and T3 both of which regulate metabolism. The TSH test measures the level of TSH in blood.

> ## NURSING ALERT
>
> The healthcare provider will likely order the thyroid hormone tests along with the TSH test.

What Is Being Measured?

- TSH level in blood

How Is the Test Performed?

- See "How to Collect Blood Specimen From a Vein" in Appendix A.

Rationale for the Test

- Assess
  - For hyperpituitarism
  - Treatment of hyperpituitarism
  - For hypopituitarism
  - Treatment of hypopituitarism
  - For hypothalamus disorder
  - The underlying cause of hyperthyroidism
  - The underlying cause of hypothyroidism

Nursing Implications

- Assess if the patient
  - Is taking Dopamine, Tegretol, Coumadin, aspirin, heparin, corticosteroids, lithium, levodopa, propylthiouracil, or Tapazole
  - Is pregnant
  - Is stressed
  - Has had an iodine dye X-ray 4 weeks before the test

Understanding the Results

- The thyroid hormone test results are available in 3 days. The laboratory determines normal values based on calibration of testing equipment with a control test. Test results are reported as high, normal, or low based on the laboratory's control test.
- Normal test results
  - Adults: 0.4 to 4.5 mIU/L
  - Newborn: 3 to 18 mIU/L
- High levels may indicate
  - Hypothyroidism
  - Pituitary gland tumor
  - Hashimoto thyroiditis
- Low levels may indicate
  - Hyperthyroidism
  - Goiter
  - Toxic nodule tumor
  - Graves disease
  - Pituitary gland damage

Teach the Patient

- Explain
  - Why sample is taken.
  - That the healthcare provider may ask the patient to refrain from taking Dopamine, Tegretol, Coumadin, aspirin, heparin, corticosteroids, lithium, levodopa, propylthiouracil, or Tapazole before the test.

11. Testosterone

The pituitary gland releases LH that stimulates the release of testosterone by the adrenal glands, testes, and ovaries. Testosterone in blood is unbound (called free) or bound to the sex hormone-binding globulin (SHBG) protein in blood. The testosterone test measures the level of testosterone in blood.

What Is Being Measured?

- TSH level in blood

How Is the Test Performed?

- See "How to Collect Blood Specimen From a Vein" in Appendix A.

Rationale for the Test

- Assess
  - The underlying cause of infertility
  - The underlying cause of erectile dysfunction
  - The underlying cause of osteoporosis in men
  - For precocious puberty (boys)
  - For the underlying cause of hirsutism in women
  - For the underlying cause of irregular menstruation
  - Treatment of prostate cancer

Nursing Implications

- Assess if the patient
  - Is taking birth control pills, digoxin, Aldactone, corticosteroids, testosterone, estrogen, barbiturates, or seizure medication
  - Has hyperthyroidism or hypothyroidism
  - Is obese

Understanding the Results

- The testosterone hormone test results are available in 2 days. The laboratory determines normal values based on calibration of testing equipment with a control test. Test results are reported as high, normal, or low based on the laboratory's control test.
- Normal test results
  - Bound testosterone
    - Men
      - Older than 19 years: 280 to 1080 ng/dL
      - 16 to 19 years: 250 to 910 ng/dL

- 14 to 15 years: 170 to 540 ng/dL
- 10 to 13 years: Less than 300 ng/dL
- 7 months to 9 years: Less than 30 ng/dL
  - Women
    - Older than 16 years: Less than 70 ng/dL
    - 14 to 15 years: Less than 60 ng/dL
    - 10 to 13 years: Less than 40 ng/dL
    - 7 months to 9 years: Less than 30 ng/dL
  - Unbound testosterone: 0.3 to 2.0 pg/mL
- High levels may indicate
  - Testicular cancer
  - Adrenal gland cancer
  - Ovarian cancer
  - Polycystic ovary syndrome (PCOS)
  - Precocious puberty (boys)
- Low levels may indicate
  - Klinefelter syndrome
  - Cirrhosis
  - Alcohol abuse
  - Testicle disorder
  - Pituitary gland damage

Teach the Patient

- Explain
- Why the sample is taken.
- That the healthcare provider may ask the patient to refrain from taking birth control pills, digoxin, Aldactone, corticosteroids, testosterone, estrogen, barbiturates, or seizure medication before the test.

Summary

Hormones are biochemical messengers that signal glands and organs how to behave. Hormones are created, stored, and excreted by glands in response to the amount of hormones in the bloodstream.

Generally, there is a balance of hormones. At times, hormones can become imbalanced caused by a gland excreting too much of a hormone. When this occurs, a different hormone is excreted into the bloodstream by a different gland, causing a decrease in the production and excretion of the initial hormone.

There are times when an imbalance of hormones is caused by a disease. The disease causes an under- or overproduction of specific hormones. Endocrine tests are ordered by the healthcare provider to assist in determining the source of the disease.

QUIZ

1. **Why might the practitioner request a sample be taken from the inferior petrosal sinus near the pituitary gland for the ACTH test?**
   A. To determine if the pituitary gland is producing CRH
   B. To determine if the pituitary gland is producing ACTH
   C. To determine if the pituitary gland is producing Cortisol
   D. To determine if the adrenal gland is producing Cortisol

2. **What is dexamethasone?**
   A. Dexamethasone is medication that signals the pituitary gland to release ACTH.
   B. Dexamethasone is medication that signals the pituitary gland that there is no cortisol in the blood.
   C. Dexamethasone is medication that signals the pituitary gland that there is a high level of cortisol in the blood.
   D. Dexamethasone is medication that signals the pituitary gland that there is a low level of cortisol in the blood.

3. **Why is the ACTH may be difficult to interpret?**
   A. ACTH levels vary by the minute.
   B. ACTH levels are normally low.
   C. ACTH levels are normally high.
   D. ACTH levels cannot be calculated.

4. **What happens when there is a high level of cortisol in blood?**
   A. Suppresses ACTH
   B. Increases dexamethasone levels

C. Increases ACTH

D. Indicates that the patient is intoxicated

5. **Renin signals the release of?**

    A. Aldosterone

    B. Cortisol

    C. Phenytoin

    D. Dexamethasone

6. **What might the practitioner do if the patient has a high cortisol level?**

    A. Order a 24-hour urine free cortisol test.

    B. Diagnose the patient with Cushing Syndrome.

    C. Diagnose the patient with hyperthyroidism.

    D. Diagnose the patient with uncontrolled diabetes.

7. **When is Luteinizing hormone measured?**

    A. Assess for sarcoidosis

    B. Assess for the underlying cause of infertility

    C. Assess for pituitary gland tumor

    D. Assess for acromegaly

8. **What is the purpose of the TSH test?**

    A. To assess the underlying cause of hyperthyroidism

    B. To assess the underlying cause of hypothyroidism

    C. To assess the treatment of hypopituitarism

    D. All of the above

9. **What is the purpose of the parathyroid hormone?**

    A. Converts vitamin D to an active form

    B. Increases absorption of calcium by the intestine

    C. Causes the kidneys to retain calcium

    D. All of the above

10. **What is the reason for ordering the estrogen level test?**

    A. To assess for estrogen-producing tumors

    B. To assess the effect of fertility therapy

    C. To assess for fetal birth defects

    D. All of the above

ANSWERS

1. B. To determine if the pituitary gland is producing ACTH.
2. C. Dexamethasone is medication that signals the pituitary gland that there is a high level of cortisol in the blood.
3. A. ACTH levels vary by the minute.
4. A. Suppresses ACTH.
5. A. Aldosterone.
6. D. Order a 24-hour urine free cortisol test.
7. B. Assess for the underlying cause of infertility.
8. D. All of the above.
9. D. All of the above.
10. D. All of the above.

chapter 9

Tumor Markers

LEARNING OBJECTIVES

1 Cancer Antigen 125 (CA-125)

2 Carcinoembryonic Antigen (CEA)

3 Prostate-Specific Antigen (PSA)

KEY WORDS

Complex prostate-specific antigen (cPSA)

Cystoscopy

Metastasized

Prostate-specific antigen density (PSAD)

Prostatitis

Transrectal ultrasound (TRUS)

An uncontrollable growth of abnormal cells in the body is called a tumor. A tumor that is unable to spread to other parts of the body is called benign (noncancerous) and remains in one location. Although a benign tumor does not spread, the size of the tumor may affect nearby areas such as pressuring or compressing a blood vessel. A tumor that is able to spread to other parts of the body is called malignant (cancerous) and can invade surrounding tissues and travel throughout the body using the lymphatic and circulatory systems. This tumor has metastasized. Cells in a malignant tumor do not have chemical properties to anchor the cells to the original site.

A tumor marker is a substance produced by the tumor that is found in blood and other bodily fluids. It may be normal cells made by the tumor at higher than normal levels. It is usually a protein or a pattern of changes to the DNA caused by the tumor. Tumor markers are usually related to a specific type of tumor. There is no generalized tumor marker that is associated with any tumor. Not every type of tumor has a tumor marker.

A high level of a tumor marker does not mean that the patient has a tumor. The tumor marker suggests a tumor is present. Other tests including a biopsy must be performed to confirm the diagnosis. Tumor markers assist the practitioner in determining the type of tumor and the choice of treatment and are also used to monitor treatment.

The presence of a tumor marker does not mean that the patient has cancer. Conditions other than cancer can also generate the tumor marker. Likewise, the absence of a tumor marker does not mean that the patient is cancer free because many times early stages of cancer do not produce a tumor marker.

In addition to tumor markers, a patient's blood can also be tested for cancer genomics. Cancer genomics are mutation of specific genes, which is called a risk marker. A risk marker indicates that a patient is at higher than normal risk for developing cancer; however, there is no sign of cancer as yet. Conversely, the presence of the tumor marker indicates a possibility that a tumor is present.

In this chapter you will learn about these tests.

1. Cancer Antigen 125

Cancer antigen 125 (CA-125) is a protein attached to the ovarian cancer cells and other cancer cells. The CA-125 test measures the level of the CA-125 in the blood.

> **NURSING ALERT**
>
> The CA-125 test is not used to screen patients for ovarian cancer. This test cannot differentiate between a benign or malignant ovarian tumor. The healthcare provider may order testing of peritoneal fluid and the chest to assess if CA-125 is present.

What Is Being Measured?

- CA-125 protein level in blood

How Is the Test Performed?

- See "How to Collect Blood Specimen From a Vein" in Appendix A.

Rationale for the Test

- Screen for
  - Ovarian cancer
  - Other types of cancers
- Assess the effectiveness of cancer treatment.

Nursing Implications

- Assess if the patient
  - Has undergone abdominal surgery in the previous 3 weeks
  - Has undergone chemotherapy recently
  - Has undergone a radioactive scan recently
  - Is pregnant
  - Is menstruating

Understanding the Results

- Test results are available in 3 days. The laboratory determines normal values based on calibration of testing equipment with a control test. Test results are reported as high, normal, or low based on the laboratory's control test.
- Normal CA-125 range: Less than 35 U/mL
- High CA-125 values may indicate
  - Ovarian cancer
  - Cancer of the endometrium
  - Cancer of the fallopian tubes
  - Liver cancer
  - Breast cancer
  - Lung cancer
  - Colon cancer
  - Pancreatic cancer
  - Esophageal cancer
  - Stomach cancer
  - Cancer of the peritoneum
  - Lymphoma
  - Pancreatitis
  - Hepatitis
  - Cirrhosis
  - Lupus
  - Endometriosis
  - Pelvic inflammatory disease
  - Uterine fibroids
  - Menstruation
  - Pregnancy

NURSING ALERT

A high level of CA-125 might be found months before other diagnostic tests, indicating the return of previously treated ovarian cancer.

Teach the Patient

- Explain
  - Why blood sample is taken
  - That this test is not used to screen for ovarian cancer
  - That a positive result does not differentiate between a benign or malignant ovarian tumor

2. Carcinoembryonic Antigen

The carcinoembryonic antigen (CEA) is a protein present during fetal development that terminates at birth. The CEA is produced in certain types of cancers. The CEA test measures the level of CEA antigen in blood.

> ### NURSING ALERT
>
> The CEA is not used to screen for early detection of a cancer and diagnose cancer. Most cancers do not cause high levels of the CEA. The healthcare provider may order a test of peritoneal fluid and cerebrospinal fluid to determine if the cancer has metastasized.

What Is Being Measured?

- CEA protein level in blood

How Is the Test Performed?

- See "How to Collect Blood Specimen From a Vein" in Appendix A.

Rationale for the Test

- Screen for cancer
- Assess
  - Effectiveness of cancer treatment
  - Success of surgery to remove the cancer

Nursing Implications

- Assess if the patient
  - Smokes, since it can affect the test result
  - Has undergone chemotherapy recently
  - Has undergone a radioactive scan recently
  - Is pregnant
  - Is menstruating

Understanding the Results

- Test results are available in 3 days. The laboratory determines normal values based on calibration of testing equipment with a control test. Test results are reported as high, normal, or low based on the laboratory's control test.
- Normal CEA range
  - Nonsmoker: Less than 3 ng/mL
  - Smoker: Less than 5 ng/mL
- High CEA values may indicate
  - Colon cancer
  - Rectal cancer
  - Lung cancer
  - Breast cancer
  - Pancreatic cancer
  - Ovarian cancer
  - Cancer has returned following treatment. Successful treatment results in CEA levels returning to normal within 6 weeks of treatment.
  - Cancer has metastasized
  - Pancreatitis
  - Kidney failure
  - Cirrhosis
  - Peptic ulcer
  - Chronic obstructive pulmonary disease (COPD)
  - Inflammatory bowel disease
  - Crohn disease

> **NURSING ALERT**
>
> CEA may be normal although the patient has cancer.

Teach the Patient

- Explain
  - Why the blood sample is taken
  - That further testing is likely if there is a positive result
  - That a negative result does not rule out cancer

3. Prostate-Specific Antigen

The prostate gland releases prostate-specific antigen (PSA) in low amounts. Increased amounts are released with an enlarged prostate gland, prostatitis, prostate cancer, and from injury resulting from a digital rectal examination, cystoscopy, or sexual activity. The PSA test measures the level of PSA in blood.

> **NURSING ALERT**
>
> PSA test is performed in conjunction with a digital rectal examination. The healthcare provider may also order the prostate-specific antigen density (PSAD) test to compare the PSA value to the prostate gland size, the prostate-specific antigen velocity (PSAV) test to determine if the PSA increases over time, the complex PSA (cPSA) to detect prostate cancer, and the transrectal ultrasound (TRUS) to measure the size of the prostate gland.

> **NURSING ALERT**
>
> The PSA level can be normal in a patient who has prostate cancer.

What Is Being Measured?

- PSA level in blood

How Is the Test Performed?

- Do not ejaculate 48 hours before the test.
- See "How to Collect Blood Specimen From a Vein" in Appendix A.

Rationale for the Test

- Screen for prostate cancer.
- Assess the treatment of prostate cancer.

Nursing Implications

- Assess if the patient
  - Has ejaculated 48 hours before the test
  - Has a urinary tract infection (UTI)
  - Has been catheterized within the past 8 weeks
  - Has prostatitis
  - Has undergone a prostate biopsy in the past 8 weeks
  - Is taking Avodart, finasteride, Cytoxan, Neosar, methotrexate, or diethylstilbestrol

Understanding the Results

- The PSA test results are available quickly.
- Normal test results (maximum level):
  - Younger than 50 years: 2.5 ng/mL
  - 51 to 60 years: 3.5 ng/mL
  - 61 to 70 years: 4.5 ng/mL
  - Older than 70 years: 6.5 ng/mL
- Higher levels may indicate
  - Prostate cancer
  - Benign prostatic hypertrophy (BPH)
  - Prostatitis
  - Recent catheterization
  - Injury

Teach the Patient

- Explain
  - Why sample is taken

- That further testing is necessary if there is a high level of PSA in the blood. This does not mean that the patient has prostate cancer.
- That a normal level of PSA does not mean that the patient is free from prostate cancer

Summary

Tumor marker tests assess the patient's blood for proteins that are frequently present if a tumor is present. These substances are secreted either by the tumor or by other cells in response to the presence of the tumor.

The existence of a tumor marker in the patient's blood does not necessarily mean that he/she has a tumor since the same proteins can be produced by other disorders. The existence of a tumor marker simply indicates that the healthcare provider needs to examine the patient more closely for other signs of tumor.

Conversely, the absence of a tumor marker in the patient's blood does not necessarily mean that a tumor is absent. A tumor might be present, but its growth is at an early stage when tumor markers have yet to be produced.

Tests are also performed on the patient's blood to identify risk markers. A risk marker is a mutation of specific genes that can later result in a tumor. The patient with a risk marker may not develop a tumor, but it is a risk for possibly developing a tumor.

QUIZ

1. **What is antigen 125?**
   A. A protein attached to the ovarian cancer cells and other cancer cells
   B. An enzyme attached to the ovarian cancer cells and other cancer cells
   C. An enzyme attached to the colon cancer cells
   D. An enzyme attached to the liver cancer cells

2. **The CA-125 test is used to**
   A. Screen for ovarian cancer
   B. Differentiate between benign or malignant ovarian tumor
   C. Screen for colon cancer
   D. None of the above

3. **Why the CA-125 test ordered following treatment for cancer?**

   A. A low level of CA-125 might be found months before other diagnostic tests indicating the return of cancer.

   B. A high level of CA-125 confirms that treatment is successful.

   C. A high level of CA-125 might be found months before other diagnostic tests indicating the return of cancer.

   D. A high level of CA-125 confirms that the tumor is benign.

4. **The CEA protein test is used to**

   A. Detect cancer early

   B. Diagnose cancer

   C. Assess the effectiveness of cancer treatment

   D. All of the above

5. **What conditions might affect the results of the PSA test?**

   A. A urinary tract infection

   B. Catheterized within the past 8 weeks

   C. Taking Avodart

   D. All of the above

6. **Successful treatment of cancer may be indicated when the results in CEA level is**

   A. Normal within 6 weeks of treatment

   B. Normal within 4 weeks of treatment

   C. Normal within 2 weeks of treatment

   D. Elevated within 6 weeks of treatment

7. **What may affect the results of the CA-125 test?**

   A. Chemotherapy recently

   B. Menstruating

   C. Radioactive scan recently

   D. All of the above

8. **What should you tell a patient who has a positive CEA test result?**

   A. A positive result will require further tests.

   B. The patient will undergo chemotherapy.

   C. The patient will undergo radiation treatments.

   D. The patient will be admitted to the hospital.

9. **Give three reasons for administering the CEA test.**

A. Screening for cancer, assessing cancer treatment, and identifying the location of the tumor for surgery

B. Screening for cancer, assessing cancer treatment, and for diagnosing cancer

C. Screening for cancer, assessing cancer treatment, and assessing for the success of surgery to remove the tumor

D. None of the above

10. **Why would the prostate-specific antigen density (PSAD) test be ordered?**

A. To diagnose prostate cancer

B. To compare the PSA value to the prostate gland size

C. To confirm the magnetic resonance imaging (MRI) diagnosis of prostate cancer

D. None of the above

ANSWERS

1. A. A protein attached to the ovarian cancer cells and other cancer cells.
2. D. None of the above.
3. C. A high level of CA-125 might be found months before other diagnostic tests indicating the return of cancer.
4. C. Assess the effectiveness of cancer treatment.
5. D. All of the above.
6. A. Normal within 6 weeks of treatment.
7. D. All of the above.
8. A. A positive result will require further tests.
9. C. Screening for cancer, assessing cancer treatment, and assessing the success of surgery to remove the tumor.
10. B. To compare the PSA value to the prostate gland size.

chapter 10

Pregnancy, Infertility, and Genetic Tests

LEARNING OBJECTIVES

1. Antisperm Antibody Test
2. α-Fetoprotein (AFP)
3. Follicle-Stimulating Hormone (FSH)
4. Human Chorionic Gonadotropin (hCG) Hormone
5. Inhibin A Test
6. Prolactin
7. Phenylketonuria (PKU) Test
8. Tay-Sachs Test
9. Sickle Cell Test
10. Hemochromatosis (HFE) Gene Test

KEY WORDS

Amniocentesis	Menstrual cycle
Down syndrome	Multiple of median
Lactogenesis	Tube defect
Luteinizing hormone	Unconjugated estriol (uE3)

Pregnancy tests determine if the patient is pregnant based on hormone levels in her blood such as the high levels of prolactin (increase lactation), hCG (produced after the placenta is implanted), and AFP (a substance made by the liver of the fetus). Infertility tests are ordered by the practitioner to assess why the patient is unable to become pregnant.

Genetic testing is ordered by the practitioner before the patient becomes pregnant and at the request of the patient to determine if the patient and the patient's partner is a carrier of a genetic disease. If genetic testing is positive, then genetic counseling is usually done to help the patient and his/her partner make an informed decision about becoming pregnant. Genetic testing is also ordered early in the pregnancy especially if the pregnancy was unplanned. Results of genetic testing indicate if the fetus will develop a genetic disease.

In this chapter you will learn about these tests.

1. Antisperm Antibody Test

An immune system response can be caused by semen, resulting in antibodies attaching to and killing sperm causing immunologic infertility. These antibodies can be in blood, vaginal fluids, or semen. Antibodies can be made in a man if his sperm comes in contact with his immune system as a result of testicular injury, prostate gland infection, vasectomy, or other surgeries that expose sperm to the immune system. Semen from her partner's sperm can cause an allergic reaction in a woman.

What Is Being Measured?

- Antisperm antibodies

How Is the Test Performed?

- A blood sample is taken from a female patient (See "How to Collect Blood Specimen From a Vein" in Appendix A).
- A semen sample is obtained.
  - Ejaculation should not occur for a 2-day period before and should not have taken place any more than 5 days before the test.
  - Collect semen samples after blood and vaginal fluid samples are taken.
  - Samples cannot be taken by engaging in sexual intercourse and withdrawal during ejaculation. Vaginal fluid may mix with the sperm.
  - A semen sample is collected through masturbation.
    - Urinate.
    - Wash and rinse your hands and penis.
    - Collect the semen in a sterile cup.
    - Do not use lubricants or condoms.
    - Take sample to the laboratory within 30 minutes.

Rationale for the Test

- Assess if
  - Antisperm antibodies are in blood, vaginal fluid, or semen.
  - Infertility maybe caused by immunologic infertility.

NURSING ALERT

Some healthcare providers disagree about the usefulness of the test since treatment is the same regardless of the test results.

Nursing Implications

- Male patients may be embarrassed about collecting a sample.
- Confer with the healthcare provider if masturbation is against the patient's religious beliefs.

Understanding the Results

- Negative test results: Antisperm antibodies are not found.
- Positive test results: Antisperm antibodies are found.

Teach the Patient

- Explain why the test is ordered.
- Explain to male patients
  - Do not ejaculate for 2 days before the test, and ejaculation should not have taken place any more than 5 days before the test.
  - How to collect a semen sample.
  - That a sample is collected through masturbation and not by engaging in sexual intercourse.
  - Do not use lubricants or condoms when collecting the sample.
  - Ask the patient to consult his healthcare provider if masturbation is against his religious beliefs.
  - Take the sample to the laboratory within 30 minutes.

2. α-Fetoprotein

α-Fetoprotein (AFP) is produced by the fetal liver and is detectable in a pregnant woman's blood. The level of AFP rises gradually in 14 weeks of gestation and continues to rise until around the 34th week of gestation when the AFP level gradually decreases.

A high or low level of AFP is a sign that there may be a problem with the fetal development. The AFP test is commonly administered as part of a maternal serum triple or quadruple screening test, which, along with other factors including the pregnant woman's age, is used to estimate the chances of birth defects.

The maternal serum triple screening test examines levels of

- AFP
- β-hCG
- uE3 (estrogen)

The maternal serum quadruple screening test examines levels of

- The same substance as the maternal serum triple screening test
- The hormone inhibin A

A healthcare provider may also administer the AFP test in nonpregnant women and in children and men to assess for a number of other diseases that cause a high level of AFP in the blood. These diseases include lymphoma, Hodgkin disease, ovarian cancer, testicular cancer, renal cell cancer, and pancreatic cancer. One-half of the patients diagnosed with these cancers have normal AFP test results.

What Is Being Measured?

- The level of AFP in the blood

How Is The Test Performed?

- The test is performed between 15 and 20 weeks of gestation.
- The patient is weighed before the blood sample is drawn. The results of the test are evaluated based on the patient's weight.
- Estimate the gestation.
- Assess if the patient is a diabetic who requires insulin injections to manage the diabetes.
- The patient's race is noted. Normal values of AFP are higher in African-American women and lower in Asian women.
- See "How to Collect Blood Specimen From a Vein" in Appendix A.

Rationale for the Test

- Assess for
  - Fetal neural tube defects
  - Spinal bifida
  - Anencephaly
  - Edward syndrome (trisomy 18)
  - Down syndrome (trisomy 21)
  - Omphalocele
  - Hepatoma in patients who have chronic hepatitis B or cirrhosis
  - Lymphoma
  - Hodgkin disease
  - Renal cell cancer

- Ovarian cancer
- Testicular cancer
- Pancreatic cancer
- Effectiveness of cancer treatment

Nursing Implications

- Assess
  - If the patient smokes. Smoking increases the AFP level in the blood.
  - If the patient is an insulin-dependent diabetic.
  - The patient's weight.
  - The gestational age of the fetus.
  - The patient's race.
  - If the patient has undergone a test, involving radioactive tracers in the previous 2 weeks since this might affect the test results.
- If high levels of AFP are detected, the healthcare provider will likely order an ultrasound and/or amniocentesis.
- Ease the patient's concerns. Tell the patient that the AFP test results provide a sign of a disease or medication condition, but are not used to make a definitive diagnosis. AFP levels can be high, but the fetus may be normal.

Understanding the Results

- The result is available quickly. The laboratory determines normal values based on calibration of testing equipment with a control test. Test results are reported as high, normal, or low based on the laboratory's control test.
- Generally the normal range
  - Pregnant women 12 to 22 weeks' gestation: 19 to 75 IU/mL or 7 to 124 mcg/L or 7 to 124 ng/mL
  - Nonpregnant women and men: 0 to 6.4 IU/mL or 0 to 20 mcg/L or 0 to20 ng/mL
- High levels may indicate
  - Neural tube defect
  - Omphalocele (abdominal organs are outside of the abdomen wall; repaired by surgery)

- Multiple fetuses
- Dead fetus
- Incorrect gestational age
- Alcohol abuse
- Cirrhosis
- Hepatitis B
- Lymphoma, Hodgkin disease, ovarian cancer, testicular cancer, renal cell cancer, and pancreatic cancer
- Low levels may indicate
  - Down syndrome (60% accuracy). Accuracy increases to 80% with the maternal serum triple screening test.
  - Incorrect gestational age.

NURSING ALERT

An ultrasound confirms the gestational age. If the gestational age is different than the estimated gestational age, the AFP is adjusted using the multiple of median (MoM) factor. An AFP value that is 0.5 to 2.5 times the multiple of median factor is considered normal.

NURSING ALERT

A normal AFP level does not rule out neural tube defects or Down syndrome. Likewise, an abnormal AFP level is not an indication of a definitive diagnosis. Additional testing such as an ultrasound or amniocentesis will likely be ordered for abnormal results. The patient may have an abnormal AFP level in their blood and a normal AFP level in the amniocentesis indicating low risk to the fetus.

Teach the Patient

- Explain
  - Why blood sample is taken.
  - That weight, race, and gestational age is used to assess the test results.
  - That there is no special preparation required for the test.

- That an abnormal test request does not mean there are developmental problems with the fetus. The test result is one of several signs that help the healthcare provider reach a diagnosis.
- That a neural tube defect is not related to the mother's age. Neural tube defects occur without a family history of this problem.

3. Follicle-Stimulating Hormone

The follicle-stimulating hormone (FSH) is produced by the pituitary gland and controls sperm production by the testes and egg production in the ovaries. The FSH level is constant in men and changes with the menstrual cycle in women, with the highest level occurring during ovulation. The FSH test measures the level of the FSH in blood.

> **NURSING ALERT**
>
> The healthcare provider may order the luteinizing hormone blood test, estrogen blood test, and the progesterone blood test in addition to the FSH test. The healthcare provider may order a sperm count or assessment of the patient's ovarian reserve.

What Is Being Measured?

- FSH level in blood

How Is the Test Performed?

- A blood sample may be taken each day for a period ordered by the healthcare provider if the patient experiences menstrual cycle problems or is unable to become pregnant.
- See "How to Collect Blood Specimen From a Vein" in Appendix A.

Rationale for the Test

- Assess
  - For the underlying cause of infertility
  - For abnormal menstrual periods
  - For precocious puberty

- The function of the pituitary gland
- Abnormal development of sexual organs

Nursing Implications

- Assess
  - The patient's age. Test results depend on the patient's age.
  - If the patient uses herbal or natural substances.
  - The first day of the patient's last menstrual period. Test results depend on her menstrual cycle.
  - Which day the patient experiences the heaviest bleeding during the menstrual period.
  - If the patient has undergone a radioactive tracer in the previous 7 days before the test.
  - If the patient has taken digitalis, cimetidine, levodopa, clomiphene, birth control pills, estrogen, or progesterone 4 weeks before the test, since these medications may affect the test results.

Understanding the Results

- FSH test results are available in 1 day. The laboratory determines normal values based on calibration of testing equipment with a control test. Test results are reported as high, normal, or low based on the laboratory's control test.
- Normal FSH range
  - Menstruating
    - Follicular/luteal phase: 5 to 20 IU/L
    - Midcycle peak: 30 to 50 IU/L
  - Postmenopause: Greater than 49 IU/L
  - Men: 5 to 15 IU/L
  - Children before puberty: Less than 7 IU/L
- High FSH may indicate
  - Women
    - Polycystic ovary syndrome (PCOS)
    - Ovarian failure before 40 years of age
    - Menopause

- Men
  - Abnormal testicle functionality
  - Klinefelter syndrome
- Children
- Start of puberty
- Low FSH may indicate
  - Women
    - Loss of ovulation
  - Men
    - Testicles not producing sperm
  - Malnutrition
  - Hypothalamus disorder
  - Pituitary gland disorder
  - Stress

Teach the Patient

- Explain
- Why blood sample is taken.
- That several blood samples may be necessary, one each for a period, ordered by the healthcare provider if the patient experiences menstrual cycle problems or is unable to become pregnant.
- That the healthcare provider may ask the patient to stop taking digitalis, cimetidine, levodopa, clomiphene, birth control pills, estrogen, or progesterone for 4 weeks prior to the test.

4. Human Chorionic Gonadotropin

When a fertilized egg implants into the uterine wall, the placenta begins development. By the ninth day, the placenta produces Human Chorionic Gonadotropin (hCG) hormone, which is detectable in the patient's blood. The hCG test measures the level of hCG in blood. The level of the hCG hormone is used as a sign of pregnancy, which is confirmed by other tests. In a normal pregnancy, the level of the hCG hormone increases until 16 weeks of gestation and then gradually decreases until birth when no hCG hormone is detectable.

A lower level of hCG hormone might indicate an ectopic pregnancy and a higher level may indicate multiple fetuses. The hCG hormone test is typically ordered as part of a maternal serum screening test that is administered after 15 weeks' gestation.

NURSING ALERT

The level of the hCG hormone can be detected before the patient misses her menstrual period and as early as 6 days after attachment of the egg. The hCG hormone test is also available as a urine test (home pregnancy test), which determines if the hCG hormone is present but does not measure the hormone level. The hCG hormone level is high 4 weeks following an abortion.

NURSING ALERT

The hCG hormone can also be produced by a molar pregnancy, choriocarcinoma (uterine cancer), ovarian cancer, or other tumors. Testicular cancer also produces the hCG hormone in men. A normal hCG hormone level does not rule out cancer.

What Is Being Measured?

- The hCG level in blood

How Is the Test Performed?

- See "How to Collect Blood Specimen From a Vein" in Appendix A.

Rationale for the Test

- Assess
  - For pregnancy
  - For ectopic pregnancy
  - For molar pregnancy
  - Treatment of molar pregnancy
  - For testicular cancer
  - For choriocarcinoma

Nursing Implications

- Assess if the patient
  - Has received hCG hormone infertility treatment prior to administering the test
  - Has taken Anergan, Phenergan, Prorex, diuretics, heparin, Ambien, Mellaril, Serentil, Stelazine, or Compazine

Understanding the Results

- The hCG hormone test results are available quickly. The laboratory determines normal values based on calibration of testing equipment with a control test. Test results are reported as high, normal, or low based on the laboratory's control test.
- Normal hCG hormone level may indicate
  - Men: Less than 5 IU/L
  - Nonpregnant women: Less than 5 IU/L
  - Pregnant women
    - 24 to 28 days' gestation: 5 to 100 IU/L
    - 4 to 5 weeks' gestation: 50 to 500 IU/L
    - 5 to 6 weeks' gestation: 100 to 10,000 IU/L
    - 14 to 16 weeks' gestation: 12,000 to 270,000 IU/L
    - After 16 weeks' gestation: Levels decrease
- High hCG hormone level may indicate
  - Men
    - Lung cancer
    - Pancreatic cancer
    - Colon cancer
    - Liver cancer
    - Testicular cancer
  - Nonpregnant women
    - Lung cancer
    - Pancreatic cancer
    - Colon cancer

- Liver cancer
- Ovarian cancer
- Choriocarcinoma
- Pregnant women
  - Multiple fetuses
  - Down syndrome
  - Molar pregnancy
  - Incorrect gestational estimate
- Low hCG hormone level may indicate
  - Pregnant women
  - Ectopic pregnancy
  - Incorrect gestational estimate
  - Fetal death
  - Risk for spontaneous abortion

Teach the Patient

- Explain
  - Why sample is taken.
  - That the hCG hormone blood test confirms a home urine pregnancy test; however, other tests are necessary to confirm the pregnancy.
  - That the healthcare provider may ask the patient to refrain from taking hCG hormone infertility treatment, Anergan, Phenergan, Prorex, diuretics, heparin, Ambien, Mellaril, Serentil, Stelazine, or Compazine for several weeks prior to the test.

5. Inhibin A Test

Inhibin A hormone is secreted by the placenta and the level of the hormone is measured by the hormone inhibin A test. The hormone inhibin A test is a component of the quadruple screen tests that is administered at the 20th week of gestation to determine if there is a risk of birth defect(s) in the fetus such as Down syndrome. The quadruple screen test also includes the AFP test, β-hCG test, and the unconjugated estriol (uE3) test.

> ### NURSING ALERT
> The hormone inhibin A test is not used to diagnose the potential birth defects. Further testing is required if the hormone inhibin A test is abnormal.

What Is Being Measured?

- Inhibin A hormone level in blood

How Is the Test Performed?

- See "How to Collect Blood Specimen From a Vein" in Appendix A.

Rationale for the Test

- Assess risk for Down syndrome and other birth defects.

Nursing Implications

- Assess if the patient
  - Smokes
  - Is obese
  - Is a diabetic

Understanding the Results

- The inhibin A hormone test results are available quickly.
- High inhibin A hormone level may indicate
  - Birth defect. Additional testing is required for positive diagnosis.

Teach the Patient

- Explain
  - Why sample is taken.
  - Abnormal test results do not necessarily mean there is a birth defect. Further testing might be ordered by the healthcare provider.

6. Prolactin

Prolactin is a hormone produced by the pituitary gland that increases during pregnancy, causing an increase in milk production and enlargement of the mammary glands. A high level of progesterone that occurs during pregnancy prevents milk from ejecting. Progesterone levels fall after delivery. Sucking on the nipple by the newborn causes ejection of milk from the breast, which simulates release of prolactin thus causing lactogenesis, resulting in increased production of milk. Prolactin levels return to normal after delivery if the mother is not breast-feeding. The prolactin test measures the level of prolactin in the blood.

What Is Being Measured?

- Prolactin level in blood

How Is the Test Performed?

- Avoid eating or drinking 12 hours before the test.
- Take the blood sample 3 hours after the patient awakens. Prolactin levels are normally higher in the morning.
- Rest for 30 minutes before taking the blood sample.
- Avoid stimulating the nipples for 1 day prior to the test.
- See "How to Collect Blood Specimen From a Vein" in Appendix A.

Rationale for the Test

- Assess for
  - Prolactinoma (pituitary gland tumor)
  - Underlying cause of amenorrhea
  - Underlying cause of infertility
  - Underlying cause of nipple discharge
  - Erectile dysfunction

Nursing Implications

- Assess if the patient
  - Exercised 12 hours prior to the test
  - Is under emotional stress

- Has difficulty sleeping
- Has undergone a radioactive tracer test 1 week prior to the test
- Is taking tricyclic antidepressants, birth control pills, phenothiazines, hypertension medication, or cocaine
- Has stimulated her nipples within 1 day prior to the test

Understanding the Results

- The prolactin test results are available quickly. The laboratory determines normal values based on calibration of testing equipment with a control test. Test results are reported as high, normal, or low based on the laboratory's control test.
- Normal prolactin test results
  - Pregnant women: 20 to 400 ng/mL
  - Nonpregnant women: Less than 25 ng/mL
  - Men: Less than 20 ng/mL
- High prolactin level may indicate
  - Prolactinoma
  - Idiopathic hyperprolactinemia
  - Hypothyroidism
  - Cirrhosis
  - Kidney disease

Teach the Patient

- Explain
- Why blood sample is taken.
- That the blood sample must be taken 3 hours after the patient awakens.
- That the patient must avoid simulating the nipples for 1 day prior to the test.
- That the patient will be asked to rest for 30 minutes before the blood sample is taken.
- That the healthcare provider may ask the patient to refrain from taking tricyclic antidepressants, birth control pills, phenothiazines, hypertension medication, or cocaine 12 hours prior to the test.
- Avoid eating or drinking 12 hours before the test.

7. Phenylketonuria Test

Phenylalanine is an amino acid in breast milk, formula, dairy products, and meats. The body requires the phenylalanine hydroxylase enzyme to metabolize phenylalanine into tyrosine. Phenylketonuria (PKU) is a genetic disorder whereby the patient is missing the phenylalanine hydroxylase enzyme and is therefore unable to metabolize phenylalanine, causing a buildup of phenylalanine level in the blood thus resulting in mental retardation and seizures. The PKU test measures the level of the phenylalanine hydroxylase enzyme in blood. Newborns are administered the PKU test between 12 and 28 hours after birth and again 1 week after birth.

> **NURSING ALERT**
>
> Infants older than 6 weeks of age may be administered a PKU urine test if a PKU test was not performed at birth. Newborns who are ill are retested 3 weeks after birth.

What Is Being Measured?

- Measures the level of the phenylalanine hydroxylase enzyme in blood

How Is the Test Performed?

- The newborn should ingest formula or breast milk for 48 hours prior to the test.
- See "How to Collect Blood Specimen From a Heel Stick" in Appendix A.

> **NURSING ALERT**
>
> The healthcare provider may order a blood sample taken from a vein to confirm a positive PKU test result that used a sample from a heel stick.

Rationale for the Test

- Assess for PKU.

Nursing Implications

- Assess if the
  - Newborn ingested formula or breast milk for 48 hours prior to the test.
  - Newborn was born prematurely.
  - Patient has vomited prior to the test.
  - Patient is taking antibiotics.

Understanding the Results

- The PKU test results are available quickly.
- Normal PKU test results: Less than 3 mg/dL.
- High PKU test results may indicate
  - PKU

Teach the Patient

- Explain
  - Why a blood sample is taken.
  - To the parents that the newborn must ingest formula or breast milk for 48 hours prior to the test.
  - That the test may be repeated 1 week after birth.

8. Tay-Sachs Test

Hexosaminidase A is an enzyme that metabolizes ganglioside, which is a fatty acid. If the hexosaminidase A is not present, ganglioside accumulates in the brain and nerve cells, resulting in neural damage. This is referred to as Tay-Sachs disease, which is an inherited disease. The Tay-Sachs test measures the amount of hexosaminidase A in the blood.

> **NURSING ALERT**
>
> The healthcare provider may order an amniocentesis or the chorionic villus sampling of the placenta to determine if the fetus has the hexosaminidase A enzyme.

NURSING ALERT

A positive result will be confirmed by genetic testing.

What Is Being Measured?

- Hexosaminidase A enzyme in blood

How Is the Test Performed?

- See "How to Collect Blood Specimen From a Vein" in Appendix A.

Rationale for the Test

- Assess
  - For Tay-Sachs disease
  - If the female patient is carrying the Tay-Sachs trait

Nursing Implications

- Assess if the female patient
  - Has had a blood transfusion 90 days prior to the test
  - Is taking birth control pills
  - Is pregnant

Understanding the Results

- The creatinine blood level test and creatinine clearance test results are available quickly. The laboratory determines normal values based on calibration of testing equipment with a control test. Test results are reported as high, normal, or low based on the laboratory's control test.
- Normal test results:
  - Total hexosaminidase: 10.4 to 23.8 U/L
  - Percentage of blood level: 56% to 80%
- One-half of the normal level may indicate: Patient is a carrier of the Tay-Sachs trait.

- No hexosaminidase A enzyme may indicate
  - Tay-Sachs disease
  - Sandhoff disease (missing hexosaminidase A and hexosaminidase B)

Teach the Patient

- Explain
  - Why a blood sample is taken.
  - That the test results may indicate the patient carries the Tay-Sachs trait and genetic counseling is recommended.
  - That the healthcare provider may ask the patient to refrain from taking birth control pills prior to the test.

9. Sickle Cell Test

Normal red blood cells contain hemoglobin A. In sickle cell disease, red blood cells contain hemoglobin S, which causes the red blood cell to form a sickle shape, therefore called sickled blood cells. Sickle cell disease is an autosomal recessive disease in which the sickle cell gene must be inherited from both parents. Patients with sickled blood cells can experience a sickle cell crisis when sickled blood cells block blood vessels, resulting in decreased blood flow. Sickled blood cells are destroyed faster than normal red blood cells leading to sickle cell anemia. The sickle cell test determines if the patient has sickled blood cells.

> **NURSING ALERT**
>
> The healthcare provider may order the high performance liquid chromatography (HPLC) test to examine the patient's DNA for the sickle cell gene. Sickle cell disease is more prevalent in African-Americans. Healthcare providers commonly test newborns for the sickle cell trait, although infants younger than 6 months can have false-negative test results since they have fetal hemoglobin in their blood and, therefore, the sickle cell test is repeated after 6 months of age. The healthcare provider may order the sickle cell test for a genus using chorionic villus sampling (CVS) or amniocentesis.

> **NURSING ALERT**
>
> The patient should undergo genetic counseling if he/she has the sickle cell trait or sickle cell disease.

What Is Being Measured?

- Existence of sickled blood cells

How Is the Test Performed?

- See "How to Collect Blood Specimen From a Vein" in Appendix A.

Rationale for the Test

- Assess for
  - Sickle cell trait
  - Sickle cell disease

Nursing Implications

- Assess if the patient
  - Has received a blood transfusion within 3 months before the test is administered
  - Should undergo genetic counseling if the test result is positive for sickle cell trait or sickle cell disease

Understanding the Results

- The sickle cell test results are available quickly.
- Normal sickle cell test results: Normal hemoglobin presence.
- Abnormal sickle cell test results:
  - Sickle cell trait: One-half of red blood cells contain hemoglobin A and the other half contains hemoglobin S.
  - Sickle cell disease: Nearly all red blood cells contain hemoglobin S.

Teach the Patient

- Explain
  - Why sample is taken.
  - That the patient should receive genetic counseling if the sickle cell trait or sickle cell disease is present.

10. Hemochromatosis Gene Test

The hemochromatosis (HFE) gene increases the absorption of iron (HFE), which causes a buildup of iron in the liver, heart, blood, joints, skin, and pancreas, resulting in joint pain, weight loss, and decreased energy. This can lead to arrhythmia, cirrhosis, diabetes, heart failure, arthritis, and change in skin color. The HFE gene test determines if the patient has the HFE gene.

> ## NURSING ALERT
>
> The healthcare provider will order the test if close family members have HFE. The healthcare provider might order the ferritin level test and transferring saturation test to measure the level of iron in the patient's blood.

> ## NURSING ALERT
>
> Existence of the HFE gene means that the patient has an increased chance of having HFE, but does not mean that the patient has HFE. It is advised that the patient consult a genetic counselor before the test is administered to discuss the risk of developing HFE.

What Is Being Measured?

- Existence of the HFE gene in blood

How Is the Test Performed?

- See "How to Collect Blood Specimen From a Vein" in Appendix A.

Rationale for the Test

- Screen for presence of the HFE gene.
- Assess
  - Underlying cause of HFE. If positive, other tests for HFE are not necessary.
  - Treatment of HFE.

Nursing Implications

- Assess if the patient
  - Has received a blood transfusion within 1 week before the test is administered
  - Has undergone genetic counseling prior to the test
- The HFE gene test may not rule out the existence of the HFE gene. The test detects the most common HFE gene mutation, but not all mutations.

Understanding the Results

- The HFE gene test results are available in 2 weeks.
- Normal HFE gene test result (negative): No mutation found.
- Abnormal HFE gene test result (positive): Mutation found. The patient has a risk of developing HFE.

Teach the Patient

- Explain
  - Why sample is taken.
- That the patient should receive genetic counseling prior to the test.
- That a positive test result does not mean that the patient will develop HFE. It means that the patient is at risk for developing HFE.

Summary

Enzymes, protein, hormones, and antibodies in a blood sample give healthcare providers clues to the underlying cause of infertility and to the existence or the risk for genetic disorders.

Infertility is sometimes caused by an immune system response to semen, where semen is recognized as an antigen, causing antibodies to attack and kill the sperm. Identifying the antisperm antibody in blood, vaginal fluids, or semen enables healthcare providers to find the cause of infertility.

The AFP level in blood is examined between 15 and 20 weeks of gestation for clues of genetic disease in the fetus. An unusually high or low level is a sign that further examination is necessary. Hormones in blood samples can indicate infertility, pregnancy, Down syndrome, and tumor.

QUIZ

1. **Why would some practitioners not order the antisperm antibody test?**
   A. Infertility maybe caused by immunologic infertility.
   B. Treatment is the same regardless of the test results.
   C. There is no treatment.
   D. Sampling is unreliable.

2. **Why is the AFP test administered?**
   A. Estimate the chances of birth defects
   B. Estimate the gender of the fetus
   C. Estimate the fetal liver function
   D. Estimate the uE3 level

3. **What does the practitioner do with the AFP test results if the ultrasound gestation age is different from the estimated gestation age?**
   A. Multiply the test results by 10.
   B. Adjust the test results using the multiple of median (MoM) factor.
   C. Multiply the test results by 15.
   D. Repeat the test.

4. **Why might the practitioner order a FSH test?**
   A. Assess the underlying cause of precocious puberty.
   B. Assess the function of the pituitary gland.
   C. Assess the underlying cause of abnormal menstrual periods.
   D. All of the above.

5. **The presence of hCG in a blood sample may indicate**
   A. Pregnancy
   B. Ectopic pregnancy
   C. Testicular cancer
   D. All of the above

6. **How would you respond to a patient who reports that a home urine pregnancy test is positive?**
   A. You are pregnant.
   B. Home pregnancy test assess for hCG hormone.
   C. Home pregnancy tests must be confirmed with other tests before the practitioner will know that you are pregnant.
   D. Home pregnancy tests are unreliable.

7. **Why is a quadruple screen test administered at the 20th week of gestation?**
   A. To determine the position of the number of fetuses
   B. To determine the position of the fetus
   C. To determine the gender of the fetus
   D. To determine if there is a risk of birth defects

8. **What is Tay-Sachs disease?**
   A. Accumulation of fatty acid in the brain and nerve cells
   B. No accumulation of fatty acid in the brain and nerve cells
   C. The presence of Hexosaminidase A enzyme in the newborn
   D. Accumulation of protein in the brain and nerve cells

9. **What is a function of progesterone?**
   A. Prevents milk from ejecting
   B. Causes lactogenesis
   C. Increases the production of milk
   D. Eases the ability for the newborn to be fed

10. **What might also produce the hCG hormone besides the placenta?**
    A. Molar pregnancy
    B. Choriocarcinoma
    C. Testicular cancer
    D. All of the above

ANSWERS

1. B. Treatment is the same regardless of the test results.
2. A. Estimate the chances of birth defects.
3. B. Adjust the test results using the multiple of median (MoM) factor.
4. D. All of the above.
5. D. All of the above.
6. C. Home pregnancy tests must be confirmed with other tests before the practitioner will know that you are pregnant.
7. D. To determine if there is a risk of birth defects.
8. A. Accumulation of fatty acid in the brain and nerve cells.
9. A. Prevents milk from ejecting.
10. D. All of the above.

chapter 11

Simple X-ray Imaging

KEY WORDS

Bitewing	Panoramic
Cartilage	Periapical
Lead apron	Photographic film
Ligaments	Soft tissue
Nonpalpable cysts	Tendons
Occlusal	X-ray beam
Orthopantogram	

Simple X-ray imaging is a cost-effective noninvasive radiological test that enables the practitioner to view inside the body. Although a simple X-ray provides a primitive view when compared with a CT scan and an MRI, these images provide sufficient information in some cases to rule out a diagnosis, make a diagnosis or serve as justification for ordering more expensive imaging tests such as a CT scan or an MRI.

Radiology imaging based on X-rays is founded on the principle that X-rays are absorbed by dense objects and pass through lesser dense objects. Dense objects such as bone appear white on the X-ray image, lesser dense objects such as air appear black, and fluid and fat appear as a lighter shade of gray.

There are various simple X-ray tests that a practitioner can order, each focusing on a particular area of the body. You will learn about each of these tests in this chapter.

1. How an X-ray Is Taken

The patient is positioned between the X-ray gun and a piece of photographic film. The X-ray gun focuses the X-ray beam at the area of the body that is being examined. A portion of the X-ray beam passes through the body striking the photographic film, leaving a black area on the photographic film. Another portion of the X-ray beam is absorbed by bone and other dense tissues in the body, which appear as shades of gray on the photographic film depending on the density of the tissues. Areas that are not being X-rayed are protected by a lead apron, where possible, to prevent radiation from reaching those areas.

Teach the Patient

- Explain
  - X-ray may not be taken if the patient is pregnant.
  - The level of radiation will not have any long-term effects on the patient.
  - The healthcare provider may require specific preparation depending on the part of the body being X-rayed.
  - Any jewelry in the vicinity of the X-ray site must be removed.
  - A radiologist is usually the healthcare professional who reads the X-ray.
  - The patient may be required to remove clothing and wear a gown during the X-ray.
  - The patient will be asked to lie still and hold his/her breath while the X-ray is being taken.
  - The X-ray room is cool.
  - The patient may feel uncomfortable while positioning for the X-ray.
- Assess
  - If the patient has signed a consent form.

2. Abdominal X-ray

An abdominal X-ray shows the position, size, and shape of the stomach, diaphragm, liver, spleen, and large and small intestines.

> **NURSING ALERT**
>
> Ovaries are not protected by a lead apron during the X-ray because of their location at the site of the X-ray. Abdominal X-rays cannot detect ulcers or bleeding.

What Is Being Examined?

- The position, size, and shape of the stomach, diaphragm, liver, spleen, and large and small intestines
- Position of nasogastric tube, nephrostomy tube, V-P shunt, or dialysis catheter

How Is the Test Performed?

- The patient may be asked to stand between the X-ray machine and the photographic film or to lie on his/her back or side on the X-ray table.
- When the patient lies on his/her back
  - A lead apron is placed over the lower pelvic area to protect the area from X-ray beam.
  - The X-ray machine is positioned over the abdomen.
  - The patient is asked to lie still and hold his/her breath while the X-ray is being taken.
  - An X-ray is taken.
- When the patient is asked to stand between the X-ray machine and the photographic film
  - The patient is asked to stand still and hold his/her breath when the X-ray is being taken.
  - An X-ray is taken.
- See "How an X-ray Is Taken" as discussed earlier in the chapter.

Rationale for the Test

- Assess
  - Underlying cause of abdominal or flank pain.

- Confirmation of position of nasogastric tube, nephrostomy tube, V-P shunt, or dialysis catheter
- Location of an ingested foreign body
- Underlying cause of vomiting and nausea
- For intestine blockage
- For perforation in the intestines or stomach

Nursing Implications

- Assess if the patient
  - Is pregnant. An ultrasound is ordered instead of an X-ray to protect the fetus from radiation exposure.
  - Has taken Pepto-Bismol (bismuth) or barium 4 days prior to the test. Bismuth and barium might obstruct the X-ray beam.
  - Has an empty bladder.

Understanding the Results

- The test takes 10 minutes and the results are ready within 15 minutes or 2 days depending on the patient's condition.
- Normal test results indicate
  - Normal position, size, and shape of the stomach, diaphragm, liver, spleen, and large and small intestines
  - No growths
  - Normal amounts of air, fluid, or stool
- Abnormal test results indicate
  - Abnormal position, size, and shape of the stomach, diaphragm, liver, spleen, and large and small intestines
  - Blockage
  - Perforation in the intestine or stomach (Conn syndrome)
  - Abnormal amounts of air, fluid, or stool
  - Kidney stones
  - Gallstones
  - Foreign object located
  - Growths

Teach the Patient

- Explain
  - Why X-ray is being taken.
  - What the patient can expect in the X-ray room.
  - That the patient should not take Pepto-Bismol (bismuth) or barium 4 days prior to the test.
  - That the patient will need to empty his/her bladder before the test.

3. Extremity X-ray

An extremity X-ray shows damage to hands, wrists, arms, feet, ankles, knees, hip, or legs.

> **NURSING ALERT**
>
> The healthcare provider may order a bone scan, CT scan, or MRI if the X-ray does not reveal a disorder.

> **NURSING ALERT**
>
> The healthcare provider may not order an X-ray if the results of the X-ray would not alter treatment of the disorder.

What Is Being Examined?

- Bones of the hands, wrists, arms, feet, ankles, knees, hip, or legs

How Is the Test Performed?

- The patient sits, stands, or lies down depending on extremity being examined.
- The extremity is positioned in front of the X-ray machine and is held in place by an apparatus if necessary.
- An X-ray is taken.
- See "How an X-ray Is Taken" as discussed earlier in the chapter.

> **NURSING ALERT**
>
> The healthcare provider may order opposing extremities X-rayed to make a comparison.

Rationale for the Test

- Assess for
  - Fracture
  - Dislocation
  - Tumors
  - Deformities/degeneration
  - Fluid around joints
  - Growth
  - The underlying cause of pain in the extremity
  - Alignment following treatment
  - Infection
  - Foreign objects

Nursing Implications

- Assess if the patient
  - Is pregnant. An ultrasound is ordered instead of an X-ray if the patient is pregnant to protect the fetus from radiation exposure.
  - Remained still during the X-ray.

Understanding the Results

- The test takes 10 minutes and the results are ready within 15 minutes or 2 days depending on the patient's condition.
- Normal test results indicate
  - No fracture
  - No dislocation
  - No tumors
  - No deformities

- No fluid around joints
- Normal growth
- Extremity is aligned
- No infection
- No foreign objects
- Abnormal test results indicate
  - Signs of fracture
  - Signs of dislocation
  - Signs of tumors
  - Signs of deformities
  - Signs of fluid around joints
  - Abnormal growth
  - Extremity misaligned
  - Signs of infection
  - Signs of foreign objects

Teach the Patient

- Explain
  - Why X-ray is being taken.
  - What the patient can expect in the X-ray room.
  - That the patient will need to hold the extremity still while the X-ray is being taken.

4. Spinal X-ray

The spine consists of 33 vertebrae, nearly all separated by a disc that absorbs shock related to movement. There are four types of spinal X-rays:

- Cervical spine: 7 vertebrae in the cervical area of the spine
- Thoracic spine: 12 vertebrae in the thoracic area of the spine
- Lumbosacral spine: 5 vertebrae in the lumbar area of the spine and 5 vertebrae in the sacrum area
- Sacrum/coccyx: 5 vertebrae in the sacrum area and 4 vertebrae in the coccyx area

> **NURSING ALERT**
>
> A disc is cartilage.

> **NURSING ALERT**
>
> Strained back muscles or ligaments are not visible on an X-ray.

What Is Being Examined?

- Structure and position of the spine

How Is the Test Performed?

- The patient lies on an X-ray table.
- The X-ray machine is positioned over the site.
- The patient is asked to lie still and hold his/her breath while the X-ray is being taken.
- An X-ray is taken (up to 5 X-rays may be taken).
- See "How an X-ray Is Taken" discussed earlier in the chapter.

> **NURSING ALERT**
>
> If the patient has a cervical collar, an X-ray will be taken and read to determine if the cervical collar can be removed without causing further injury.

Rationale for the Test

- Assess for
  - Fracture
  - Dislocation
  - Tumors
  - Deformities/degeneration
  - Curvature of the spine
  - Bone spurs

- The underlying cause of weakness, pain, or numbness
- Alignment following treatment

Nursing Implications

- Assess if the patient
  - Is pregnant. An ultrasound is ordered instead of an X-ray if the patient is pregnant to protect the fetus from radiation exposure.
  - Is morbidly overweight, since this can blur details of the X-ray.
  - Has taken Pepto-Bismol (bismuth) or barium 4 days prior to the test. Bismuth and barium might obstruct the X-ray beam.
  - Can remain still during the X-ray.

Understanding the Results

- The test takes 15 minutes and the results are ready within 15 minutes or 2 days depending on the patient's condition.
- Normal test results indicate
  - No fracture
  - No dislocation
  - No tumors
  - No deformities/degeneration
  - Spine is aligned
  - No bone spurs
- Abnormal test results indicate
  - Signs of fracture
  - Signs of dislocation
  - Signs of tumors
  - Signs of deformities/degeneration
  - Spine is misaligned
  - Signs of bone spurs

Teach the Patient

- Explain
  - Why X-ray is being taken.

- What the patient can expect in the X-ray room.
- That the patient should not take Pepto-Bismol (bismuth) or barium 4 days prior to the test.
- That the patient will need to lie still while the X-ray is being taken.

5. Mammogram

A mammogram is an X-ray that detects palpable and nonpalpable cysts or masses in the breast and is used to screen for signs of breast cancer. Suspicious masses are biopsied to determine if the mass is cancerous.

NURSING ALERT

A mammogram can be performed on a patient who has had breast implants. A mammogram cannot be performed if the patient is breast-feeding. A breast ultrasound determines if a mass is a cyst or solid mass. A digital mammogram is considered to have the same accuracy as an X-ray mammogram. The healthcare provider may order the breast cancer (BRCA) gene test if there is a history of breast cancer in the patient's family.

NURSING ALERT

A mammogram is not normally performed if the patient is pregnant. If the mammogram must be performed, a lead apron is placed over the patient's abdomen.

NURSING ALERT

The healthcare provider must provide the patient with the original mammogram images if requested.

What Is Being Examined?

- The breast for signs of cysts or solid masses

How Is the Test Performed?

- Remove all powders, deodorant, ointments, or perfume from the breast since these may appear on the X-ray image.

- Schedule the mammogram for within 2 weeks after the end of the patient's menstrual period to reduce tenderness of her breasts.
- Remove the patient's clothes above the waist and provide her with a gown.
- The patient stands or sits.
- Each breast is placed on the X-ray plate.
- A second plate is placed on top of the breast.
- The breast is compressed.
- The patient is asked to hold her breath while the X-ray is taken.
- X-ray images are taken from the top and side of the breast.
- See "How an X-ray Is Taken" as discussed earlier in the chapter.

Rationale for the Test

- Assess
  - If the patient has cysts, solid masses, or calcification in the breast
  - Underlying cause of breast discomfort

Nursing Implications

- Assess if the patient
  - Is pregnant
  - Is breast-feeding
  - Has breast implants
  - Removed all powders, deodorant, ointments, or perfume from the breast since these may appear on the X-ray image
- Assess if the mammogram was scheduled for 2 weeks after the end of the patient's menstrual period to reduce tenderness of her breasts
- Identify the location of any previous breast biopsies.

Understanding the Results

- The test takes 15 minutes and the results are ready within 15 minutes or 10 days depending on the patient's condition.
- Normal test results indicate
  - No cyst
  - No solid mass

- Normal tissue
- Clear ducts
- Abnormal test results indicate
  - Signs of cyst
  - Signs of solid mass
  - Signs of calcification

NURSING ALERT

A normal mammogram does not rule out breast cancer. Results may be difficult to interpret if the patient is obese.

Teach the Patient

- Explain
  - Why mammogram is being taken.
  - The procedure for taking the mammogram.
  - That the breast is compressed to obtain the best possible view of the breast.
  - That the test will be uncomfortable but not painful.
  - That the patient should not use powders, deodorant, ointments, or perfume on the breasts on the day of the mammogram.
  - That the patient should schedule the mammogram for within 2 weeks after the end of her menstrual period to reduce tenderness of the breasts.

6. Chest X-ray

A chest X-ray shows the position, size, and shape of the collarbone, breastbone, heart, airway, lungs, thoracic spine, ribs, lymph nodes, and blood vessels.

NURSING ALERT

The healthcare provider may also order an echocardiogram (ECG), ultrasound, MRI, or a CT scan.

What Is Being Examined?

- The position, size, and shape of the collarbone, breastbone, heart, airway, lungs, thoracic spine, ribs, lymph nodes, and blood vessels

How Is the Test Performed?

- Remove the patient's clothes above the waist and provide her with a gown.
- The patient stands or sits or lies down on the X-ray plate.
- The patient is asked to hold his/her breath while the X-ray is being taken.
- X-ray images are taken from the front and side.
- See "How an X-ray Is Taken" as discussed earlier in the chapter.

Rationale for the Test

- Assess
  - For pulmonary disease or disorders
  - The underlying cause of chest pain or respiratory problems
  - The underlying cause of cardiac problems
  - A chest injury
  - Positioning of a medical device
- Identify foreign objects in the airway and esophagus.

Nursing Implications

- Assess if the patient
  - Is pregnant
  - Is able to hold his/her breath
  - Has removed all jewelry in the thoracic area since these may appear on the X-ray image
  - Is obese
- Assess scars in the thoracic area that might appear on the X-ray.

Understanding the Results

- The test takes approximately 15 minutes and the results are ready within 15 minutes or 2 days depending on the patient's condition.

- Normal test results indicate
  - Normal position, size, and shape of the collarbone, breastbone, heart, airway, lungs, thoracic spine, ribs, lymph nodes, and blood vessels.
  - No abnormal fluid seen.
  - Medical device is in the proper position.
- Abnormal test results indicate
  - Abnormal position, size, and shape of the collarbone, breastbone, heart, airway, lungs, thoracic spine, ribs, lymph nodes, and blood vessels.
  - Abnormal fluid seen.
  - Medical device is not in the proper position.

Teach the Patient

- Explain
- Why X-ray is being taken.
- The procedure for taking the X-ray.
- That the patient should remove all jewelry in the thoracic area.

7. Dental X-ray

Dental X-rays are used to assess the condition of the patient's jaw, mouth, and teeth. There are four types of dental X-rays:

- Panoramic (orthopantogram): This assesses the temporomandibular joints, the jaw, sinuses, teeth, and nasal area for tumors, fractures, cysts, and impacted teeth, but not cavities.
- Occlusal: This assesses the palate and lower portions of the mouth for fractures, cleft palate, abscesses, tumors, cysts, and immature teeth.
- Bitewing: This is a single view of the upper and lower back teeth and is used to assess the formation of teeth, bone loss, infection, and tooth decay.
- Periapical: This is a view of a tooth and used to assess abscesses, tumors, cysts, and the overall status of the patient's teeth.

What Is Being Examined?

- The temporomandibular joints, the jaw, sinuses, teeth, mouth, and nasal area

How Is the Test Performed?

- The patient sits.
- The patient bites down on the X-ray film carrier that holds the X-ray film.
- X-ray image is taken.
- In a panoramic X-ray, the patient places his/her head in the arm of the X-ray machine and arm rotates while taking the X-ray image.
- See "How an X-ray Is Taken" as discussed earlier in the chapter.

Rationale for the Test

- Assess
  - For cysts, tumors, abscesses
  - The underlying cause of mouth and sinus pain
  - The health of teeth
  - The position of teeth
  - For abnormal structures in the mouth and jaw

Nursing Implications

- Assess if the patient
  - Is pregnant
  - Is able to open his/her mouth enough to insert the X-ray film carrier in the mouth
  - Has foreign objects in his/her mouth such as body piercing, retainers, dentures, braces, or bridges

Understanding the Results

- The test takes a few minutes and the results are ready within 15 minutes.
- Normal test results indicate
  - Normal position, size, and shape of the temporomandibular joints, the jaw, sinuses, teeth, mouth, and nasal area
- Abnormal test results indicate
  - Tooth decay
  - Abnormal position, size, and shape of the temporomandibular joints, the jaw, sinuses, teeth, mouth, and nasal area

Teach the Patient

- Explain
  - Why X-ray is being taken.
  - The procedure for taking the X-ray.

8. Facial X-ray

A facial X-ray is used to assess facial bones, sinuses, and the orbital cavity.

> **NURSING ALERT**
>
> The healthcare provider may also order a CT scan.

What Is Being Examined?

- The facial bones, sinuses, and the orbital cavity

How Is the Test Performed?

- The patient sits.
- The patient must remove eye glasses and body piercing in the area of the X-ray.
- The patient must hold his/her head still. A brace may be provided to stabilize the patient's head.
- X-ray image is taken.
- See "How an X-ray Is Taken" as discussed earlier in the chapter.

Rationale for the Test

- Assess for
  - Cysts, tumors, abscesses
  - The underlying cause of sinus pain
  - Fractures
  - Foreign objects

Nursing Implications

- Assess if the patient
  - Is pregnant
  - Is able to sit still for the X-ray
  - Has a prosthetic eye
  - Has a neck injury
  - Has body piercing in the area being X-rayed
  - Has removed eye glasses

Understanding the Results

- The test takes 30 minutes and the results are ready within 15 minutes.
- Normal test results indicate
  - Normal position, size, and shape of bones in the face and the orbital cavity
- Abnormal test results indicate
  - Inflammation
  - Infection
  - Abnormal position, size, and shape of bones in the face and the orbital cavity
  - Cysts, tumors, abscesses
  - Foreign object

Teach the Patient

- Explain
  - Why X-ray is being taken.
  - Procedure for taking the X-ray.

9. Skull X-ray

A skull X-ray is used to assess the skull and sinuses.

> **NURSING ALERT**
>
> The healthcare provider may also order a CT scan.

What Is Being Examined?

- The skull and sinuses

How Is the Test Performed?

- The patient sits still.
- The patient must remove eye glasses and body piercing in the area of the X-ray.
- The patient must hold his/her head still. A brace may be provided to stabilize the patient's head.
- X-ray image is taken. Several images are taken: front, back, top, and sides.
- See "How an X-ray Is Taken" as discussed earlier in the chapter.

Rationale for the Test

- Assess for
  - Cysts, tumors, abscesses
  - The underlying cause of sinus pain
  - Fractures
  - Foreign objects

Nursing Implications

- Assess if the patient
  - Is pregnant
  - Is able to sit still for the X-ray
  - Has a prosthetic eye
  - Has a neck injury
  - Has body piercing in the area being X-rayed
  - Has removed eye glasses

Understanding the Results

- The test takes 30 minutes and the results are ready within 15 minutes.
- Normal test results indicate
  - Normal position, size, and shape of bones in the skull and the orbital cavity

- Abnormal test results indicate
  - Inflammation
  - Infection
  - Abnormal position, size, and shape of bones in the skull
  - Cysts, tumors, abscesses
  - Foreign object

Teach the Patient

- Explain
  - Why X-ray is being taken.
  - The procedure for taking the X-ray.

Summary

X-rays, although primitive to today's CT or CAT scans, and MRI, provide a cost-effective method of viewing the inside of the body without opening the skin. There are many types of X-ray tests, which you learned about in this chapter. Each works basically the same way.

An X-ray is absorbed by dense material such as bone and passes through less dense material such as soft tissue. The X-ray beam passes through the patient and onto photographic film located on the opposite side of the patient.

The photographic film turns black when struck by the X-ray beam. Those areas of the photographic film that are not struck by the X-ray beam appear gray. As a result, dense objects in the patient's body appear as shades of gray on the photographic film. Any unexpected gray area on the photographic film requires additional assessment by the healthcare provider.

QUIZ

1. **Why should the patient avoid taking Pepto-Bismol (bismuth) prior to an X-ray?**
   A. Bismuth might prevent the patient from remaining still during the X-ray.
   B. Bismuth might absorb the X-ray beam.
   C. Bismuth might obstruct the X-ray beam.
   D. Bismuth might enhance the X-ray beam.

2. **An X-ray is not to be ordered if**
   A. The results of the X-ray would not alter the treatment
   B. The patient is older than 7 years
   C. The patient is older than 82 years
   D. The patient has not been diagnosed with a bone disorder

3. **What would you do if the patient arrived for an X-ray wearing a cervical collar?**
   A. Remove the cervical collar and take the X-ray.
   B. Keep the cervical collar in place when taking the X-ray.
   C. Reschedule the X-ray.
   D. Ask the patient if the cervical collar can be removed.

4. **What would you do if a patient who is breast-feeding is scheduled for a mammogram?**
   A. Cancel the mammogram.
   B. Procedure with the mammogram.
   C. Cover the patient's breasts with a lead apron.
   D. Make sure that the patient is finished breast-feeding for the day before taking the mammogram.

5. **What should you tell the patient not to use prior to a mammogram?**
   A. Deodorant
   B. Ointments
   C. Powders
   D. All of the above

6. **The patient asks why the practitioner ordered orthopantogram. What is your best response?**
   A. To assess temporomandibular joints
   B. To assess sinuses
   C. To assess jaw
   D. All of the above

7. **During what type of X-ray might the patient be placed in a brace for the X-ray?**
   A. Facial X-ray
   B. Orthopantogram
   C. Periapical
   D. Occlusal

8. **What would you expect if the practitioner ordered a mammogram and the patient is pregnant?**

   A. Cancel the mammogram.

   B. Reschedule the mammogram until the third trimester.

   C. Reschedule the mammogram until the second trimester.

   D. Place a lead apron over the patient's abdomen.

9. **What is the best way to avoid tenderness of the breasts in a mammogram?**

   A. Schedule the mammogram during the second week of patient's menstrual period.

   B. Schedule the mammogram during the patient's menstrual period.

   C. Schedule the mammogram for within 2 weeks after the end of the patient's menstrual period.

   D. Schedule the mammogram for within 3 weeks after the end of the patient's menstrual period.

10. **What would concern the practitioner if the patient is morbidly overweight before taking a spinal X-ray?**

    A. Details in the X-ray can be blurred by the additional weight.

    B. The patient may break the X-ray machine.

    C. The patient may not be able to withstand the test.

    D. The patient is unable to be moved during the X-ray.

ANSWERS

1. C. Bismuth might obstruct the X-ray beam.
2. A. The results of the X-ray would not alter the treatment.
3. B. Keep the cervical collar in place when taking the X-ray.
4. A. Cancel the mammogram since a mammogram is not administered if the patient is breast-feeding.
5. D. All of the above.
6. D. All of the above.
7. A. Facial X-ray.
8. D. Place a lead apron over the patient's abdomen.
9. C. Schedule the mammogram within 2 weeks after the end of the patient's menstrual period.
10. A. Details in the X-ray can be blurred by the additional weight.

chapter 12

Computed Tomography Scan

LEARNING OBJECTIVES

1. Full-Body CT Scan
2. CT Scan of the Head
3. CT Scan of the Spine

KEY WORDS

Computed tomography
Contrast material
CT myelogram
Intrathecal space
Intrathecally
Intravenous pyelogram

Iodine dye
Kidneys, ureters, and bladder (KUB)
Positron emission tomograph (PET)
Shellfish allergy
Temporomandibular disorder

A computed tomography (CT, CAT) scan is a radiology imaging test that creates detailed images of structures within the body using a doughnut-shaped X-ray machine. The patient lies within the doughnut-shaped scanner and an X-ray beam rotates around him/her creating an image that represents a thin slice of him/her. Each rotation takes less than 1 second.

All sliced images are stored on a computer. The computer is used to reassemble sliced images of the patient enabling the healthcare provider to identify any abnormalities. Typically, the healthcare provider will print the image of any slices that indicate an abnormality, which is then saved with the patient's chart.

The patient may be administered contrast material such as iodine dye. The contrast material makes structures within the patient's body stand out on the computer by differentiating them with white, black, and shades of gray. Contrast material is administered intravenously or into joints or cavities of the body. The patient may also be asked to ingest other kinds of contrast material.

A CT scan may be used for staging cancer to assess if the cancer has spread to other sites in the body. CT scans are also used to identify masses or tumors, as well as fluid and the infection process. CT scans guide the healthcare provider when performing a procedure such as a biopsy.

You will learn about different types of CT scans in this chapter.

1. Full-Body CT Scan

A full-body CT scan creates an image of the patient's entire body. A healthcare provider orders a full-body CT scan if it is suspected that the patient may have disorders throughout the body and the healthcare provider is unable to narrow the disorder to specific areas of the body. This situation may occur if the patient is involved in a severe motor vehicle accident.

> ## NURSING ALERT
>
> Typically, a healthcare provider orders a CT scan for a specific part of the body rather than ordering a full-body scan. A full CT scan is time consuming and usually provides more than enough information necessary for the healthcare provider to diagnose the patient's disorder. Some healthcare providers feel that a full-body scan identifies benign growths and other disorders that do not adversely affect the patient but could lead to additional tests and surgery that are unnecessary.

The result of a CT scan is commonly compared with the results of a positron emission tomograph (PET) to identify cancer.

> ## NURSING ALERT
>
> Determine if the patient is allergic to shellfish or iodine. Contrast material may contain iodine and other substances that could cause the patient to have an allergic reaction. Also determine if the patient will be administered a sedative to relax her/him during the CT scan. If so, make sure that the patient does not drive any vehicle following the CT scan until the sedative has worn off.

What Is Being Examined?

- Head
- Thorax
- Abdomen
- Kidneys, ureters, and bladder (KUB)
- Intravenous pyelogram for urinary tract blockage
- Liver
- Pancreas
- Bile ducts
- Gallbladder
- Adrenal glands
- Spleen
- Pelvis (ovaries, fallopian tubes, uterus, prostate gland)
- Extremities

How Is the Test Performed?

- Depending on the nature of the CT scan, the patient may be administered an enema or asked not to eat after midnight prior to the CT scan.
- If contrast material is required for the test, then the patient is administered the contrast material before the test. The method for administering the contrast material depends on the nature of the CT scan.
  - Approximately 40 minutes before the test, the patient may be asked to ingest contrast material.
  - Contrast material may be administered in a vein or in a cavity, such as the bladder or rectum, immediately before the test.
- The patient removes jewelry and clothes and is given a gown to wear during the test.
- The patient lies on the CT scanner table.
- The patient must lie still during the test.
- The patient will be in the CT room alone.
- The CT scan technician is in the next room observing through a window.
- The patient and the CT scan technician are able to converse during the test using an intercom.
- The CT scanner table moves into the opening of the CT scanner.
- The CT scanner moves around the patient when taking images of him/her.
- The patient hears a clicking sound as the CT scanner moves.
- The CT scan can take up to 2 hours.
- A radiologist, who is a medical doctor, interprets the results of the CT scan and writes a report that is given to the patient's healthcare provider.
- The patient is asked to drink large amounts of water and other fluids for 24 hours following the CT scan to flush the contrast material from the body.

Rationale for the Test

- Assess for
  - Growths
  - Obstructions
  - Inflammation or infection

- Foreign objects
- Bleeding
- Fluid collection
- Pulmonary embolism

Nursing Implications

- Assess if the patient
  - Has allergies (shellfish, iodine).
  - Is breast-feeding since contrast material can pass to the baby in breast milk. The patient should give formula to the baby instead of breast milk for 2 days following the CT scan if contrast material is administered.
  - Has heart disorder, asthma, thyroid or kidney disorders, or diabetes.
  - Takes Glucophage.
  - Has taken Pepto-Bismol 4 days prior to the CT scan.
- Determine if the patient
  - Is claustrophobic
  - Can lie still during the test

Understanding the Results

- The results are available within 2 days.
- Normal test results indicate
  - Normal size of organs and blood vessels
  - No blockages
  - No bleeding
  - No abnormal fluid collection
  - No growths
  - No inflammation
- Abnormal test results indicate
  - Abnormal size of organs and blood vessels
  - Blockages
  - Bleeding

- Abnormal fluid collection
- Growths
- Inflammation

Teach the Patient

- Explain
- Why the CT scan is being administered.
- The CT scan test.
- Why contrast material may be administered.
- That the contrast material may leave a metallic taste and that the patient may feel flushed when the contrast material is administered IV.
- That the healthcare provider may ask the patient to stop taking Glucophage several days before the CT scan, since there might be a reaction with contrast material.
- That some patients may be allergic to the contrast material and that the healthcare team is ready to take measures to reverse any adverse reaction to the contrast material.
- That the healthcare provider may ask the patient to stop breast-feeding for 2 days following the CT scan if contrast material is administered.
- That the patient will be asked to drink a large amount of water for 24 hours following the CT scan if contrast material is administered.
- That the healthcare provider may administer a sedative prior to the test if the patient is unable to relax during the test. If a sedative is administered, the patient should arrange to be driven home following the test.

2. CT Scan of the Head

The patient's head is placed into the CT scanner as it takes sliced images of the skull, brain, and other parts of the head. The healthcare provider may order a perfusion CT. A perfusion CT is used to determine the blood supply to areas of the brain. Contrast material is administered IV. Areas of the brain that receive blood are highlighted on the computer image by the contrast material. Areas without blood flow are not highlighted.

What Is Being Examined?

- Head
- Brain
- Eyes
- Ears
- Nose
- Mouth
- Sinuses

How Is the Test Performed?

- See "Full-Body CT Scan" discussed earlier in this chapter.
- The CT scan of the head takes approximately 30 minutes.

Rationale for the Test

- Assess for
  - Growths
  - Obstructions
  - Inflammation or infection
  - Foreign objects
  - Bleeding
  - Fluid collection
  - Headache
  - Vertigo
  - Vision problem
  - Broken bones
  - The result of facial surgery
  - Temporomandibular disorder
  - Paget disease
  - Stroke
  - Reasons for change in the level of consciousness
- Provide baseline images before surgery

Nursing Implications

- See "Full-Body CT Scan" discussed earlier in this chapter.
- Assess if the patient
  - Has removed glasses, contact lenses, and hearing aids

Understanding the Results

- The results are available within 2 days.
- Normal test results indicate
  - Normal-sized skull, brain, ventricles, blood vessels, eyes, ears, sinuses
  - No blockages
  - No bleeding
  - No abnormal fluid collection
  - No foreign objects
  - No ischemia
- Abnormal test results indicate
  - Abnormal-sized skull, brain, ventricles, blood vessels, eyes, ears, sinuses
  - Blockages
  - Inflammation
  - Growth
  - Fluid collection
  - Foreign objects

Teach the Patient

- See "Full-Body CT Scan" discussed earlier in this chapter.
- Explain
  - That contrast material may be administered intravenously and flows throughout blood vessels in the brain, showing areas of the brain that are receiving blood and are not receiving blood.

3. CT Scan of the Spine

The CT scan of the spine creates images of the cervical, thoracic, and lumbo-sacral spine. All 33 vertebrae and discs are pictured along with the cerebrospinal fluid (CSF). During the scan, the CT scanner can be tilted to follow the curvature of the spine. Depending on the purpose of the scan, the healthcare provider may require that contrast material be administered intrathecally into the spinal canal.

What Is Being Examined?

- Vertebrae
- Discs
- CSF

How Is the Test Performed?

- See "Full-Body CT Scan" discussed earlier in this chapter.
- The healthcare provider may order a CT myelogram. A CT myelogram requires that a sample of CSF be removed for microscopic examination before contrast material is administered. Contrast material is then administered in the intrathecal space around the spinal cord.
- If a CT myelogram is performed, the patient lies on his/her stomach. An area of the lumbar spine is anesthetized and contrast material is injected. The CT table is tilted to help distribute the contrast material throughout the spine.
- After a CT myelogram, the patient is asked to keep his/her head raised to prevent seizures and headaches.

Rationale for the Test

- Assess for
  - Growths
  - Obstructions
  - Narrowing of the spinal canal
  - Deformities
  - Fractures
  - Inflammation and infection
  - Bone compression
  - Osteoporosis
  - Congenital defects

Nursing Implications

- See "Full-Body CT Scan" discussed earlier in this chapter.

Understanding the Results

- The results are available within 2 days.
- Normal test results indicate
  - Normal size of vertebrae, discs, and spinal canal
  - No blockages
  - No inflammation or infection
- Abnormal test results indicate
  - Abnormal size of vertebrae, discs, and spinal canal
  - Blockages
  - Inflammation or infection
  - Osteoporosis, arthritis
  - Spinal stenosis
  - Growths

Teach the Patient

- See "Full-Body CT Scan" discussed earlier in this chapter.
- Tell the patient to contact his/her healthcare provider if he/she experiences
  - A headache that lasts more than 1 day or a severe headache following the CT scan
  - A temperature of 101.1°F or greater
  - Numbness, pain, or weakness in extremities
  - Irritability
  - Difficult bowel movements or trouble urinating
- Explain that the patient
  - Should keep his/her head raised following the CT scan to avoid headaches.
  - May experience nausea and vomiting following the CT scan.
  - In rare situations may experience a seizure following the CT scan and if this occurs, should seek emergency medical help immediately.

Summary

A computed tomography (CT) scanner uses X-rays to create detailed images of the inside of a patient's body on a computer screen enabling a radiologist to identify abnormalities inside the patient.

A patient lies on a table that is slowly inserted into the doughnut-shaped CT scanner. The X-ray beam rotates around the patient creating a thin image of the cross-section of the body in less than 1 second.

Each slice is stored on a computer and is reassembled, enabling the radiologist to examine slices in sequence for any abnormality. If an abnormality is found, the relative slices can be printed and saved in the patient's chart.

Depending on the nature of the CT scan, the patient may be administered contrast material. Contrast material such as an iodine dye causes areas of the body affected by this material to be highlighted on the computer image. Areas of the body unaffected by the contrast material are not highlighted, possibly indicating a blockage.

QUIZ

1. **Why would you ask the patient to drink a large amount of water following a CT scan?**

   A. To disperse X-rays

   B. To flush the contrast material

   C. To avoid cramps

   D. To concentrate X-rays

2. **A patient anxious about a CT scan may be administered:**

   A. Amphetamine

   B. Adderall

   C. Dexedrine

   D. A sedative.

3. **You are sending the patient for a CT scan and patient tells you she is allergic to shellfish. What do you do?**

   A. Send the patient for the CT scan.

   B. Reschedule the CT scan.

   C. Notify the healthcare provider and radiologist.

   D. Cancel the CT scan.

4. **Can a patient who is breast-feeding receive a CT scan?**

   A. Yes, however the patient should use formula instead of breast-feeding for 2 days following the CT scan if contrast material is administered.

   B. Yes, if a lead apron is placed over the patient's abdomen.

   C. No, the CT scan might affect the fetus.

   D. No, if contrast material is not administered.

5. **Should you ask the patient to stop taking Glucophage before a CT scan?**

   A. Yes, Glucophage may react with contrast material.

   B. Yes, Glucophage reacts to X-rays.

   C. No, Glucophage reacts to MRI.

   D. No, if contrast material is administered before the CT scan.

6. **What would you tell the patient who asks you purpose of a perfusion CT?**

   A. Perfusion CT determines if the patient has osteoporosis.

   B. Perfusion CT determines results of the KUB.

   C. Perfusion CT assesses blood supply to the brain.

   D. Perfusion CT assesses the function of the lymph system.

7. **Where is contrast material administered in a CT myelogram?**

   A. Muscle

   B. In the intrathecal space

   C. Nerve

   D. Legs

8. **What do you want the patient to do after a CT scan of the spine with contrast material?**

   A. Lie on the right side of her back.

   B. Lie on her stomach with her head facing left.

   C. Bend over with her head down.

   D. Keep her head elevated.

9. **What should the patient do if she experiences a seizure following the CT scan?**

   A. Call her healthcare provider immediately.

   B. Call for emergency medical care immediately.

   C. Lie down on her bed.

   D. Keep her head elevated.

10. **The patient reports weakness in the extremities following a CT scan. What should you do first?**
    A. Call her practitioner.
    B. Call the radiologist.
    C. Ask the patient to lie down.
    D. Call for emergency medical help immediately.

ANSWERS

1. B. To flush the contrast material.
2. D. A sedative.
3. C. Notify the healthcare provider and radiologist.
4. A. Yes, however the patient should use formula instead of breast-feeding for 2 days following the CT scan if contrast material is administered.
5. A. Yes, Glucophage may react with contrast material.
6. C. Perfusion CT assesses blood supply to the brain.
7. B. In the intrathecal space.
8. D. Keep her head elevated.
9. B. Call for emergency medical care immediately.
10. C. Ask the patient to lie down.

chapter 13

Magnetic Resonance Imaging and Positron Emission Tomography Scan

LEARNING OBJECTIVES

1. Abdominal MRI
2. Breast MRI
3. Head MRI
4. Knee MRI
5. PET Scan
6. Shoulder MRI
7. Spinal MRI

KEY WORDS

BRCA1	Magnetic resonance angiogram (MRA)
BRCA2	Magnetic resonance spectroscopy
Cervical spine	Open MRI
Claustrophobic	Photon
Closed MRI	Positron
Contrast material	Radioactive
Diffusion–perfusion imaging	Sciatica
Gadolinium	Shellfish allergy
Glucagon	Spinal disc disorders
Iodine allergy	Spinal stenosis
Lumbosacral spine	Thoracic spine

Magnetic resonance imaging (MRI) is a radiology imaging test that uses pulsating radio waves in a magnetic field to produce an image of inside the patient's body. The patient lies on his/her back on a table. A coil is placed around the area of the patient that is being scanned and a belt is placed around him/her to detect breathing. The table moves into the magnetic field and the belt triggers the MRI scan so that breathing does not interfere with capturing the image.

A clanking/tapping noise is heard while the MRI scans the patient. The patient may listen to music through headphones to block out the noise.

There are two main types of MRI machines; one is closed the other is open. In the closed machine, the patient's body is entirely enclosed while only a portion of the body is enclosed in an open machine.

The healthcare provider may order that contrast material be administered to the patient prior to the MRI. The contrast material highlights areas of the body that are being studied and may be ingested or administered intravenously.

The MRI produces digital images that are displayed on a computer screen and can be stored for further review by the patient's healthcare team. The MRI creates images that are more detailed than images produced by a CT scan, X-ray, or ultrasound.

No metal objects should be on or inside the patient during an MRI, including credit cards. Information on the credit card might be erased by the MRI's magnetic field. An X-ray may be ordered to determine if there is any metal inside the patient before the MRI is administered, especially if he/she was in an accident where metal fragments might be embedded throughout the body.

However, dental fillings are usually permitted although the patient is likely to feel tingling in the mouth during the MRI. The patient may experience skin irritation if he/she has iron pigment tattoos.

A positron emission tomography (PET) scan is a nuclear medicine test that creates a roadmap of blood flow in the patient's body, enabling the healthcare provider to visualize abnormal blood flow to his/her tissues and organs.

A radioactive chemical called a tracer and a special camera that detects the tracer inside the patient's body are the keys to a PET scan. The healthcare provider administers the tracer into the patient's veins prior to the scan. The tracer gives off positrons, which are very small charged particles that can be detected by the PET scan camera. The PET scan camera takes a series of images, each capturing the position of positrons in the body. These images are stored and replayed on a computer screen.

These images show the tracer containing blood as the blood makes its way into organs and tissues, giving the healthcare provider a clear picture of blood flow within the body.

In this chapter you will learn about different kinds of MRI tests and PET scan.

1. Abdominal MRI

An abdominal MRI produces detailed images of organs, structures, and tissues contained within the abdomen. The healthcare provider may order that the patient be administered contrast material prior to the MRI to highlight parts of the abdomen on the MRI image. This enables the healthcare provider to identify any subtle abnormalities that may exist in the abdomen.

What Is Being Examined?

- Abdominal organs, structures, and tissues

How Is the Test Performed?

- The patient is assessed for any metal that might be on or inside his/her body. The healthcare provider determines if the presence of any metal may require cancellation of the MRI.

- An assessment is made to determine if the patient can be administered contrast material over a 2-minute period, if required for the MRI. Contrast material is either ingested or administered IV, causing a flushing feeling for the patient. Contrast material may or may not be used if the patient is allergic to shellfish or iodine or if he/she has kidney abnormalities or sickle cell anemia, depending on the type of contrast material that the healthcare provider plans to use for the test.

- An assessment is made to determine if the patient is claustrophobic. If so, then the healthcare provider may administer a sedative to the patient or schedule the test to be performed using an open MRI machine.
- The patient removes all clothing and wears a gown during the MRI.
- The patient may be given headphones to avoid hearing the clanking/tapping noise created by the MRI.
- The patient may be administered glucagon to reduce intestinal movement during the test.
- The patient lies on his/her back on the MRI table.
- A coil is placed on top of the patient's abdomen.
- A belt is cinched around the abdomen to detect the patient's breathing patterns.
- The table is moved into the MRI machine as images are taken of the abdomen.
- Images are viewed during and after the MRI is completed to assist the healthcare provider reach a diagnosis.

Rationale for the Test

- Assess
  - The size of abdominal organs and structures
  - The existence of a growth
  - For a blockage
  - The existence of fluid within the abdomen
  - For inflammation
  - Blood flow

Nursing Implications

- Determine if the patient has any metal on or inside his/her body.
- Assess if the patient
  - Has eaten or drunk before the MRI is administered. Some MRI studies require that the patient refrain from eating or drinking 12 hours before the test is administered.

- Is allergic to shellfish, iodine, or contrast material.
- Is pregnant.
- Is claustrophobic.
- Has kidney disease.
- Is wearing any medication patches.
- Can lie still during the test.

Understanding the Results

- The test takes 60 minutes and the results are ready immediately if the test is performed by the healthcare provider or within a few hours if a technician performs the test.
- Normal test results indicate
  - Normal size of abdominal organs and structures
  - No growth(s)
  - No blockage
  - No fluid within the abdomen
  - No inflammation
  - Normal blood flow
- Abnormal test results indicate
  - Unusual size of abdominal organs and structures.
  - The existence of a growth.
  - A blockage is identified.
  - Fluid exists within the abdomen.
  - Inflammation or infection is present.
  - Unusual blood flow.

Teach the Patient

- Explain
- Why MRI is being taken.
- What the patient will experience during the MRI.
- That no metal can be on or inside the patient during the MRI.
- That the patient will not feel any pain during the procedure, although he/she may feel a tingling sensation if he/she has metal fillings in his/her teeth.

- That the patient may be administered a sedative if he/she is claustrophobic.

- That some patients who are allergic to shellfish and iodine may also be allergic to contrast material. If the patient is allergic to contrast material, the healthcare provider will discuss the risk and benefit of administering the contrast material. If the patient agrees that the benefits outweigh the risk, then the healthcare provider may administer medication that counteracts the allergic reaction to the contrast material.

- That the patient may be asked to drink contrast material or that the contrast material may be administered by IV, causing a flushing feeling.

- That the patient may be asked to refrain from eating or drinking 12 hours before the MRI.

2. Breast MRI

A breast MRI produces detailed images of the breast that provide more information to the healthcare provider than a breast ultrasound or traditional mammography. Healthcare providers order breast MRIs typically when other tests such as a mammography indicate an abnormality. If the abnormality is inflammation, a growth, or blood flow to breast tissues, the healthcare provider may administer contrast material to enhance the image of those areas of the breast.

Women who are positive for the BRCA1 or BRCA2 gene or whose family members developed breast cancer before the age of 50 are considered high risk for developing breast cancer and may be recommended for annual breast MRIs to detect early signs of breast cancer.

The healthcare provider may also order annual breast MRIs for women who normally have dense breast tissue. An MRI is better suited to examine dense breast tissue than an ultrasound test.

What Is Being Examined?

- Breasts

How Is the Test Performed?

- The patient is assessed for any metal that might be on or inside her body. The healthcare provider determines if the presence of any metal may require cancellation of the MRI.

- An assessment is made to determine if the patient can be administered contrast material over a 2-minute period, if required for the MRI.

Contrast material is either ingested or administered IV, causing a flushing feeling for the patient. Contrast material may not be used if the patient is allergic to shellfish and iodine or if she has kidney abnormalities or sickle cell anemia.

- An assessment is made to determine if the patient is claustrophobic. If so, then the healthcare provider may administer a sedative to the patient or schedule the test to be performed using an open MRI machine.
- The patient removes all clothing and wears a gown during the MRI.
- The patient may be given headphones to block out the clanking/tapping noise created by the MRI.
- The patient lies on her back on the MRI table.
- A coil is placed on top of the patient's chest area.
- A belt is cinched around the patient to detect the patient's breathing patterns.
- The table is moved into the MRI machine as images of the breasts are taken.
- Images are viewed during and after the MRI is completed to assist the healthcare provider in reaching a diagnosis.

Rationale for the Test

- Assess
  - For infection
  - The existence of a growth
  - For inflammation
  - Blood flow
  - Women who are at a high risk for breast cancer
  - Women who normally have dense breast tissue
  - Breast cancer treatment
  - Breast implants

Nursing Implications

- Determine if the patient has any metal on or inside her body.
- Assess if the patient
  - Is allergic to shellfish, iodine, or contrast material

- Is pregnant
- Is claustrophobic
- Has kidney disease
- Is wearing any medication patches
- Can lie still during the test

Understanding the Results

- The test takes 60 minutes and the results are ready immediately if the test is performed by the healthcare provider or within a few hours if a technician performs the test.
- Normal test results indicate
  - No growth(s)
  - No blockage
  - No infection
  - No inflammation
  - Normal blood flow
  - Breast implant correctly positioned
- Abnormal test results indicate
  - The existence of a growth
  - Breast implants improperly positioned
  - Inflammation or infection is present
  - Unusual blood flow or blockage

Teach the Patient

- Explain
- Why MRI is being taken.
- What the patient will experience during the MRI.
- That no metal can be on or inside the patient during the MRI.
- That the patient will not feel any pain during the procedure, although she may feel a tingling sensation if she has metal fillings in her teeth.
- That the patient may be administered a sedative if she is claustrophobic.

- That some patients who are allergic to shellfish and iodine may also be allergic to contrast material. If the patient is allergic to contrast material, the healthcare provider will discuss with her the risk and benefits of administering the contrast material. If the patient agrees that the benefits outweigh the risk, then the healthcare provider may administer medication that counteracts the allergic reaction to the contrast material.

- That the contrast material may be administered IV causing a flushing feeling.

3. Head MRI

An MRI of the head is ordered to produce images of the brain and blood vessels that supply blood to the brain to determine the underlying cause of headache, assess for head injury, or determine if the patient has abnormal blood flow or a disorder that affects the brain. Unlike an ultrasound, the head MRI is a closed procedure and does not require that the patient's skull be opened.

There are three types of MRIs used to assess the brain:

- Magnetic resonance spectroscopy: Assesses changes in brain chemistry caused by disease

- Magnetic resonance angiogram (MRA): Assesses speed, direction, and flow of blood in the brain

- Diffusion–perfusion imaging: Assesses inflammation, tumors, and stroke and evaluates the fluid content of the brain

> ## NURSING ALERT
>
> Healthcare providers may order an MRI with gadolinium containing contrast material. Gadolinium can cause nephrogenic fibrosing dermopathy in patients who have kidney failure.

What Is Being Examined?

- Brain

How Is the Test Performed?

- The patient is assessed for any metal that might be on or inside his/her body. The practitioner determines if the presence of any metal may require cancellation of the MRI.
- An assessment is made to determine if the patient can be administered contrast material, if required for the MRI. Contrast material is administered IV, causing a flushing feeling for the patient. Contrast material may not be used if the patient is allergic to shellfish and iodine or if he/she has kidney abnormalities or sickle cell anemia.
- An assessment is made to determine if the patient is claustrophobic. If so, then the healthcare provider may administer a sedative to the patient or schedule the test to be performed using an open MRI machine.
- The patient removes all clothing and wears a gown during the MRI.
- The patient may be given headphones to block out the clanking/tapping noise created by the MRI.
- The patient lies on his/her back on the MRI table.
- A belt is placed on the patient to detect his/her breathing patterns.
- The table is moved into the MRI machine as images are taken of the brain.
- Images are viewed during and after the MRI is completed to assist the healthcare provider reach a diagnosis.

Rationale for the Test

- Assess
  - For infection
  - The existence of a growth
  - For inflammation
  - Blood flow
  - For stroke
  - For suspected head injury
  - For hydrocephaly
  - For multiple sclerosis (MS)
  - For Alzheimer disease
  - For Parkinson disease
  - For Huntington disease

Nursing Implications

- Determine if the patient has any metal on or inside his/her body.
- Assess if the patient
  - Is allergic to shellfish, iodine, or contrast material
  - Is pregnant
  - Is claustrophobic
  - Has kidney disease
  - Is wearing any medication patches
  - Can lie still during the test

Understanding the Results

- The test takes 60 minutes and the results are ready immediately if the test is performed by the healthcare provider or within a few hours if a technician performs the test.
- Normal test results indicate
  - No growth(s)
  - No blockage
  - No infection
  - No inflammation
  - Normal blood flow
- Abnormal test results indicate
  - The existence of a growth
  - Inflammation or infection is present
  - Unusual blood flow or blockage

Teach the Patient

- Explain
- Why MRI is being taken.
- What the patient will experience during the MRI.
- That no metal can be on or inside the patient during the MRI.
- That the patient will not feel any pain during the procedure, although he/she may feel a tingling sensation, if he/she has metal fillings in his/her teeth.

- That the patient may be administered a sedative if he/she is claustrophobic.
- That some patients who are allergic to shellfish or iodine may also be allergic to contrast material. If the patient is allergic to contrast material, the healthcare provider will discuss with him/her the risk and benefit of administering the contrast material. If the patient agrees that the benefits outweigh the risk, then the healthcare provider may administer medication that counteracts the allergic reaction to the contrast material.
- That the contrast material may be administered IV, causing a flushing feeling.

4. Knee MRI

A knee MRI produces detailed images of structures and tissues contained within the knee. These images enable the healthcare provider to identify any abnormalities that may exist in the knee including damage to tendons, ligaments, cartilage, and fluid. The healthcare provider may order a knee MRI to assess if the patient requires arthroscopy of the knee.

What Is Being Examined?

- Knee structures and tissues

How Is the Test Performed?

- The patient is assessed for any metal that might be on or inside his/her body. The healthcare provider determines if the presence of any metal may require cancellation of the MRI.
- An assessment is made to determine if the patient can be administered contrast material, if required, for the MRI. Contrast material is administered IV causing a flushing feeling for the patient. Contrast material may not be used if the patient is allergic to shellfish or iodine or if he/she has kidney abnormalities or sickle cell anemia.
- An assessment is made to determine if the patient is claustrophobic. If so, the healthcare provider may administer a sedative to the patient or schedule the test to be performed using an open MRI machine.
- The patient removes all clothing and wears a gown during the MRI.
- The patient may be given headphones to blockout the clanking/tapping noise created by the MRI.

- The patient lies on his/her back on the MRI table.
- A coil is placed on top of the patient's knee.
- A belt is cinched around the patient to detect his/her breathing patterns.
- The table is moved into the MRI machine as images are taken of the abdomen.
- Images are viewed during and after the MRI is completed to assist the healthcare provider reach a diagnosis.

Rationale for the Test

- Assess
  - The knee structures and tissues
  - The existence of a growth
  - For arthritis
  - Tendons, ligaments, cartilage, meniscus
  - If arthroscopy is required

Nursing Implications

- Determine if the patient has any metal on or inside his/her body.
- Assess if the patient
  - Is allergic to shellfish, iodine, or contrast material
  - Is pregnant
  - Is claustrophobic
  - Has kidney disease
  - Is wearing any medication patches
  - Can lie still during the test
  - Has had prior knee surgeries requiring metal devices to be implanted in the knee

Understanding the Results

- The test takes 60 minutes and the results are ready immediately if the test is performed by the healthcare provider or within a few hours if a technician performs the test.

- Normal test results indicate
  - Normal structures and tissues in the knee
  - No growth(s)
  - No blockage
  - No fluid within the knee
  - No inflammation
  - Normal blood flow
- Abnormal test results indicate
  - Unusual structures and tissues in the knee.
  - The existence of a growth.
  - A blockage is identified.
  - Fluid exists within the knee.
  - Inflammation or infection is present.
  - Unusual blood flow.

Teach the Patient

- Explain
  - Why MRI is being taken.
  - What the patient will experience during the MRI.
  - That no metal can be on or inside the patient during the MRI.
  - That the patient will not feel any pain during the procedure, although he/she may feel a tingling sensation if he/she has metal fillings in his/her teeth.
  - That the patient may be administered a sedative if he/she is claustrophobic.
  - That some patients who are allergic to shellfish and iodine may also be allergic to contrast material. If the patient is allergic to contrast material, the healthcare provider will discuss with him/her the risk and benefits of administering the contrast material. If the patient agrees that the benefits outweigh, the risk, then the healthcare provider may administer medication that counteracts the allergic reaction to the contrast material.
  - That the patient may be administered contrast material IV, causing a flushing feeling.

5. PET Scan

The PET scan is ordered to study blood flow and metabolic activity within a patient's body. Healthcare providers frequently combine results from the PET scan with the CT scan results to obtain a thorough understanding of how well tissues and organs are being infused with blood.

> **NURSING ALERT**
>
> Sometimes a CT scan is performed along with a PET scan. The tracer contains low-level radiation that will rarely lead to tissue damage. The tracer is flushed from the patient's body within 24 hours following the scan. It is rare that a patient will have an allergic reaction to the tracer. The practitioner may order a single photon emission computed tomography (SPECT) to determine if a patient with chest pain is at risk for cardiac arrest.

What Is Being Examined?

- Blood flow and metabolic activity of tissues and organs

How Is the Test Performed?

- The patient is administered the tracer intravenously.
- The patient lies on a table.
- The patient may be given a blindfold or earplugs to wear during the scan.
- Electrocardiogram (ECG) electrodes are placed on the patient if his/her heart is being studied.
- The PET scan camera moves around the patient.
- The patient might be asked to tell a story or read during the scan if his/her brain is being studied.
- The healthcare provider or PET scan technician is outside the PET scan room and is able to speak to the patient through an intercom and see him/her through a window.
- Patients must drink lots of fluid for a full day to flush the tracer from their bodies.

Rationale for the Test

- Assess
  - Blood flow to organs and tissues
  - Metabolic activity or organs
  - For stroke and transient ischemic attack (TIA)
  - For multiple sclerosis
  - For Parkinson disease and Alzheimer disease
  - For epilepsy
  - For coronary artery disease
  - For the presence of cancer and if the cancer has metastasized

Nursing Implications

- The patient will likely be asked to withhold medications for 24 hours before the PET scan.
- The healthcare provider may ask the patient to decrease the dose of insulin if he/she is a diabetic.
- Assess if the patient
  - Has ingested caffeine or alcohol 24 hours before the PET scan
  - Eaten 8 hours before the PET scan
  - Is pregnant
  - Is breast-feeding
  - If the patient signed a consent form prior to the PET scan
  - Can lie still during the test

Understanding the Results

- The test takes 3 hours and the results are ready immediately if the test is performed by the healthcare provider or within a few hours if a technician performs the test.
- Normal test results indicate
  - Normal blood flow
  - No growth
  - No blockage
  - Normal metabolic activity

- Abnormal test results indicate
  - Unexpected blood flow
  - The existence of a growth
  - A blockage
  - Unusual metabolic activity

Teach the Patient

- Explain
- Why PET scan is being taken.
- What the patient will experience during the PET scan.
- That the patient will not feel any pain during the procedure.
- That the patient may be administered a sedative if he/she is claustrophobic.
- The patient must refrain from ingesting alcohol, caffeine, and tobacco for 24 hours prior to the PET scan.
- That the patient may be asked to stop taking or to reduce the dose of medication prior to the PET scan.
- That the PET scan may not be administered if the patient is pregnant or breast-feeding.
- That the healthcare provider may administer a sedative prior to the PET scan if the patient is anxious and unable to lie still for the test.
- That the healthcare provider may ask the patient to tell a story or read during the PET scan, and ECG electrodes may be attached to the his/her body during the test.

6. Shoulder MRI

The shoulder MRI is ordered to show the healthcare provider detailed images of inside the shoulder including ligaments, cartilages, muscles, bone structure within the shoulder, and fluid. These images are more detailed than can be achieved using ultrasound and CT scans and are commonly ordered to assess shoulder pain that is unexplained by other signs or symptoms.

What Is Being Examined?

- Shoulder structures and tissues

How Is the Test Performed?

- The patient is assessed for any metal that might be on or inside his/her body. The healthcare provider determines if the presence of any metal may require cancellation of the MRI.

- An assessment is made to determine if the patient can be administered contrast material, if required, for the MRI. Contrast material is administered IV, causing a flushing feeling for the patient. Contrast material may not be used if the patient is allergic to shellfish or iodine or if he/she has kidney abnormalities or sickle cell anemia.

- An assessment is made to determine if the patient is claustrophobic. If so, then the healthcare provider may administer a sedative to the patient or schedule the test to be performed using an open MRI machine.

- The patient removes all clothing and wears a gown during the MRI.

- The patient may be given headphones to block out the clanking/tapping noise created by the MRI.

- The patient lies on his/her back on the MRI table.

- A coil is placed on the patient's shoulder.

- A belt is cinched around the patient to detect his/her breathing patterns.

- The table is moved into the MRI machine as images are taken of the shoulder.

- Images are viewed during and after the MRI is completed to assist the healthcare provider reach a diagnosis.

Rationale for the Test

- Assess
  - The shoulder structures and tissues
  - The existence of a growth
  - For arthritis
  - Tendons, ligaments, cartilage, bones, muscles
  - For rotator cuff disorders
  - If arthroscopy is required

Nursing Implications

- Determine if the patient has any metal on or inside his/her body
- Assess if the patient
  - Is allergic to shellfish, iodine, or contrast material
  - Is pregnant
  - Is claustrophobic
  - Has kidney disease
  - Is wearing any medication patches
  - Can lie still during the test
  - Has had prior knee surgeries requiring metal devices to be implanted in the shoulder or other parts of the body

Understanding the Results

- The test takes 60 minutes and the results are ready immediately if the test is performed by the healthcare provider or within a few hours if a technician performs the test.
- Normal test results indicate
  - Normal structures and tissues in the shoulder
  - No growth(s)
  - No blockage
  - No fluid within the shoulder
  - No inflammation
  - Normal blood flow
- Abnormal test results indicate
  - Unusual structures and tissues in the shoulder.
  - The existence of a growth.
  - A blockage is identified.
  - Fluid exists within the shoulder.
  - Inflammation or infection is present.
  - Unusual blood flow.
  - Rotator cuff disorders.
  - Ligament and tendon tear or injury.

Teach the Patient

- Explain
- Why MRI is being taken.
- What the patient will experience during the MRI.
- That no metal can be on or inside the patient during the MRI.
- That the patient will not feel any pain during the procedure, although he/she may feel a tingling sensation if he/she has metal fillings in his/her teeth.
- That the patient may be administered a sedative if he/she is claustrophobic.
- That some patients who are allergic to shellfish and iodine may also be allergic to contrast material. If the patient is allergic to contrast material, the healthcare provider will discuss with him/her the risk and benefits of administering the contrast material. If the patient agrees that the benefits outweigh the risk, then the healthcare provider may administer medication that counteracts the allergic reaction to the contrast material.
- That the patient may be administered contrast material IV, causing a flushing feeling.

7. Spinal MRI

The spinal MRI shows detailed images of the patient's spine. This includes the cervical spine, thoracic spine, and lumbosacral spine. The spinal MRI helps the healthcare provider assess if the patient has spinal disc disorders, spinal stenosis, as well as tumors or arthritis. The healthcare provider also orders a spinal MRI to assess unexplained spinal pain.

What Is Being Examined?

- Spine

How Is the Test Performed?

- The patient is assessed for any metal that might be on or inside his/her body. The healthcare provider determines if the presence of any metal may require cancellation of the MRI.

- An assessment is made to determine if the patient can be administered contrast material, if required, for the MRI. Contrast material is administered IV, causing a flushing feeling for the patient. Contrast material may not be used if the patient is allergic to shellfish or iodine or if he/she has kidney abnormalities or sickle cell anemia.

- An assessment is made to determine if the patient is claustrophobic. If so, then the healthcare provider may administer a sedative to the patient or schedule the test to be performed using an open MRI machine.

- The patient removes all clothing and wears a gown during the MRI.

- The patient may be given headphones to block out the clanking/tapping noise created by the MRI.

- The patient lies on his/her back on the MRI table.

- A belt is cinched around the patient to detect his/her breathing patterns.

- The table is moved into the MRI machine as images are taken of the shoulder.

- Images are viewed during and after the MRI is completed to assist the healthcare provider reach a diagnosis.

Rationale for the Test

- Assess
  - The spinal structures and tissues
  - For ruptured disc
  - For sciatica
  - For spinal stenosis
  - Growths
  - For arthritis
  - For damaged nerves

Nursing Implications

- Determine if the patient has any metal on or inside his/her body.
- Assess if the patient
  - Is allergic to shellfish, iodine, or contrast material
  - Is pregnant
  - Is claustrophobic

- Has kidney disease
- Is wearing any medication patches
- Can lie still during the test
- Has had prior surgeries where metal devices might have been implanted in the shoulder or other parts of the body

Understanding the Results

- The test takes 60 minutes and the results are ready immediately if the test is performed by the healthcare provider or within a few hours if a technician performs the test.
- Normal test results indicate
  - Normal structures and tissues in the spine
  - No growth(s)
  - No blockage
  - No inflammation
  - Normal blood flow
  - No damaged nerves
- Abnormal test results indicate
  - Unusual structures and tissues in the spine.
  - The existence of a growth.
  - A blockage is identified.
  - Inflammation or infection is present.
  - Ruptured disc.
  - Sciatica.
  - Spinal stenosis.
  - Arthritis.

Teach the Patient

- Explain
  - Why MRI is being taken.
  - What the patient will experience during the MRI.
  - That no metal can be on or inside the patient during the MRI.

- That the patient will not feel any pain during the procedure, although he/she may feel a tingling sensation if he/she has metal fillings in his/her teeth.

- That the patient may be administered a sedative if he/she is claustrophobic.

- That some patients who are allergic to shellfish or iodine may also be allergic to contrast material. If the patient is allergic to contrast material, the healthcare provider will discuss with him/her the risk and benefits of administering the contrast material. If the patient agrees that the benefits outweigh, the risk, then the healthcare provider may administer medication that counteracts the allergic reaction to the contrast material.

- That the patient may be administered contrast material IV, causing a flushing feeling.

Summary

There are times when healthcare providers require seeing inside the patient's body at a higher resolution than is provided by the CT scan and ultrasound scan. In these situations, the healthcare provider may order an MRI.

An MRI uses pulsating radio waves in a magnetic field to produce an image of inside the patient's body. A coil and a belt are placed on the patient. The coil is placed over the area being scanned and the belt detects the patient's breathing, assuring that breaths do not interfere with taking the MRI image.

The patient lies on a table that is moved into the MRI machine. The MRI machine creates a clanking/tapping noise as images are taken. Some patients may be disturbed by this noise; therefore, headphones are provided to block out the noise. Contrast material may be administered to the patient prior to the MRI to highlight areas of the body that are being studied.

Some patients feel claustrophobic and become anxious when placed inside the MRI machine. The healthcare provider may administer a sedative to relax the patient prior to the scan or may schedule an open MRI, which is less enclosed than a traditional MRI machine.

The MRI generates digital images of the inside of the patient's body on a computer screen. Those images are stored for review by the patient's healthcare team.

No metal objects can be on or inside the patient during an MRI. However, dental fillings are permitted, although the patient is likely to feel tingling in his/her mouth during the MRI. The patient may also experience skin irritation if he/she has iron pigment tattoos.

A PET scan creates an image of a radioactive tracer as the tracer travels throughout the patient's bloodstream creating a roadmap of the bloodstream for the healthcare provider.

Prior to the scan, the tracer is usually administered into the patient's vein. As the tracer moves along with blood, it gives off tiny charged particles called positrons that are detected by the PET scan camera. These images are then stored and replayed on a computer, enabling the healthcare provider to study blood flow to organs and tissues and to assess the patient's metabolic activities.

QUIZ

1. **Can a patient with metal dental fillings undergo an MRI?**
    A. No, the MRI metal alert alarm sounds.
    B. Yes, but the patient may experience a tingling sensation in his/her mouth.
    C. No, there is a risk that the fillings will be extracted by the MRI.
    D. Yes, but a plastic cap must be placed over each filling.

2. **Can a patient receive an MRI with contrast if the patient is allergic to shellfish?**
    A. No, the MRI must be cancelled.
    B. The practitioner will evaluate the benefit and risk of continuing with the MRI.
    C. Yes, the MRI continues as scheduled.
    D. Yes, but a crash-cart must be standing by before continuing with the MRI.

3. **Why would a woman who is positive for BRCA1 receive annual MRI scan?**
    A. The patient is at high risk for breast cancer and the MRI provides highly detailed views of the patient's breasts.
    B. BRCA1 interferes a normal mammogram is necessary.
    C. Only radio waves can penetrate the BRCA1 so an MRI is not necessary.
    D. A positive BRCA1 means that the patient is not at risk for cancer and does not need an MRI scan.

4. **Can a patient who is claustrophobic undergo an MRI scan?**
    A. Yes, the patient can be given a sedative.
    B. Yes, the patient can be scheduled for an open MRI.
    C. Yes, the MRI should not be cancelled.
    D. All of the above.

5. **How are images taken in coordination with the patient's breathing?**

   A. Metal transducers are placed on the patient's body.

   B. Plastic transducers are placed inside the patient's body.

   C. A belt is placed around the patient's chest.

   D. Plastic transducers are placed both on and inside the patient's body.

6. **What is used to assess the speed, direction, and flow of blood?**

   A. MRI

   B. MRA

   C. X-ray

   D. All of the above

7. **The patient tells you she is fearful that the tracer will destroy her tissues. How should you respond?**

   A. Explain that the tracer contains a very low dose of radiation that remains in the body for 24 days after the test and causes minor tissue damage.

   B. Explain that the tracer contains a very low dose of radiation that is flushed from the body within 24 hours of the test and rarely causes any tissue damage.

   C. Explain that the tracer contains the same amount of radiation as the sun and causes no more than a minor sunburn.

   D. You won't feel anything.

8. **What test is used to assess changes in the brain chemistry caused by disease?**

   A. Magnetic resonance spectroscopy

   B. MRA

   C. Diffusion–perfusion imaging

   D. MRI

9. **Why should a patient with kidney disease avoid being administered contrast material prior to an MRI?**

   A. The patient might have difficulty excreting the contrast material.

   B. The contrast material contains metallic elements.

   C. Patients with kidney disease should never receive an MRI.

   D. None of the above.

10. **What does a patient wear during an MRI?**

    A. The patient removes all clothing and wears a gown during the MRI.

    B. The patient needs only to expose the area of the body that is being assessed.

    C. The patient removes all clothing during the MRI.

    D. The patient can remain in street clothes during the MRI.

ANSWERS

1. B. Yes, but the patient may experience a tingling sensation in his/her mouth.
2. B. The practitioner will evaluate the benefit and risk of continuing with the MRI.
3. A. The patient is at high risk for breast cancer and the MRI provides highly detailed views of the patient's breasts.
4. D. All of the above.
5. C. A belt is placed around the patient's chest.
6. B. MRA.
7. B. Explain that the tracer contains a very low dose of radiation that is flushed from the body within 24 hours of the test and rarely causes any tissue damage.
8. A. Magnetic resonance spectroscopy.
9. A. The patient might have difficulty excreting the contrast material.
10. A. The patient removes all clothing and wears a gown during the MRI.

chapter 14

Ultrasound Scan

343

KEY WORDS

Color Doppler
Conductive gel
Continuous-wave Doppler
Duplex Doppler
Latex allergy
Power Doppler

Sonohysterogram
Transabdominal
Transrectal
Transvaginal
Valsalva maneuver

An ultrasound scan creates an image of organs and structures inside the body using sound waves similar in concept to the way in which ship crews are able to identify underwater objects while on the surface of the water.

High-frequency sound waves are transmitted by a transducer that is placed on the patient's skin. Sound waves penetrate the skin, bounce off organs and structures in the patient's body, and are detected by the transducer.

Sound waves detected by the transducer are translated into an image that appears on the ultrasound screen. The healthcare provider can then measure organs and structures that appear on the image to determine any abnormality.

Images can either be printed and included in the patient's chart or can be stored on a computer. An ultrasound can detect a growth but cannot differentiate between one that is malignant or benign, which is determined by a biopsy. An ultrasound can differentiate between a solid growth and a fluid-filled cyst.

An ultrasound scan is commonly ordered instead of a CT scan or MRI because it is less expensive and in many situations provides the healthcare provider with sufficient information to assist in diagnosis.

In this chapter you will learn about different kinds of ultrasound scans.

1. Benign Prostatic Hyperplasia Ultrasound

Middle-aged men might experience the urgency to void, hesitancy waiting for the urinary stream, or a weak urinary stream. These may be signs of an enlarged prostate that places pressure on the bladder and blocks the urinary stream. Noncancerous, enlarged prostate is referred to as benign prostatic hyperplasia (BPH) or hypertrophy. An ultrasound is used to assist the health-care provider diagnose the condition.

The BPH ultrasound is also used to help guide the healthcare provider when taking a biopsy of the prostate, which is commonly performed if the patient's prostate-specific antigen (PSA) level is elevated.

NURSING ALERT

The healthcare provider may also evaluate the bladder and the kidneys while performing the BPH ultrasound to determine urinary retention and kidney stones that may block urinary flow.

NURSING ALERT

The BPH ultrasound cannot determine if urinary flow is blocked by the prostate.

What Is Being Examined?

- The prostate gland

How Is the Test Performed?

- The ultrasound transducer is either inserted into the rectum (transrectal ultrasound [TRUS]) or placed on the patient's abdomen (transabdominal ultrasound).
- An image of the prostate, kidneys, and bladder appears on the screen.
- The healthcare provider estimates the size of the prostate and determines if there is any urinary retention or blockage.

Rationale for the Test

- Assess
  - The size of the prostate
  - Urinary retention
  - A urinary blockage
- Guide the healthcare provider when taking a biopsy of the prostate.

Nursing Implications

- Assess if the patient can lie still during the test.

Understanding the Results

- The test takes 30 minutes and the results are ready immediately if the test is performed by the healthcare provider or within a few hours if a technician performs the test.
- Normal test results indicate
  - Prostate is an acceptable size
  - Kidneys show no obstruction
  - No urine or an acceptable volume of urine in the bladder
- Abnormal test results indicate
  - Enlarged prostate
  - Enlarged kidneys
  - Kidney obstruction
  - Enlarged bladder
  - Significant volume of urine in bladder

Teach the Patient

- Explain
- Why ultrasound is being taken.
- That clear gel will be placed on the ultrasound site to increase the conduction of sound.
- That the patient will not feel any pain.
- That the patient must lie still during the test.

2. Transvaginal Ultrasound and Hysterosonogram

When a woman has difficulty conceiving, the healthcare provider may perform a transvaginal ultrasound or a hysterosonogram, which is also known as a sonohysterogram. These scans enable the healthcare provider to assess ovarian follicle development and the endometrium. This assessment may help the healthcare provider determine when to perform intrauterine insemination.

> **NURSING ALERT**
>
> The transvaginal ultrasound is the preferred method rather than the transabdominal ultrasound for assessing the uterine lining and follicle growth.

> **NURSING ALERT**
>
> The transvaginal ultrasound may not display scars or small tumors.

What Is Being Examined?

- The uterus
- Uterine lining
- The endometrial cavity
- Ovarian follicle development

How Is the Test Performed?

- The patient may be required to have an empty bladder prior to the scan or a full bladder depending on what is being examined.
- The ultrasound transducer is inserted into the vagina.
- The healthcare provider performs the ultrasound scan from within the vagina.
- When preparing for a hysterosonogram, the uterus is filled with fluid prior to insertion of the transducer into the vagina.

Rationale for the Test

- Assess
  - The uterus
  - The fallopian tubes
  - Ovaries
  - The endometrial cavity
  - Uterine lining
  - Ovarian follicle development

- To schedule intrauterine insemination
- To guide the healthcare provider when removing follicles

Nursing Implications

- Assess if the patient
  - Can lie still during the test
  - Has an empty bladder prior to the test

Understanding the Results

- The test takes 30 minutes and the results are ready immediately if the test is performed by the healthcare provider or within a few hours if a technician performs the test.
- Normal test results indicate
  - No growths.
  - No scar tissue.
  - The uterus is a normal shape.
  - The fallopian tubes are not blocked.
  - Ovaries are normal size.
  - The endometrial cavity is normal shape.
  - Uterine lining is normal size.
- Abnormal test results indicate
  - Few follicles
  - Uterine fibroids
  - Ovarian cysts
  - Hydrosalpinx
  - Thick uterine lining
  - Deformed uterine lining
  - Enlarged uterus
  - Abnormal fallopian tubes

Teach the Patient

- Explain
  - Why ultrasound is being taken.

- That the patient must have an empty bladder before the scan.
- That the patient will not feel any pain.
- That the patient must lie still during the test.
- That the transducer is inserted into the vagina.
- That the uterus will be filled with fluid if the healthcare provider orders a hysterosonogram.

3. Testicular Ultrasound

A healthcare provider may order a testicular ultrasound if the patient shows signs and symptoms of testicular abnormalities or infertility. The testicular ultrasound displays an image of the patient's testicles and scrotum including the epididymis, which is the coiled tube behind the testicle that collects sperm. The testicular ultrasound also displays an image of the vas deferens, which is the tube that connects the prostate gland to the testicles.

What Is Being Examined?

- The testicles
- The scrotum
- The epididymis
- The vas deferens

How Is the Test Performed?

- A conductive gel is placed on the transducer or on the scrotum.
- The transducer is placed on the scrotum and moved around to capture the image.
- The patient may be asked to hold his breath for a few seconds while the image is being taken.

Rationale for the Test

- Assess
  - The testicles
  - The epididymis
  - The vas deferens

- The scrotum
- The spermatic cord
- For hydroceles and spermatoceles
- Guide the healthcare provider when performing a testicular biopsy.

Nursing Implications

- Assess
  - If the patient can lie still during the test.
  - If the patient has open skin in the scrotum.
- A consent form must be signed if the patient is undergoing a testicular biopsy.
- The patient must remove all clothing from the waist down.
- Towels are used to lift the scrotum.
- Wipe the conductive gel from the patient's skin when the test is completed.

Understanding the Results

- The test takes 30 minutes and the results are ready immediately if the test is performed by the healthcare provider or within a few hours if a technician performs the test.
- Normal test results indicate
  - No growths.
  - The testicles are of normal shape.
  - The epididymitis does not show inflammation or blockage.
  - The spermatic cord is not twisted.
  - There is no fluid in the scrotum.
- Abnormal test results indicate
  - There is a growth on one or both testicles.
  - There is inflammation, infection, or blockage in the epididymis.
  - The spermatic cord is twisted.
  - There is fluid in the scrotum.

Teach the Patient

- Explain
  - Why ultrasound is being taken.

- That the patient will not feel any pain.
- That the patient must lie still during the test.
- That the patient will have to remove all clothing from the waist down.
- That towels are used to lift the scrotum.
- That conductive gel is placed on the scrotum and it will be wiped off after the test is completed.
- That the transducer is placed on and moved around the scrotum.
- That a consent form must be signed if the patient is undergoing a testicular biopsy.

4. Abdominal Ultrasound

An abdominal ultrasound is ordered to view upper abdominal organs and structures. These include the liver, gallbladder, spleen, pancreas, and kidneys. It is also ordered to assist the healthcare provider in assessing the abdominal aorta, which is the artery located at the back of the chest and abdomen that supplies blood to the legs, abdomen, and organs in the lower portion of the body.

NURSING ALERT

The healthcare provider may order an ultrasound of specific organs or structures within the abdomen if the abdominal ultrasound shows an abnormal condition in the abdomen.

What Is Being Examined?

- Liver
- Gallbladder
- Bile ducts
- Spleen
- Pancreas
- Kidneys
- Abdominal aorta

How Is the Test Performed?

- The patient must remove jewelry from the abdominal area.
- The patient should eat a fat-free dinner the night before the test.
- The patient should avoid eating 12 hours before the test to prevent gas from building up in the intestines.
- The patient may be asked to drink 6 glasses of water 1 hour before the test.
- The patient must remove all clothing from the waist down.
- A conductive gel is placed on the abdomen.
- The transducer is placed on the abdomen and moved around to capture the image.
- The healthcare provider may push on the abdomen to move organs within the abdominal cavity to get a clearer view of other organs.
- The patient may be asked to change position during the test.
- The patient may be asked to hold his/her breath for a few seconds.

Rationale for the Test

- Assess
  - Liver
  - Gallbladder
  - Bile ducts
  - Spleen
  - Pancreas
  - Kidneys
  - Abdominal aorta
- Guide the healthcare provider when taking a biopsy or when performing a paracentesis.

Nursing Implications

- Assess if the patient
  - Can lie still during the test
  - Has had a barium enema for an upper GI test 2 days prior to the ultrasound scan

- Has had a barium enema for a lower GI test 2 days prior to the ultrasound scan
- Has removed jewelry from the abdominal area
- Has eaten a fat-free dinner the night before the test
- Has not eaten 12 hours before the ultrasound scan
- Has drunk 6 glasses of water 1 hour before the ultrasound scan
- Has an open wound in the abdominal area
- Is obese
- Has signed a consent form when undergoing a biopsy.
- Has removed all clothing from the waist down.
- Wipe the conductive gel from the patient's skin when the test is completed.

Understanding the Results

- The test takes 60 minutes and the results are ready immediately if the test is performed by the healthcare provider or within a few hours if a technician performs the test.
- Normal test results indicate
  - No growths
  - All organs are normal shape
  - No inflammation or blockage of the bile ducts
- Abnormal test results indicate
  - There is a growth on one or multiple organs.
  - There is inflammation, infection, or blockage of the bile ducts.
  - The aorta is enlarged.
  - Fluid appears in the abdomen.

Teach the Patient

- Explain
- Why ultrasound is being taken.
- That the patient will not feel any pain.
- That the patient must lie still during the test.
- That the patient will have to remove all clothing from the waist down.

- That the patient will need to remove jewelry from the abdominal area.
- That the patient should eat a fat-free dinner the night before the test.
- That the patient should avoid eating for 12 hours before the test.
- That the patient may be asked to drink 6 glasses of water 1 hour before the test.
- That the healthcare provider may push on the abdomen to move organs within the abdominal cavity to get a clearer view of other organs.
- That the patient may be asked to change position during the test.
- That the patient may be asked to hold his/her breath for a few seconds while the ultrasound is being taken.
- That conductive gel is placed on the abdomen and it will be wiped off after the test is completed.
- That the transducer is placed on and moved around the abdomen.
- That a consent form must be signed if the patient is undergoing a biopsy.

5. Breast Ultrasound

The breast ultrasound creates an image of all areas of the breast, including portions of the breast that are near the chest. A mammogram typically doesn't show images of the breast that are near the chest. A breast ultrasound is sometimes performed on younger women whose breast tissues are dense, making it difficult to see breast abnormalities on a mammogram.

A healthcare provider frequently orders a breast ultrasound to assess a lump identified by either palpation or from a mammogram. The breast ultrasound can distinguish between a solid mass and a cyst. If it is a solid mass, then the healthcare provider performs a biopsy to determine if the mass is benign or malignant.

NURSING ALERT

A breast ultrasound does not replace an annual mammogram.

What Is Being Examined?

- The breast

How Is the Test Performed?

- The patient must remove jewelry from the breast area.
- The patient must remove clothing above the waist.
- A conductive gel is placed on the transducer before placing it on the breast.
- The transducer is placed on the breast and moved around to capture the image.

Rationale for the Test

- Assess
  - A mass found on palpation or by a mammogram
  - The breast of a younger woman whose breast tissues are dense
  - Silicone breast implants
  - Breast pain
- Guide the healthcare provider when taking a biopsy or when draining a cyst.

Nursing Implications

- Assess if the patient
  - Can lie still during the test
  - Has removed jewelry from the breast area
  - Has an open wound in the breast area
- A consent form must be signed if the patient is undergoing a biopsy or a cyst drainage.
- The patient must remove all clothing above the waist.
- Wipe the conductive gel from the patient's skin when the test is completed.

Understanding the Results

- The test takes 30 minutes and the results are ready immediately if the test is performed by the healthcare provider or within a few hours if a technician performs the test.
- Normal test results indicate
  - No mass found

- Normal-shaped breasts
- No inflammation
- Abnormal test results indicate
  - There is a cyst.
  - There is a solid mass.
  - There is inflammation or infection.

Teach the Patient

- Explain
- Why ultrasound is being taken.
- That the patient will not feel any pain.
- That the patient must lie still during the test.
- That the patient will have to remove all clothing from the waist up.
- The patient will need to remove jewelry from the breast area.
- That conductive gel is placed on the breast and it will be wiped off after the test is completed.
- That the transducer is placed on and moved around the breast.
- That a consent form must be signed if the patient is undergoing a biopsy or drainage of a cyst.

6. Cranial Ultrasound

A cranial ultrasound creates images of the brain and ventricles. Since ultrasound cannot penetrate bone, a cranial ultrasound is performed on babies up to 18 months old, whose cranium has yet to form. A cranial ultrasound is commonly used in premature newborns to assess complications of the premature birth.

A cranial ultrasound is also performed on adults during brain surgery to visualize any masses in the brain. The ultrasound is able to capture the image because a portion of the patient's cranium is removed during surgery, enabling the ultrasound to penetrate the brain tissue.

What Is Being Examined?

- Brain
- Ventricles

How Is the Test Performed?

- On babies
  - Feed the baby near the time of the ultrasound scan to keep the baby still and comfortable during the scan.
  - Place the baby on his/her back or have the parent hold the baby.
  - The transducer is placed on and moved around the fontanelle.
- On adults
  - A portion of the cranium is removed in surgery.
  - The transducer is placed on and moved around the exposed brain.

Rationale for the Test

- Assess for
  - Babies
  - Why the baby has an abnormally large head
  - For encephalitis
  - For meningitis
  - For hydrocephalus
  - For periventricular leukomalacia (PVL)
  - For intraventricular hemorrhage (IVH)
- Adults
  - Brain mass

Nursing Implications

- Assess if
  - Baby can lie still during the test.
  - Parent can hold the baby still during the test.
  - Baby's cranium has closed.

Understanding the Results

- The test takes 30 minutes and the results are ready immediately.
- Normal test results indicate
  - No mass or cyst found

- Normal-shaped brain
- No inflammation
- No bleeding
- There is no excessive cerebrospinal fluid (CSF)
- Abnormal test results indicate
  - There is a mass or cyst
  - There is inflammation or infection
  - There is bleeding
  - There is excessive CSF

Teach the Patient

- Explain
- Why ultrasound is being taken.
- That the patient will not feel any pain.
- That the patient must lie still during the test and the parent can hold the baby during the test.
- That conductive gel is placed on the fontanelle and it will be wiped off after the test is completed.
- That the transducer is placed on and moved around the fontanelle.
- That the test will be conducted during surgery, if the patient is an adult.

7. Doppler Ultrasound

A Doppler ultrasound is used to assess blood flow through the blood vessels. There are four types of Doppler ultrasound:

- Continuous-wave: Produces a pulsating, audible sound reflecting pulsating blood through a blood vessel.
- Duplex: Produces an image of the blood vessel along with a computer-generated graph, which indicates the speed and direction of blood flow.
- Color: Produces an image of the blood vessel with the speed and direction of blood flow represented by colors on the image.
- Power: Similar to the color Doppler; however, the power Doppler is 5 times as sensitive in detecting blood flow.

What Is Being Examined?

- Blood flow in blood vessels

How Is the Test Performed?

- The patient should remove all jewelry around the site of the blood vessel.
- The patient will remove all clothing around the site of the blood vessel.
- A conductive gel is placed on the skin that covers the blood vessel.
- The transducer is placed over and moved around the blood vessel.
- If the extremities are being tested, the healthcare provider may test both extremities to compare the results. Furthermore, the test may be performed with the patient both lying and sitting. The healthcare provider may also place the blood pressure cuff on the extremities during the test.
- The patient may be asked to perform the Valsalva maneuver by pinching his/her nose, closing his/her mouth, and then exhaling.
- If arteries in the neck are being tested, the patient will place his/her head on a pillow.

Rationale for the Test

- Assess for
  - Narrow blood vessels
  - Blood clots (deep vein thrombosis)
  - Atherosclerosis
  - Stroke
- Use of mapping in vein grafts

Nursing Implications

- Assess if the
  - Patient can lie still during the test.
  - Patient has smoked cigarettes or chewed tobacco or otherwise ingested nicotine 2 hours before the test. Nicotine constricts blood vessels resulting in a false test result.
  - Patient can perform the Valsalva maneuver.

- Patient is obese, since this can interfere with the test.
- Patient has arrhythmias, which may alter blood flow through unobstructed blood vessels.

Understanding the Results

- The test takes 60 minutes and the results are ready immediately.
- Normal test results indicate
  - No blood clots
  - Normal blood flow and pulse
- Abnormal test results indicate
  - There is a blockage in blood flow.
  - There is an abnormal pulse.
  - There is abnormal shape of blood vessels.

Teach the Patient

- Explain
- Why ultrasound is being taken.
- That the patient will not feel any pain.
- That the patient must lie still during the test.
- That conductive gel is placed on the skin over the blood vessel and it will be wiped off after the test is completed.
- That the transducer is placed on and moved around the skin over the blood vessel.
- That patient should avoid smoking, chewing tobacco, or otherwise ingesting nicotine 2 hours before the test.
- That the healthcare provider may ask the patient to perform the Valsalva maneuver.
- That arrhythmias may provide a false test result.

8. Fetal Ultrasound

A fetal ultrasound produces an image (sonogram) of the fetus, the placenta, and amniotic fluid during pregnancy. The healthcare provider orders a fetal ultrasound to determine the size, position, and sex of the fetus and to identify any abnormalities prior to birth.

There are two types of fetal ultrasound tests:

- Transabdominal: The ultrasound transducer is placed on the patient's abdomen.
- Transvaginal: The ultrasound transducer is covered in a latex sheath and inserted into the vagina.

> ## NURSING ALERT
>
> Verify that the patient is not allergic to latex if the healthcare provider is performing a transvaginal ultrasound. A normal fetal ultrasound does not rule out fetal abnormalities or problems with the placenta and amniotic fluid.

What Is Being Examined?

- The fetus
- The placenta
- Amniotic fluid

How Is the Test Performed?

- Transabdominal ultrasound
  - The patient should remove all jewelry around the abdomen.
  - The patient will remove all clothing around the abdomen.
  - Early pregnancy: The patient needs a full bladder and must drink a large volume of water and avoid urinating until the test is completed. The water moves the intestines away from the uterus. If the patient is unable to maintain a full bladder, the healthcare provider may order the insertion of a urinary catheter through her urethra and fill the bladder with sterile water.
  - Late pregnancy: The patient does not need a full bladder since the intestines are repositioned by fetal growth.
  - The patient lies on her back.
  - A conductive gel is placed on the abdomen.
  - The transducer is placed over and moved around the abdomen.
  - If the patient becomes short of breath, the healthcare provider may raise the head of the bed or place the patient on her side.

- Transvaginal ultrasound
  - The patient does not need a full bladder for this test.
  - The patient lies on her back with hips raised.
  - Verify before the test that the patient is not allergic to latex.
  - The healthcare provider places a transducer covered with a latex sheath into the vagina to capture the image.

Rationale for the Test

- Assess
  - Progress of the pregnancy
  - The gestational age of the fetus
  - For fetal defects
  - The number of fetuses
  - The placenta
  - The amniotic fluid
  - The fetal position
  - The cervix
- Detection of ectopic pregnancy

Nursing Implications

- Assess if the patient
  - Can lie still during the test
  - Has a full bladder if a transabdominal ultrasound is being performed
  - Is allergic to latex if a transvaginal ultrasound is being performed
  - Is obese

Understanding the Results

- The test takes 60 minutes or less and the results are ready immediately.
- Normal test results indicate
  - Expected fetal gestation
  - Normal placenta
  - Expected volume of amniotic fluid
  - No birth defects

- Abnormal test results indicate
  - Underdeveloped or abnormally developed fetus
  - Unexpected fetal position
  - Placenta previa
  - Molar pregnancy
  - Suspected birth defect discovered
  - Unexpected volume of amniotic fluid

Teach the Patient

- Explain
  - Why ultrasound is being taken.
  - That the patient will not feel any pain.
  - That the patient must lie still during the test.
  - That the patient will require a full bladder. If the patient is unable to drink a sufficient volume of water, then a urinary catheter will be inserted and sterile water will be placed into her bladder (transabdominal).
  - That the patient will not urinate until after the test is concluded (transabdominal).
  - That conductive gel is placed on the skin over the abdomen and it will be wiped off after the test is completed (transabdominal).
  - That the transducer is placed on and moved around the abdomen (transabdominal).
  - That the ultrasound transducer may be covered in a latex sheath and inserted into the patient's vagina (transvaginal).
  - That if the patient feels short of breath during the test, the head of the bed will be raised or she will be repositioned on her side (transvaginal).
  - That a normal fetal ultrasound does not rule out abnormalities with the fetus, placenta, or amniotic fluid.

9. Pelvic Ultrasound

A pelvic ultrasound creates images of the bladder, ovaries, uterus, cervix, fallopian tubes, prostate gland, and seminal vesicles. There are three types of pelvic ultrasound tests.

- Transabdominal: The transducer is moved along the abdomen.
- Transrectal: The transducer is inserted into the rectum.
- Transvaginal: The transducer is covered with a latex sheath and inserted in the vagina.

> **NURSING ALERT**
>
> Verify that the patient is not allergic to latex before a transrectal or transvaginal ultrasound is performed.

What Is Being Examined?

- Bladder
- Ovaries
- Uterus
- Cervix
- Fallopian tubes
- Prostate gland
- Seminal vesicles

How Is the Test Performed?

- Transabdominal ultrasound
  - The patient removes all jewelry from below the waist.
  - The patient will remove all clothing from below the waist.
  - The patient will be required to fill his/her bladder to push the intestines away from the pelvic organs. If the patient is unable to drink water, the healthcare provider will insert a catheter into the patient's bladder and infuse sterile water.
  - The patient will be required to sign a consent form if the ultrasound is used to guide the healthcare provider to take a biopsy.
  - The patient lies on his/her back.
  - A conductive gel is placed on the abdomen.
  - The transducer is placed over and moved around the abdomen.

- Transrectal ultrasound
  - The patient is given an enema an hour before the test.
  - Verify that the patient is not allergic to latex.
  - A latex sheath is placed over the ultrasound transducer.
  - The patient lies on his/her left side with knees bent.
  - The ultrasound transducer is lubricated and then inserted into the patient's rectum to capture the image.
- Transvaginal ultrasound
  - The patient should avoid drinking fluids 4 hours before the test.
  - The patient lies on her back with hips raised.
  - Verify before the test that the patient is not allergic to latex.
  - The healthcare provider places a transducer covered with a latex sheath into the vagina to capture the image.

Rationale for the Test

- Assess
  - The cause of urinary disorders
  - The bladder
  - For growths
  - For pelvic inflammatory disease (PID)
  - For placement of intrauterine device (IUD)
  - The size of pelvic organs and structures
  - The fetal position
  - For the cause of infertility
- Guide the healthcare provider when performing a biopsy.

Nursing Implications

- Assess if the patient
  - Has ingested contrast material 2 days before the ultrasound
  - Can lie still during the test
  - Has a full bladder (transabdominal)

- Is allergic to latex (transrectal or transvaginal)
- Has removed jewelry and clothing from below the waist
- Signed a consent if the ultrasound is used for a biopsy
- Has been given an enema 1 hour before the test (transrectal)
- Can lie on left side and bend knees (transrectal)
- Has not drunk fluids 4 hours before the test (transvaginal)
- Is obese

Understanding the Results

- The test takes 30 minutes or less and the results are ready immediately.
- Normal test results indicate
  - Pelvic organs are normal size
  - No growth
  - No blockages
  - Intrauterine device is in the expected position
- Abnormal test results indicate
  - Unexpected size of one or more pelvic organs.
  - Growths are seen.
  - Inflammation and infection noticed.
  - Unexpected fluid.
  - Blockage found.
  - Intrauterine device is not in the expected position.

Teach the Patient

- Explain
- Why ultrasound is being taken.
- That the patient will not feel any pain.
- That the patient must lie still during the test.
- That the patient cannot ingest contrast material 2 days before the test.
- That the patient will require a full bladder. If the patient is unable to drink a sufficient volume of water, then a urinary catheter will be inserted and sterile water will be placed into the bladder (transabdominal).

- That the patient will not urinate until after the test is concluded (transabdominal).
- That the patient will be given an enema 1 hour before the test (transrectal).
- That the patient must avoid drinking 4 hours before the test (transvaginal).
- That conductive gel is placed on the skin over the abdomen and it will be wiped off after the test is completed (transabdominal).
- That the transducer is placed on and moved around the abdomen (transabdominal).
- That the ultrasound transducer may be covered in a latex sheath and inserted into the rectum or vagina (transrectal or transvaginal).
- That if she feels short of breath during the test, the head of the bed will be raised or that she will be repositioned on her side (transvaginal).

10. Thyroid and Parathyroid Ultrasound

The thyroid and parathyroid ultrasound is used to create an image of the thyroid and the parathyroid glands. The thyroid gland produces thyroxine that controls body's metabolism. The parathyroid gland produces the parathyroid hormone (PTH) that controls body's calcium and phosphorus balance in the blood.

NURSING ALERT

The thyroid and parathyroid ultrasound enables the healthcare provider to assess the size of these glands but not the production of hormones.

What Is Being Examined?

- Thyroid gland
- Parathyroid gland

How Is the Test Performed?

- The patient removes all jewelry from the head and neck area.
- The patient may be asked to remove all clothing from above the waist.

- The patient lies on his/her back and a pillow is placed under his/her shoulders.
- A conductive gel is placed on the neck.
- The healthcare provider may place a bag filled with water or a sponge of gel over the patient's throat to increase conductivity.
- The transducer is placed over and moved around the neck. The patient may be asked to turn his/her head.

Rationale for the Test

- Assess
  - The size of the thyroid gland
  - The size of the parathyroid gland
  - For growths
- Guide the healthcare provider when performing a biopsy.

Nursing Implications

- Assess if the patient
  - Can lie still during the test
  - Has removed jewelry and clothing from above the waist
  - Signed a consent if the ultrasound is used for a biopsy
  - Can move his/her head
  - Is obese

Understanding the Results

- The test takes 30 minutes and the results are ready immediately.
- Normal test results indicate
  - Thyroid is normal size
  - Parathyroid is normal size
  - No growth
- Abnormal test results indicate
  - Unexpected size of thyroid or parathyroid
  - Growths are seen

Teach the Patient

- Explain
  - Why ultrasound is being taken.
  - That the patient will not feel any pain.
  - That the patient must lie still during the test.
  - That conductive gel is placed on the skin over the neck, and it will be wiped off after the test is completed.

Summary

High-frequency sound waves penetrate the patient's body. Some waves are reflected and others pass through the body. The reflected waves are received by a transducer and passed through to a computer that generates an image on the screen.

The healthcare provider is able to view the image and determine if there are any abnormal organs or structures in the patient's body. An ultrasound can differentiate between a fluid-filled cyst and a solid mass but cannot tell if the solid mass is benign or malignant. Only a biopsy study of the mass can make this determination.

An ultrasound is less expensive than alternative tests such as a CT scan or MRI. Although these other alternative tests provide greater detail, the ultrasound typically provides sufficient information to help the healthcare provider reach a diagnosis.

QUIZ

1. **How do you increase conductivity of sound waves across the patient's skin?**
   A. Place gel on the patient's skin over the site of the test.
   B. Place gel on the patient's body before conducting the test.
   C. Increase ambient noise.
   D. Decrease ambient noise.

2. **How do you reposition the intestine prior to an abdominal ultrasound?**
   A. Position the patient on her left side.
   B. Fill the bladder with contrast.
   C. Fill the bladder with water.
   D. Position the patient on her right side.

3. **What test is used to indicate blood flow?**

   A. Doppler ultrasound
   B. Continuous-wave Doppler
   C. Color Doppler
   D. All of the above

4. **What does a fetal ultrasound produce?**

   A. A sonogram
   B. A discogram
   C. An angiogram
   D. Dexagram

5. **What must you verify before the patient undergoes a transvaginal ultrasound?**

   A. A signed consent is received that acknowledges that conductive gel will be placed on the patient's abdomen.
   B. That the patient is over 18 years of age.
   C. That the patient is not allergic to latex.
   D. A signed consent is received that acknowledges that the transducer will be pressed down on her abdomen.

6. **What should you tell the patient if the patient is unable to drink a large volume of fluid before a transabdominal ultrasound?**

   A. The test will be cancelled.
   B. An MRI will be ordered.
   C. Sterile water is inserted into the bladder using a urinary catheter.
   D. The practitioner will order a CT scan.

7. **What should you tell a patient who is scheduled for thyroid ultrasound?**

   A. Remove all jewelry from the head and neck area.
   B. The patient may be asked to remove all clothing from above the waist.
   C. The patient lies on her back and a pillow is placed under his/her shoulders.
   D. All over the above.

8. **Why would a practitioner order a transabdominal ultrasound?**

   A. The cause of urinary disorders
   B. Pelvic inflammatory disease (PID)
   C. Placement of intrauterine device (IUD)
   D. All of the above

9. The patient tells you he is feeling relaxed since he has smoked several cigarettes in the parking lot before coming in for a Doppler ultrasound. What should you do?

   A. Notify the practitioner since nicotine constricts blood vessels and could result in a false test result.
   B. Continue with the test as scheduled.
   C. Tell the patient about the dangers of smoking.
   D. Tell the patient it is good that he is relaxed before the test.

10. What would you do if the patient feels short of breath during a transvaginal ultrasound?

   A. Reposition the patient or raise the head of the bed.
   B. Stop the test.
   C. Tell the patient to take deep breaths.
   D. Distract the patient by asking her about her children.

ANSWERS

1. A. Place gel on the patient's skin over the site of the test.
2. C. Fill the bladder with water.
3. D. All of the above.
4. A. A sonogram.
5. C. Verify that the patient is not allergic to latex.
6. C. Sterile water is inserted into the bladder using a urinary catheter.
7. D. All over the above.
8. D. All over the above.
9. A. Notify the practitioner since nicotine constricts blood vessels and could result in a false test result.
10. A. Reposition the patient or raise the head of the bed.

chapter 15

Cardiovascular Tests and Procedures

LEARNING OBJECTIVES

1. Cardiac Blood Pool Scan
2. Cardiac Calcium Scoring
3. Electrocardiogram
4. Cardiac Perfusion Scan
5. Ankle-Brachial Index
6. Echocardiogram
7. Pericardiocentesis
8. Venogram

> ## KEY WORDS
>
> Computed tomography (CT)
> Doppler echocardiogram
> Ejection fraction
> First-pass scan
> Gamma camera
> Holter monitoring
> Multigated acquisition (MUGA)
>
> Peripheral arterial disease (PAD)
> Plaque
> Stress echocardiogram
> Transesophageal echocardiogram (TEE)
> Transthoracic echocardiogram (TTE)

Cardiovascular tests are performed to assess the patient's heart and vascular system to determine if the blood is adequately being pumped and flowing throughout his/her body. These tests measure cardiac contraction, the risk for coronary artery disease, and are used to identify blockage to coronary arteries and blood vessels of the extremities.

When a blockage is identified, the healthcare provider can perform one of several procedures to restore blood flow. The blockage might be surgically removed or pressed against the wall of the blood vessel and held in place by a stent. Alternatively, the healthcare provider may surgically bypass the blocked blood vessels using a vein from the patient's leg or by using an artificial blood vessel.

In this chapter you will learn about these tests and procedures.

1. Cardiac Blood Pool Scan

The cardiac blood pool scan is a test that measures the percentage of the patient's blood that is pumped in a cardiac contraction and therefore indicates how well the heart is contracting. This is referred to as the ejection fraction.

The healthcare provider administers radioactive material called a tracer into the patient vein. A gamma camera is used to monitor the tracer as the blood flows throughout the patient's heart. The healthcare provider can use one of the following two types of cardiac blood pool scans to estimate the ejection fraction.

- Multigated acquisition (MUGA): This is also known as gated scan. Each contraction of the heart triggers the gamma camera to take a picture of the heart, which is stored in a computer. These images are then placed back on the computer screen showing cardiac contractions. The healthcare provider may perform the MUGA scan twice—first without medication and the second after giving the patient nitroglycerin. Nitroglycerin dilates arteries and veins, reducing the amount of blood that must be pumped by the heart, which decreases the amount of oxygen requirements of the heart because the heart works less. The impact of the decreased cardiac workload should be reflected in the MUGA scan.

- First-pass: This captures images of the blood going through the heart and lungs for the first time.

NURSING ALERT

The MUGA scan is not used on children and does not provide information about heart valves and thickness of cardiac walls. The first-pass scan is used on children to assess the existence of congenital heart disease.

NURSING ALERT

The cardiac blood pool scan is not performed if the patient is pregnant.

What Is Being Examined?

- Cardiac contractions

How Is the Test Performed?

- The patient is administered the radioactive tracer into a vein.
- MUGA scan
  - A sample of blood is taken.
  - The radioactive tracer is mixed with the blood sample.
  - The blood sample is then reinjected into the patient's vein.
- It takes 4 hours for the patient's red blood cells to absorb the entire tracer. The patient may be able to leave the healthcare facility during this period.
- The patient is asked to remove dentures and jewelry before the scan is performed.
- The patient removes clothing.
- The patient lies on a table.
- An electrocardiogram (ECG) is attached to the patient.

- The patient must lie still each time a picture is taken, which can take 5 minutes.
- The gamma camera is positioned close to the patient's chest and is repositioned during the scan.
- The patient may be asked to change position or to leave the table to perform exercises and then return to the table to continue the scan. The patient may be administered nitroglycerin.
- The patient will drink lots of fluid for 2 days following the scan to flush the tracer from his/her body.
- The MUGA scan takes 3 hours to complete and the first-pass scan takes 1 hour to complete.

Rationale for the Test

- To assess ventricle contractions
- To assess cardiac blood flow
- To diagnose cardiac abnormalities

Nursing Implications

- Determine if the patient
  - Has any allergies.
  - Has recently undergone radioactive tracer scans.
  - Has an implant in the chest such as a pacemaker.
  - Is wearing comfortable clothes if the patient is asked to exercise.
  - Can lie still on his back.
  - Has recently had a barium enema.
  - Is pregnant. The cardiac blood pool scan is not performed if the patient is pregnant.
- Assess if the patient
  - Has eaten 4 hours before the scan.
  - Has ingested caffeine 6 hours before the scan.
  - Has smoked for 6 hours before the scan.
  - Has provided the healthcare provider with all medications that are being taken. Digoxin and nitrate medication can affect the scan results.

Understanding the Results

- The MUGA scan takes 3 hours and the first-pass scan takes 1 hour. Results are ready within a week of the scan.
- Normal test results indicate
  - Ejection fraction is 55% to 65%
  - Normal blood flow through the heart
  - Cardiac structures are normal and contracting normally
- Abnormal test results indicate
  - Ejection fraction is less than 55%
  - Inadequate cardiac contractions
  - Abnormal cardiac structures
  - Improper blood flow through the heart

Teach the Patient

- Explain
  - Why scan is being performed.
  - What the patient will experience during the scan.
  - That the patient will not feel any pain during the procedure except for a pinch from the needle used to administer the tracer.
  - That patient must tell the healthcare provider of any allergies, has recently undergone radioactive tracer scans, has an implant in the chest such as a pacemaker, or has recently had a barium enema.
  - That the patient cannot eat for 4 hours before the scan.
  - That the patient cannot ingest caffeine for 6 hours before the scan.
  - That the patient cannot smoke for 6 hours before the scan.
  - The healthcare provider must be informed of all medications that the patient takes.

2. Cardiac Calcium Scoring

Coronary arteries supply blood to cardiac muscles. Restricted coronary arteries decrease blood and oxygen supply to cardiac muscles. Blood flow through the coronary arteries is restricted by a plaque buildup on the coronary artery wall. Plaque contains calcium. Cardiac calcium scoring determines the level of calcium containing plaque on the coronary artery walls, using a computed tomography (CT). Images of thin sections of the heart are taken using the CT scan and are stored in a computer and reviewed by the healthcare provider to assess signs of coronary artery disease.

> **NURSING ALERT**
>
> Healthcare providers use a variety of assessment methods to determine if the patient has coronary artery disease.

> **NURSING ALERT**
>
> A patient can have a high cardiac calcium score without having coronary artery disease.

What Is Being Examined?

- Assessing the buildup of plaque containing calcium on the walls of the coronary arteries.

How Is the Test Performed?

- The patient removes all jewelry.
- The patient removes clothing above the waist.
- The patient lies on a table.
- An ECG is attached to the patient.
- The patient may be administered medication to decrease cardiac contractions if the patient's heart rate is greater than 90 beats/min.
- The patient may be administered a sedative if he/she feels claustrophobic being inside the CT machine.
- The patient will be alone in the CT room but can communicate with the CT technician using an intercom.
- The patient must lie still on a table.
- The table is slid into the CT scan.
- The patient is asked to hold breath and lie still for 30 seconds while images are taken by the CT machine.

Rationale for the Test

- To assess for coronary artery disease

Nursing Implications

- Assess if the patient
  - Is claustrophobic
  - Can lie still on the back
  - Has removed jewelry
  - Has ingested caffeine 12 hours before the test
  - Has smoked 12 hours before the test

Understanding the Results

- The cardiac calcium scoring test takes 30 minutes. Results are ready within 1 week of the scan.
- Normal test results indicate
  - Score 0 = No plaque. There is a 5% chance of developing coronary artery disease.
  - Score < 11 = 10% chance of developing coronary artery disease.
- Abnormal test results indicate
  - Score 11 to 100 = Plaque was found. The patient has mild coronary artery disease.
  - Score 101 to 400 = Plaque was found. The patient has coronary artery disease and possibly a blockage of one or more coronary arteries.
  - Score > 400 = Plaque was found. The patient has coronary artery disease and there is a 90% chance that there is a blockage of one or more coronary arteries.

Teach the Patient

- Explain
  - Why scan is being performed.
  - What the patient will experience during the scan.
  - That the patient will not feel any pain during the procedure except for a pinch from the needle used to administer a sedative, if necessary.

- That the patient will be administered a sedative if he/she feels claustrophobic being in the CT machine.
- That the patient should not ingest caffeine 12 hours before the test.
- That the patient should not smoke 12 hours before the test.

3. Electrocardiogram

An electrocardiogram (ECG) records electrical activity of the heart on paper. Electrical activity causes contractions of the heart, resulting in blood being pumped throughout the body. Any disruption of the electrical activity might cause the heart to perform less than normally, which appears on the ECG paper tracing.

Telemetry is a type of ECG that is used in a healthcare facility to constantly monitor the patient's cardiac activity. A monitoring device worn by the patient transmits cardiac electrical activity to a telemetry monitor at the nurse's station. An alarm is sounded whenever there is abnormal cardiac activity. A telemetry nurse interprets the tracing on the telemetry monitor and prints the tracing while taking appropriate action.

The Holter monitoring ECG, sometimes referred to as an ambulatory ECG, is a type of portable ECG that is attached to the patient for 24 hours. This device is worn on the patient's waist or around the shoulder, enabling the healthcare provider to detect abnormal electrical activity of the heart during activities of daily living such as when the patient exercises and when sleeping. Holter monitoring can be continuously recorded or intermittently recorded. The two types of intermittently recorded Holter monitoring are:

- Event monitor: The patient presses a button whenever a cardiac symptom occurs, causing the Holter monitor to record cardiac activity.
- Loop recorder: The Holter monitor constantly records cardiac electrical activity. The patient presses a button whenever a cardiac symptom occurs.

What Is Being Examined?

- Electrical activity of the heart

How Is the Test Performed?

- The patient removes all jewelry.
- The patient removes clothing covering the area where the ECG leads are attached to the patient.

- The patient lies on a table.
- An ECG is attached to the patient.
- The patient lies still.

Rationale for the Test

- To assess the cause of chest pain, palpitations, and other symptoms.
- To assess the effects of medication on the heart.
- To assess signs and symptoms of heart disease.
- To assess the performance of a pacemaker.

Nursing Implications

- Assess if the patient
  - Can lie still on the back
  - Has removed jewelry

Understanding the Results

- The cardiac catheterization test takes 1 hour. Results are ready immediately.
- Normal test results indicate
  - Expected electrical activity on the trace paper
- Abnormal test results indicate
  - Unexpected electrical activity on the trace paper

Teach the Patient

- Explain
  - Why ECG is being performed.
  - What the patient will experience during the procedure.
  - That the patient will not feel any pain during the procedure.
  - That the patient will be required to remove jewelry.

4. Cardiac Perfusion Scan

The cardiac perfusion scan is commonly performed to determine the volume of blood in cardiac muscle during stress and at rest. Before the test, the patient is administered a radioactive tracer into his/her vein. A camera scans the patient's heart while at rest and stores the image on a computer. The heart is then placed under stress by using medication or asking the patient to physically exercise. The heart is then scanned by the camera and images are stored on the computer. The healthcare provider then compares the images to determine if the heart is receiving sufficient blood supply.

What Is Being Examined?

- The volume of blood in heart muscle

How Is the Test Performed?

- The patient removes all jewelry.
- The patient removes clothing above the waist.
- The patient lies on a table.
- An ECG is attached to the patient.
- Radioactive tracer is injected into the patient's vein.
- The camera is placed close to the patient's chest.
- The patient must remain still while the image is taken.
- The camera is moved and the patient is asked to exercise using a treadmill or stationary bike. During exercising the patient's blood pressure is monitored by an ECG.
- If the patient is unable to exercise, then medication is administered to simulate the stress of exercise on his/her heart.
- The patient lies on the table.
- Radioactive tracer is injected into the patient's vein.
- The camera is placed close to the patient's chest.
- The patient remains still while the image is taken.
- The patient can resume normal activity following the test.

Rationale for the Test

- To assess the underlying cause of chest pain
- To assess the results of angioplasty and bypass surgery

Nursing Implications

- Assess if the patient
  - Can lie still on the back.
  - Has allergies.
  - Has taken Viagra, Cialis, or Levitra within 2 days of the procedure. These medications can cause the patient's blood pressure to fall if the patient is administered nitroglycerin during the procedure.
  - Is taking anticoagulants such as Coumadin, aspirin, or heparin.
  - Is taking Trental or Persantine.
  - Is pregnant.
  - Is breast-feeding. If so, the patient must discard breast milk collected 2 days following the test, since the breast milk will contact the radioactive tracer.
  - Has eaten or drunk 3 hours before the test.
  - Has drunk caffeine, alcohol, or smoked tobacco 1 day before the test.
  - Has removed jewelry.
  - Can exercise.
  - Recently had a heart attack or myocarditis.
  - Has a pacemaker.
  - Has an electrolyte imbalance.

Understanding the Results

- The test takes 1 hour. Results are ready within 1 week.
- Normal test results indicate
  - Normal blood volume in the cardiac muscle
- Abnormal test results indicate
  - Decreased blood volume in the cardiac muscle

Teach the Patient

- Explain
  - Why the scan is being performed.
  - What the patient will experience during the procedure.

- That the patient might feel flushed, nauseous, dizzy, or have a headache if medication is administered to place the patient's heart under stress.
- That the patient will not feel any pain during the procedure except for a pinch from the needle used to administer the tracer material.
- That the patient should not drink or eat for 3 hours before the procedure.
- That the patient should tell the healthcare provider if he/she takes Viagra, Cialis, Levitra, Coumadin, aspirin, heparin, Trental, or Persantine.
- That the patient should tell the healthcare provider during the test if the patient experiences fatigue, chest pain, shortness of breath, aching in the lower extremities, or lightheadedness, while the test is in progress.
- That the patient will be required to remove jewelry.
- That the patient may resume normal activities following the test.

> **NURSING ALERT**
>
> The patient should call emergency medical care if he/she experiences difficulty in breathing or chest pains after leaving the healthcare facility following the test.

5. Ankle-Brachial Index

The ankle-brachial index (ABI) evaluates blood circulation in the lower extremity for peripheral arterial disease (PAD). The test may also be performed to determine how well blood is flowing to the extremities after procedures or surgery. The ABI is determined by measuring the patient's blood pressure in both ankles and arms while the patient is resting.

> **NURSING ALERT**
>
> The patient may be asked to exercise. If so, the same blood pressures are taken and compared to the resting blood pressure.

What Is Being Examined?

- The patient is being screened for PAD.

How Is the Test Performed?

- The patient lies on a table.
- Blood pressure is taken in both arms and legs.
- The ABI is calculated as: ABI = ankle blood pressure + brachial blood pressure.

Rationale for the Test

- To assess for PAD
- To assess for risk for stroke

Nursing Implications

- Determine if the patient
  - Is able to have blood pressure taken in both arms and legs
  - Can lie on the back
  - Can walk on a treadmill
  - Is wearing comfortable clothes
- Assess if the patient has been diagnosed with arterial disease.

Understanding the Results

- The test takes less than 1 hour. Results are ready immediately.
- Normal
  - An index of 1 or 1.1 indicating that blood pressure in the arms and ankles is approximately the same; peripheral blood flow is unobstructed.
- Abnormal
  - 0.98: narrowing of peripheral blood flow
  - 0.80: intermittent claudication
  - 0.25: high risk for PAD

Teach the Patient

- Explain
  - Why test is being performed.
  - What the patient will experience during the test.

- That the patient will not feel any pain during the test.
- That the patient should wear comfortable clothes, since he/she will be walking on the treadmill.

6. Echocardiogram

An echocardiogram is an ultrasound scan of the patient's heart. Sound waves are transmitted by a transducer through the patient's chest to the heart. Sound waves echo off the heart and are detected by the transducer creating an image of the heart. Images are stored on a computer enabling the healthcare provider to play back images showing the beating heart. The three types of echocardiograms are

- Stress: Two sets of images of the heart are captured. The first set of images taken is of the resting heart. The second set of images is taken when the heart is under stress either following exercise or from medication.
- Transthoracic: This creates a set of views that illustrate the beating heart, which is the most common type of echocardiogram.
- Transesophageal: Under local anesthesia, the transducer is inserted down the patient's esophagus, enabling the generation of a clear image of the heart, since these images are not obscured by bones. This type of scan is commonly used to assess for vegetation on the heart valves.

What Is Being Examined?

- Cardiac function and structures

How Is the Test Performed?

- The patient removes clothing above the waist.
- The patient removes jewelry worn above the waist.
- The patient lies on a table.
- The patient is attached to an ECG.
- Stress echocardiogram
  - The patient is given a baseline ECG.
  - The patient is asked to pedal a stationary bicycle or walk on a treadmill while another ECG is taken.

- If the patient is unable to exercise, the healthcare provider will administer dobutamine to chemically stress the patient's heart.
- The patient is asked to lie on the table.
- The patient may be administered saline through a vein to help the healthcare provider assess the patient's cardiac function.
- If the healthcare provider is unable to obtain a clear view of the heart, the patient may be administered contrast material into the patient's vein. If this is done, then the patient will be placed on a mechanical ventilator to assist the patient's respiration.
- Conductive gel is placed on the left side of the patient's chest.
- A transducer is moved along the patient's chest as it generates sound waves through the body and receives reflected sound waves.
- The healthcare provider asks the patient to change position, breathe slowly, or hold breath at different times during the test.
- Reflected sound waves create an image of the heart on a computer screen.
- Transesophageal echocardiogram
  - A saline or heparin lock is inserted into the patient's arm.
  - The patient is administered medication that decreases saliva and stomach secretions.
  - The patient is administered a sedative. The patient remains conscious during the test.
  - The patient's blood oxygen level is measured by the pulse oximeter during the test.
  - The healthcare provider sprays an anesthetic over the back of the patient's throat to decrease the patient's gag reflex.
  - The patient's head is tilted forward.
  - A mouth guard is inserted into the patient's mouth to protect his/her teeth.
  - A transducer probe is inserted down into the patient's esophagus as the patient swallows. The transducer probe remains in place for 20 minutes.
  - The healthcare provider will suction excess saliva.
  - The patient is asked not to swallow during the test.
  - The transducer sends and receives sound waves and generates an image of the patient's heart.

- The transducer probe is removed once all images of the heart are captured.
- The patient is not permitted to ingest anything until the gag reflex is restored and the anesthetic wears off.

Rationale for the Test

- Assess for
  - Cardiac function
  - Cardiac abnormalities
  - Pericardial effusion
  - Valve abnormalities and vegetations
  - Ejection fraction

Nursing Implications

- Determine if the patient
  - Can lie on the back
  - Can swallow (transesophageal echocardiogram)
  - Can walk on a treadmill or pedal a stationary bicycle (stress echocardiogram)
  - Is wearing comfortable clothes
  - Has lung disease
  - Has large breasts
- Assess if the patient
  - Has eaten or drunk for 6 hours before the test
  - Has dentures
  - Has transportation home if the patient is to receive a sedative
  - Has signed a consent form
  - Has difficulty breathing
  - Has removed jewelry
  - Has removed clothing above the waist

Understanding the Results

- The transthoracic, stress, and Doppler echocardiograms each take 1 hour to perform. The transesophageal echocardiogram takes 2 hours to perform. Results are available in a week.

- Normal test results indicate
  - Normal cardiac function
  - No cardiac growth
  - No fluid buildup around the heart
  - Normal ejection fraction
- Abnormal test results indicate
  - Unexpected cardiac function
  - Cardiac growth
  - Fluid buildup around the heart
  - Heart valve vegetations or other valve abnormalities
  - Abnormal ejection fraction

Teach the Patient

- Explain
  - Why the test is being performed.
  - How the test is performed.
  - What the patient will experience during the test.
  - That the patient will not feel any pain during the test.
  - That the patient should wear comfortable clothes, since he/she will be walking on the treadmill or pedaling a stationary bicycle (stress echocardiogram).
  - That the patient will need to remove jewelry and clothing from the waist up.
  - That the patient should refrain from eating and drinking 6 hours before the test.
  - That the patient should remove all dentures prior to the test.
  - That the patient will not be able to drive for 12 hours following the test if a sedative is administered.
  - That conductive gel is wiped off the patient following the test.
  - That the patient's heart rate may increase for 15 minutes and then return to normal in 3 minutes following administration of dobutamine, if to a patient undergoing a stress echocardiogram who is unable to exercise.
  - That the patient can request to take a break during the test if he/she feels uncomfortable.

- That the patient may experience an unusual feeling in the throat if he/she is receiving a transesophageal echocardiogram.
- That the patient may feel sleepy or experience blurred vision, have trouble speaking, or have a dry mouth following the test. These should resolve shortly following the test.
- Although the patient is awake during the test, he/she probably will not remember the test itself.
- That the patient may experience hoarseness or a sore throat following a transesophageal echocardiogram. Lozenges and gargling with warm salt water will provide relief.
- That the patient should avoid drinking alcohol for a day following the transesophageal echocardiogram.
- That the patient may experience nausea.

NURSING ALERT

Prior to the test, the patient and the healthcare provider should arrange for a signal that the patient can give to the practitioner to indicate that the patient is uncomfortable during a transesophageal echocardiogram. The patient should call the healthcare provider if experiencing chest pains, difficulty swallowing, difficulty speaking, fast heartbeat, or difficulty breathing following the test.

7. Pericardiocentesis

There are disorders that cause pericardial effusion, which is the result of excess fluid buildup in the pericardium (sac around the heart). As a result, the patient may experience cardiac tamponade, which inhibits cardiac contraction and is a life-threatening emergency. The healthcare provider may perform a pericardiocentesis to remove the excess fluid, thereby restoring normal cardiac contraction. Pericardial effusion can be caused by inflammation of the pericardium because of viral, bacterial, or fungal infection, blood from an injury, or disorders such as kidney failure, hypothyroidism, or rheumatoid arthritis.

NURSING ALERT

Sometimes pericardiocentesis is performed in the emergency department.

What Is Being Examined?

- Removal of excess fluid from the pericardium

How Is the Test Performed?

- A blood test is taken prior to the procedure to determine if the patient has anticoagulation problems.
- The patient removes clothing above the waist.
- The patient removes jewelry worn above the waist.
- The patient angles his/her back on a table.
- A saline or heparin lock is inserted into the patient's arm.
- The patient is attached to an ECG.
- The patient is administered a sedative.
- The insertion site is cleaned with an antiseptic.
- The patient is administered a local anesthetic at the insertion site.
- A needle is inserted either between the patient's left ribs or below the sternum and into the pericardium guided by an echocardiogram.
- The patient may be asked to remain still or hold the breath while the needle is inserted.
- A catheter is slid over the needle into the pericardium and the needle is removed.
- The fluid is drained by the catheter.
- The catheter is removed once fluid is drained.
- Pressure is applied to the site for 5 minutes to stop bleeding.
- A chest X-ray is taken of the patient to ensure there is no collateral damage such as a collapsed lung.
- The patient may remain in the healthcare facility for observation.

Rationale for the Procedure

- Restore cardiac contraction
- Assess the source of pericardial effusion

Nursing Implications

- Determine if the patient
  - Can lie on the back

- Can respond to direction during the procedure
- Has taken anticoagulants (Coumadin, heparin) or antiplatelets (aspirin, clopidogrel)
- Has allergies
- Has recently been administered antibiotics
- Assess if the patient
  - Has eaten or drunk for 12 hours before the test
  - Has signed a consent form
  - Has removed jewelry
  - Has removed clothing above the waist

Understanding the Results

- The procedure takes 30 minutes; however, the fluid may drain for several hours following the procedure. Results from analysis of the fluid removed from the pericardium are available within 1 week.
- Normal test results indicate
  - Less than or equal to 50 mL of fluid drained
  - Normal clear/pale yellow fluid
  - No bacteria
  - No abnormal cells
  - Less than 500 white blood cells present in the fluid
- Abnormal test results indicate
  - Greater than 50 mL of fluid drained
  - Fluid appears cloudy
  - Bacteria cells found in the fluid
  - Abnormal cells found in the fluid
  - More than 500 white blood cells present in the fluid

Teach the Patient

- Explain
  - Why the procedure is being performed.
  - How the procedure is performed.
  - What the patient will experience during the procedure.

- That the patient will not feel any pain during the procedure.
- That the patient might experience an irregular heartbeat during the procedure.
- That the patient will need to remove jewelry and clothing from the waist up.
- That the patient should refrain from eating and drinking 12 hours before the test.
- That the patient may remain in the healthcare facility for observation following the procedure.
- That the patient may feel pressure as the needle is inserted.

NURSING ALERT

The patient should tell the healthcare provider if experiencing chest pain or shortness of breath during the procedure. After returning home, the patient should call emergency medical help if experiencing chest pain, trouble breathing, sweating, lightheadedness, and signs of shock. The patient should call the healthcare provider if vomiting blood, is short of breath, has a fever, or feels dizzy.

8. Venogram

A venogram produces an X-ray image of blood flowing through the patient's veins. It is used by healthcare providers to assess the function of valves in the veins and if there is deep vein thrombosis (DVT). Venograms are used to evaluate

- Extremities
- Pelvis
- Kidneys

What Is Being Examined?

- Blood flow through veins

How Is the Test Performed?

- The patient removes all jewelry.
- The patient removes clothing.

- The patient must not eat 4 hours before the test.
- The patient can drink clear fluids up to 4 hours before the test but must not drink after 4 hours.
- The patient is asked to empty his bladder.
- The patient lies on a table that may be tilted during the test.
- For extremities, an elastic band is placed around the extremity that is being examined to fill the vein with blood.
- The patient may be administered a local anesthetic at the insertion site.
- Contrast material is inserted into the patient's vein.
- For kidneys
  - A catheter is inserted into the femoral vein in the groin and guided into the vein in the patient's kidney.
  - The contrast material is administered through the catheter. The catheter is removed once the test is completed.
  - The contrast material may also be administered into the inferior vena cava.
- X-ray images are taken of the area that is being studied.
- After the test is completed, saline is inserted into the vein to help flush the contrast material.
- The patient may be administered heparin to prevent a blood clot following the test.
- A dressing is placed on the insertion site.
- The patient is asked to drink lots of water to flush the contrast material from the body.

Rationale for the Test

- To identify thrombosis
- To identify sites for filters
- To assess valves in veins

Nursing Implications

- Assess if the patient
  - Has signed a consent
  - Can lie still on the back
  - Has allergies

- Is pregnant
- Is taking Coumadin, heparin, or aspirin
- Has avoided eating or drinking for 4 hours before the test
- Has emptied his/her bladder before the test
- Has removed jewelry
- Has kidney disorder
- Has asthma
- Has diabetes

Understanding the Results

- Venogram takes 1 hour or less to perform.
- Normal test results indicate
  - Normal blood flow
  - No growth(s) in the kidney
- Abnormal test results indicate
  - Blockage of blood flow
  - Varicose veins
  - Growth(s) in the kidney

Teach the Patient

- Explain
- Why the test is being performed.
- What the patient will experience during the test.
- That the patient will not feel any pain during the test except for a pinch when the contrast material is inserted into the vein.
- That the patient may feel pins and needles in the arm or leg that is being studied, but this dissipates quickly following the test.
- That the patient will have to sign a consent form.
- That the patient must empty his/her bladder before the test.
- That the patient will be required to rest in bed for 3 hours if a kidney venogram is performed.
- That the patient should drink lots of water for a day following the procedure to flush the contrast material from the body.

> **NURSING ALERT**
>
> The patient should call the healthcare provider if after the test he/she feels pain or experiences swelling in the area that was studied, or if experiences a fever.

Summary

In order to keep tissues oxygenated and fluid balanced within the body, the cardiovascular system must function adequately. In this chapter, you learned about several cardiovascular tests that are performed to assess cardiac function and blood flow throughout the body. These tests assess cardiac contraction, the risk for coronary artery disease, and are used to identify blockage to coronary arteries and blood vessels to the extremities.

Cardiovascular disorders can result in the blockage of blood flow to the heart or other vessels in the patient's body. In this chapter you also learned about several surgical procedures that remove or press plaque against the wall of the blood vessel, which is then held in place by a stent allowing blood to flow through the vessel. Alternatively, the healthcare provider may surgically bypass the blocked blood vessels using a vein from the patient's leg or by using an artificial blood vessel.

QUIZ

1. **What test measures the ejection fraction of the heart?**
   A. Cardiac blood pool scan
   B. Venogram
   C. Pericardiocentesis
   D. ABI

2. **What is the purpose of cardiac calcium scoring?**
   A. To assess cardiac contractions
   B. To stimulate cardiac contractions
   C. To assess the buildup of plaque containing calcium on the walls of the coronary arteries
   D. To assess the workload of the heart

3. **What is an ambulatory electrocardiogram?**

   A. Holter monitor

   B. ECC

   C. ABI

   D. PAD monitor

4. **What is the purpose of ankle-brachial index?**

   A. Assess for risk for stroke.

   B. Blood pressure is taken in both arms and legs.

   C. Screened for peripheral arterial disease (PAD).

   D. All of the above.

5. **What is the most common type of echocardiogram?**

   A. Transabdominal

   B. Transesophageal

   C. Stress

   D. Transthoracic

6. **What should be done before the transesophageal echocardiogram?**

   A. Make sure that the patient can talk.

   B. Make sure that the patient can hold her breath for 5 seconds.

   C. Arrange for a signal that the patient can give to the practitioner to indicate that the patient is uncomfortable during the procedure.

   D. Arrange for the patient speak during the procedure

7. **What might be practitioner do if the patient is diagnosed with cardiac tamponade?**

   A. Perform an echocardiogram

   B. Perform a pericardiocentesis

   C. Perform an ABI

   D. Perform Holter monitoring

8. **Why should the patient avoid taking Coumadin prior to a cardiac procedure?**

   A. The patient's bleeding time increases.

   B. There is a high risk of bleeding.

   C. The healthcare provider will need to take precautions to control bleeding that might occur during the procedure.

   D. All of the above.

9. **Why would a practitioner order a venogram?**
   A. To assess blood flow through the heart
   B. To assess blood flow through veins
   C. To assess blood flow through the brain
   D. To assess blood flow through the eyes

10. **Why would a practitioner order a MUGA?**
    A. To assess cardiac contraction
    B. To assess blood flow
    C. To assess blood flow to the extremities
    D. To assess blood flow to the lungs

ANSWERS

1. A. Cardiac blood pool scan.
2. C. To assess the buildup of plaque containing calcium on the walls of the coronary arteries.
3. A. Holter monitor.
4. D. All of the above.
5. D. Transthoracic.
6. C. Arrange for a signal that the patient can give to the practitioner to indicate that the patient is uncomfortable during the procedure.
7. B. Perform a pericardiocentesis.
8. D. All of the above.
9. B. To assess blood flow through veins.
10. A. To assess cardiac contraction.

Female and Maternity Tests and Procedures

LEARNING OBJECTIVES

1. Amniocentesis
2. Biophysical Profile (BPP)
3. Breast Cancer Gene Test (BRCA)
4. Breast Ultrasound
5. Cervical Cerclage (Weak Cervix)
6. Chorionic Villus Sampling (CVS)
7. Contraction Stress Test
8. Cordocentesis
9. Cranial Ultrasound
10. Galactosemia Test
11. Karyotyping
12. Pap Smear

⑬ Sperm Penetration Tests

⑭ Sweat Test

⑮ Vaginosis Tests

KEY WORDS

Amniotic fluid volume	Chorioamnionitis
Body movement	Chorionic villi
BRCA1	Fetal anemia
BRCA2	Fetal lung development
Breathing movement	Fetal monitor

Female patients routinely undergo breast and cervical examinations for signs of cysts, growths, abnormal tissue, structural abnormalities, and infection. In this chapter you will learn about tests and procedures that are performed to test for disorders and repair of disorders.

When a mammogram reveals a suspicious growth, the healthcare provider usually orders a breast ultrasound to closely examine the growth and then possibly a breast biopsy. If the tissue sample is cancerous, the healthcare provider may perform a mastectomy. A mastectomy may be performed even if there is no sign of breast cancer. These are explored in this chapter.

The patient may decide to have her breasts altered for therapeutic or cosmetic reasons. You will learn about procedures that augment, reduce, and lift the breast in this chapter.

There are a number of tests used to examine the vulva, vagina, cervix, uterus, and fallopian tubes. Many of these tests enable the healthcare provider to take a tissue sample or perform a biopsy on abnormal tissue. If the tissue sample is identified to be cancerous, the cancerous organ is removed.

There are several tests that are performed during pregnancy and shortly after childbirth to assess the health of the fetus and newborn. In a high-risk pregnancy, the healthcare provider might perform a chorionic villus sampling or amniocentesis early on in the pregnancy to determine if the fetus has a genetic disorder or other health issues.

Amniocentesis, for example, may be suggested in high-risk pregnancies that have a high risk of birth defects. This condition is confirmed by performing a cordocentesis where a sample of blood is taken from the umbilical cord while in the womb.

Later in the pregnancy, the healthcare provider performs a biophysical profile of the fetus to determine the overall health of the fetus. This is when an assessment is made of the fetal heart rate, breathing and body movements, muscle tone, and the volume of amniotic fluid.

It is also around this same period when the mother may undergo a contraction stress test. The contraction stress test determines if the fetus is healthy enough to survive the reduced oxygen levels that are common with natural childbirth.

In some pregnancies, the woman might experience an incompetent cervix that could result in the cervix opening prior to the 37th week of gestation, causing a premature birth. In this situation, the healthcare provider is likely to perform a cervical cerclage, which temporarily closes the cervix until the mother enters labor.

If the birth is premature, the healthcare provider may perform a cranial ultrasound to determine if there were complications caused by the premature birth.

The newborn is typically administered the sweat test that helps determine if the newborn has a high level of chloride in his sweat, which may be an indication of cystic fibrosis.

You will learn about these tests and procedures in this chapter.

1. Amniocentesis

Amniotic fluid contains cells shed by the fetus. About the 16th week of gestation, the healthcare provider may perform amniocentesis, which is the removal of some amniotic fluid. Fetal cells contain the amniotic fluid which is analyzed to determine if the fetus has a birth defect. Amniocentesis is also performed during the third trimester, if there is a risk of premature birth, to determine fetal lung development and to assess if the mother has chorioamnionitis, which is an infection of the amniotic fluid.

Amniocentesis is ordered if an integrated test result is positive, indicating that the fetus has a high chance of having a birth defect. These tests include α-fetoprotein (AFP), estriol, inhibin A, and chorionic gonadotropin (hCG). It is also ordered if parents are carriers of a genetic trait that is likely to be passed on to the fetus. These include cystic fibrosis, Duchenne muscular dystrophy, sickle cell anemia, thalassemia, hemophilia, and Tay-Sachs disease.

Amniocentesis is also performed to determine if the fetus is Rh-positive when the mother has the Rh factor. This tests the amniotic fluid for increased bilirubin levels after the 20th week of gestation, which indicates that the fetal blood cells are being attacked by the mother's antibodies.

> ### NURSING ALERT
>
> Amniocentesis does not identify all birth defects. There are many birth defects that are not revealed by amniocentesis.

What Is Being Examined?

- The fetus

How Is the Procedure Performed?

- The patient will sign a consent form.
- The patient must have an empty bladder.
- The patient lies on a table with her abdomen exposed.
- The insertion site is cleaned with an antiseptic.
- The insertion site is injected with a local anesthetic.
- Conductive gel is placed on the mother's abdomen.
- A fetal monitor is placed on the mother's abdomen to monitor the fetus during the procedure.
- The mother's vital signs are monitored during the procedure.
- The healthcare provider performs a fetal ultrasound to guide insertion of the needle.
- A needle is passed through the abdomen into the uterus. It is removed and reinserted if the fetus moves close to the needle.
- Two tablespoons of amniotic fluid are drawn up from the needle into a syringe.
- The needle is removed.
- A bandage covers the insertion site.

Rationale for the Test

- Assess
  - For birth defects
  - Fetal lung development
  - For chorioamnionitis
  - For Rh antibodies

Nursing Implications

- Determine if the patient
  - Signed a consent form
  - Has emptied her bladder
  - Can lie on her back
  - Is able to lie still

Understanding the Results

- The procedure takes less than 30 minutes. Results are known within 2 weeks.
- Normal test results indicate
  - No signs of birth defect.
  - Fetal lungs are adequately developed.
  - No signs of chorioamnionitis.
- Abnormal test results indicate
  - Signs of birth defect.
  - Fetal lungs are not adequately developed.
  - The mother has chorioamnionitis.

NURSING ALERT

A normal result from amniocentesis does not rule out a birth defect.

Teach the Patient

- Explain
  - Why the test is being performed.
  - What the patient will experience during the test.
  - That the patient will not feel any pain during the test, except a pinch when the local anesthetic is administered.
  - That the patient should breath slowly during the procedure to relax her abdominal muscle.
  - That the patient may feel a cramp in the abdomen.

- That the patient may feel pulling on her abdomen when amniotic fluid is removed.
- That the patient must sign a consent form.
- That the patient must empty her bladder before the procedure.
- That the patient should avoid exercise for 24 hours following the test.
- That the patient should not have sexual intercourse for 24 hours following the test.
- That the patient should not douche or use tampons for 24 hours following the test.

> **NURSING ALERT**
>
> The patient should call her healthcare provider if she notices fluid or bloody discharge from the insertion site or if there is swelling and redness at the insertion site. She should also call her healthcare provider if she experiences fever, pain, or cramping in her abdomen.

2. Biophysical Profile

The biophysical profile (BPP) test assesses the health of the fetus and is commonly performed in the last trimester of the pregnancy, although the healthcare provider may perform this test earlier and frequently in high-risk pregnancies. The BPP test consists of a nonstress test and a fetal ultrasound. Each element of the test is graded according to Table 16.1.

What Is Being Examined?

- Fetal assessment

How Is the Procedure Performed?

- The patient refrains from smoking 2 hours before the test.
- The patient must have a full bladder except if she is near term. If the patient is unable to fill her bladder, a urinary catheter is inserted into the urethra and saline will be infused into the bladder.
- The patient lies on a table with her abdomen exposed.

TABLE 16.1	Biophysical Profile Elements				
	Nonstress Test	Breathing Movement	Body Movement	Muscle Tone	Amniotic Fluid Volume
Normal (2 points)	Two or more heart rate increases with a rate of 15 minutes or greater while the fetus moves	One or more breathing movements of 60 seconds	Three or more arm, leg, or body movements	Flexed arms and legs; head rests on chest; one or more extensions and flexions	1 cm of amniotic fluid in the uterine cavity
Abnormal (0 points)	One or more heart rate increases or the rate is not 15 minutes or greater while the fetus moves	Breathing movements of less than 60 seconds	Less than three arm, leg, or body movements	Arms, legs, and spine are extended; open hand; fetus not returning to normal position; extension and flexion is slow	Less than 1 cm of amniotic fluid in the uterine cavity

- Nonstress test
  - Conductive gel is placed on her abdomen.
  - Two belts of the fetal monitor are placed on her abdomen to measure fetal heart rate and contractions.
  - The fetal monitor constantly records the fetus during the test. The test results appear on a strip of paper.
  - The patient is asked to press a button connected to the fetal monitor each time the fetus moves and if there is a contraction.
  - The 2 belts of the fetal monitor are removed and the gel is wiped from the patient's abdomen.
- Fetal ultrasound
  - Conductive gel is applied to her abdomen.
  - A transducer is pressed against and moved about the abdomen.
  - Images of the fetus appear on a computer screen.
  - Conductive gel is wiped off the abdomen.

Rationale for the Test

- Assess
  - Fetus movement
  - Fetal heart rate

- Volume of amniotic fluid
- Muscle tone
- Breathing rate

Nursing Implications

- Determine if the patient
  - Can lie on her back
  - Is able to lie still
  - Is able to follow instructions
  - Has smoked 2 hours before the test
  - Has a full bladder
  - Is hypo- or hyperglycemic
  - Is using alcohol or narcotics

Understanding the Results

- The procedure takes less than 30 minutes. Results are known immediately.
- Normal test results indicate
  - A score of 8 or greater
- Undetermined test results indicate
  - A score of 5 to 8. The patient should be retested.
- Abnormal test results indicate
  - A score of less than 5. The healthcare provider will order different tests to further assess the fetus and mother.

Teach the Patient

- Explain
  - Why the test is being performed.
  - What the patient will experience during the test.
  - That the patient will not feel any pain during the test.
  - That the patient must not smoke 2 hours before the test.
  - That the patient must have a full bladder unless she is near term.

3. Breast Cancer Gene Test

Scientists have discovered two genes called the breast cancer genes (BRCA1, BRCA2) that if mutated are associated with breast and ovarian cancer. A woman who carries this mutated gene and has a family history of breast or ovarian cancer may have a higher than normal chance of developing these cancers. However, she also has a chance of not developing these cancers. The presence of the breast cancer gene does not mean that the woman will develop breast or ovarian cancer. The breast cancer gene test determines if the patient's BRCA1 and BRCA2 genes are mutated. If so, some patients may decide to have a mastectomy and/or oophorectomy to prevent these cancers from developing. Patients who test positive may also be advised to take tamoxifen to inhibit this gene.

> ### NURSING ALERT
>
> Male patients who have a family history of breast cancer and prostate cancer may also have this gene. These patients can also develop breast cancer and prostate cancer.

What Is Being Examined?

- Determine if the patient has the breast cancer gene.

How Is the Procedure Performed?

- The healthcare provider removes a blood sample from a vein in the patient's arm.
- The blood sample is sent to the laboratory for examination.

Rationale for the Test

- Assess the patient's chances of developing breast or ovarian cancer.
- Provide information to enable the patient to decide whether or not to take preventive measures.

Nursing Implications

- Determine if the patient
  - Has signed a consent form

- Has been taken anticoagulant medication such as Plavix, Coumadin, heparin, or aspirin
- Has undergone genetic counseling to understand the significance of this test

Understanding the Results

- The procedure takes less than 1 hour. Results are ready within 2 weeks of the procedure.
- Normal (negative) test results indicate
  - The BRCA1 and BRCA2 genes are not mutated.
- Uncertain (variant of uncertain significance VUS)
  - It is undetermined if the BRCA1 and BRCA2 genes are mutated.
- Abnormal (positive) test results indicate
  - One or both BRCA1 and BRCA2 genes are mutated.
  - Positive for endometrial hyperplasia.
  - Cancer cells were present in the sample.

NURSING ALERT

A normal result does not mean that the patient will not develop breast cancer or ovarian cancer.

Teach the Patient

- Explain
- Why the test is being performed.
- What the patient will experience during the test.
- That the patient will have to sign a consent form.
- That the patient should undergo genetic counseling before the test is administered to fully understand the significance of the test.
- A negative result does not mean that the patient will not develop breast cancer or ovarian cancer.
- A positive result does not mean that the patient will develop breast cancer or ovarian cancer. It means there is a higher probability if the patient also has a strong family trait of breast cancer or ovarian cancer.

- That the patient should undergo genetic counseling if the test result is positive or uncertain to fully understand the significance of these results.

4. Breast Ultrasound

A breast ultrasound is used to examine suspicious findings of a mammogram because ultrasound technology can differentiate between a cyst and solid tissue. Furthermore, the breast ultrasound can examine areas of the breast that are difficult to view on a mammogram.

What Is Being Examined?

- Suspicious findings of a mammogram

How Is the Procedure Performed?

- The patient removes her clothing from above the waist.
- The patient either sits or lies on a table.
- A conductive gel is placed on the ultrasound transducer.
- The ultrasound transducer is pressed on and moved around the breast.
- Images of breast tissue are displayed on a computer screen.
- Any conductive gel remaining on the breast is removed.

Rationale for the Test

- To determine if a lump in the breast is a cyst or a solid mass
- To assess suspicious results from a mammogram
- To assess the underlying cause of swelling and pain in the breast
- To guide the healthcare provider's decision to take a breast biopsy
- To assess breast implants

Nursing Implications

- Determine if the patient
  - Can sit or lie on her back

Understanding the Results

- The procedure takes less than 1 hour. Preliminary results are immediate. Complete results are available within 2 days.
- Normal test results indicate
  - Normal breast tissue
- Abnormal test results indicate
  - The lump is identified as a cyst.
  - The lump is identified as a solid mass.

Teach the Patient

- Explain
  - Why the procedure is being performed.
  - What the patient will experience during the procedure.
  - The patient may feel pain if she has a fibrocystic breast.

5. Cervical Cerclage (Weak Cervix)

If the patient has an incompetent cervix, the cervix might open prior to the 37th week of gestation and could result in premature birth. The healthcare provider may perform a cervical cerclage, which is a procedure to close the cervix, to ensure that the cervix remain closed until after the 37th week of gestation.

> **NURSING ALERT**
>
> When a cervical cerclage has been performed, the cervix must be manually opened before the patient goes into labor otherwise the healthcare provider may perform a cesarean section.

What Is Being Examined?

- Closing of incompetent cervix

How Is the Procedure Performed?

- The patient removes her clothing.
- The patient lies on a table with her feet in stirrups.

- A breathing tube is inserted into the patient's throat.
- The patient is connected to an ECG.
- The patient is connected to a pulse oximeter to measure the oxygen content of the blood.
- A speculum is placed into the vagina to spread the vaginal walls.
- If the amnion (amniotic sac) is protruding
  - A catheter is inserted through the cervix.
  - A bulb at the end of the catheter is inflated pushing the amnion into the pelvis.
- Incisions are made in the cervix.
- Tape is tied through the incisions, closing the cervix or stitches made to close the cervix.

Rationale for the Test

- To prevent premature opening of the cervix

Nursing Implications

- Determine if the patient
  - Has signed a consent form
  - Has any allergies
  - Has been taking anticoagulant medication such as Plavix, Coumadin, heparin, or aspirin
  - Can lie on her back
  - Is able to lie still
  - Has been treated for infection of the pelvis, cervix, or vagina
  - Has not eaten or drunk for 12 hours before the procedure
  - Does not have uterine contractions
  - Does not have vaginal bleeding
  - Does not have ruptured membranes

Understanding the Results

- The procedure takes less than 1 hour. Results are immediate.

- Normal test results indicate
  - The cervix is closed.
- Abnormal test results indicate
  - The healthcare provider is unable to close the cervix.

Teach the Patient

- Explain
  - Why the procedure is being performed.
  - What the patient will experience during the procedure.
  - That the patient will have to sign a consent form.
  - That the patient should not eat or drink 12 hours before the procedure.
  - Should not exercise following the procedure.
  - Should not perform any heavy lifting following the procedure.

NURSING ALERT

The patient should call her healthcare provider if she has a fever, has an odorous discharge from the vagina, experiences heavy vaginal bleeding, or has abdominal pain.

6. Chorionic Villus Sampling

The placenta contains chorionic villi, which are tiny growths that contain the same genetic material as the fetus. Chorionic villus sampling is a procedure in which a sampling of chorionic villi is biopsied between the 10th and 12th week of gestation and is examined to determine if the fetus has a genetic disorder. There are two methods used to biopsy the chorionic villus. These are

- Transabdominal: A needle is inserted through the abdomen.
- Transcervical: A catheter is inserted through the cervix.

NURSING ALERT

Chorionic villus sampling is performed earlier in gestation than amniocentesis.

What Is Being Examined?

- Genetic material of the chorionic villus

How Is the Procedure Performed?

- The patient signs a consent form.
- The patient lies on a table.
- The patient either removes her clothing below the waist or exposes her abdomen, depending on which biopsy method is used by the healthcare provider.
- Conductive gel is placed on her abdomen.
- A fetal monitor is attached to the abdomen to monitor the fetus.
- Transabdominal
  - The insertion site is cleaned with an anesthetic.
  - A local anesthetic is administered to the insertion site.
  - An ultrasound transducer is pressed on and moved around the abdomen.
  - Images of the fetus and uterus are displayed on a computer screen.
  - A needle is inserted through the abdomen.
  - A sample of the chorionic villi is removed.
  - The needle is removed.
  - The insertion site is bandaged.
- Transcervical
  - The patient places her feet in stirrups.
  - A speculum is inserted to spread apart the vaginal wall.
  - The cervix is cleaned with an antiseptic soap.
  - An ultrasound transducer is pressed on and moved around the abdomen.
  - Images of the fetus and uterus are displayed on a computer screen.
  - A catheter is inserted through the cervix.
  - A sample of the chorionic villi is removed.
  - The needle is removed.

Rationale for the Test

- To assess for fetal genetic disorder

Nursing Implications

- Determine if the patient
  - Has a full bladder
  - Has signed a consent form
  - Has allergies

Understanding the Results

- The procedure takes less than 1 hour. Results are known within 2 weeks.
- Normal test results indicate
  - Normal cells in the sample
- Abnormal test results indicate
  - Abnormal genetic material found

Teach the Patient

- Explain
  - Why the test is being performed.
  - What the patient will experience during the test.
  - That the patient will not feel any pain during the test, except for a slight pinch when the local anesthetic is administered.
  - That patient might feel cramping following the procedure.
  - That the patient may have vaginal spotting following the procedure.
  - That the patient may have a small amount of amniotic fluid leakage following the procedure.

> **NURSING ALERT**
>
> The patient should call her healthcare provider if cramping, spotting or leakage of amniotic fluid occurs 48 hours after the procedure. A call should be made if she experiences fever, swelling at the insertion site or is dizzy.

7. Contraction Stress Test

The healthcare provider usually performs a BPP test of the fetus to assess breathing, movement, muscle tone, and the volume of amniotic fluid. If the

BPP test indicates suspicious results, the healthcare provider might perform a contraction stress test.

The contraction stress test determines if the fetus will remain healthy during natural childbirth. Uterine contractions reduce oxygen to the fetus, which normally does not harm the fetus. However, some fetuses can become negatively affected by the lower oxygen level, so the healthcare provider might decide a caesarean birth.

During the contraction stress test, a fetal heart monitor is attached to the mother while she is administered oxytocin. Oxytocin is a hormone that induces uterine contractions. The fetal heart rate is expected to decelerate during a contraction and accelerate following the contraction. If the heart rate does not accelerate, then the fetus may not remain healthy during natural childbirth.

> ### NURSING ALERT
>
> This test is not usually performed if the mother has in the past had a cesarean section, placenta previa, placenta abruptio, incompetent cervix, premature rupture of the amniotic membrane, been administered magnesium sulfate, or is pregnant with multiple fetuses.

What Is Being Examined?

- The fetus's ability to remain healthy during natural childbirth

How Is the Procedure Performed?

- The patient refrains from eating or drinking 8 hours before the test.
- The patient refrains from smoking 2 hours before the test.
- The patient empties her bladder.
- The patient signs a consent form.
- The patient lies on the table with back raised, lying slightly to the left side.
- The patient exposes her abdomen.
- Conductive gel is placed on the patient's abdomen.
- Two fetal monitor straps are placed on the abdomen to record contractions and the fetal heart rate.
- The patient's vital signs are monitored.

- A baseline is measured for 10 minutes of the fetal heart rate and contractions.
- A low dose of oxytocin is administered. The dose is increased until there are three contractions, each lasting more than 45 seconds over a period of 10 minutes.
- The fetal monitor continually records the fetal heart rate and contractions during the test.
- The healthcare provider continues to observe the fetal monitor, which shows the fetal heart and contractions have returned to the baseline values.

Rationale for the Test

- Assess
  - Ability of the fetus to remain healthy during natural childbirth
  - Health of the placenta

Nursing Implications

- Determine if the patient
  - Has signed a consent form
  - Has any allergies
  - Has been taking anticoagulant medication such as Plavix, Coumadin, heparin, or aspirin
  - Can lie on her back
  - Is able to lie still
  - Is able to follow instructions
  - Has eaten or drunk 8 hours before the test
  - Has smoked 2 hours before the test
  - Has emptied her bladder

Understanding the Results

- The procedure takes less than 2 hours. Preliminary results are known immediately. Detailed results are known within 1 week.
- Normal (negative) test results indicate
  - The fetal heart rate returned to normal following the contractions.

- Abnormal (positive) test results indicate
  - The fetal heart rate showed late decelerations following the contractions.
  - Contractions were hyperstimulated lasting longer than 90 seconds.

> **NURSING ALERT**
>
> The contraction stress test may have a false-positive result.

Teach the Patient

- Explain
  - Why the test is being performed.
  - What the patient will experience during the test.
  - That the patient will not feel any pain during the procedure, except for a pinch from the needle used to administer the oxytocin.
  - That the patient cannot eat 12 hours before the open biopsy.
  - That the patient cannot smoke 2 hours before the test.
  - That the patient should empty her bladder before the test.

8. Cordocentesis

If amniocentesis or other tests reveal that the fetus might have anemia, the healthcare provider may order a cordocentesis to confirm the finding, typically in the second trimester. A cordocentesis is the sampling of fetal blood from the umbilical cord to determine if the fetus has a blood disorder or is Rh-positive. The blood sample is also used to assess the oxygen level in fetal blood.

What Is Being Examined?

- Fetal blood

How Is the Procedure Performed?

- The patient will sign a consent form.
- The patient must have an empty bladder.
- The patient lies on a table with her abdomen exposed.

- The insertion site is cleaned with an antiseptic.
- The insert site is injected with a local anesthetic.
- Conductive gel is placed on the mother's abdomen.
- A fetal monitor is placed on the mother's abdomen to monitor the fetus during the procedure.
- The mother's vital signs are monitored during the procedure.
- The healthcare provider performs a fetal ultrasound to guide insertion of the needle.
- A needle is passed through the abdomen into the umbilical cord. The needle is removed.
- A small amount of blood is drawn up from the needle into a syringe.
- The needle is removed.
- A bandage covers the insertion site.

NURSING ALERT

The healthcare provider may administer medication to temporarily stop the fetus from moving and to prevent preterm labor and infection.

Rationale for the Test

- Assess
  - For fetal anemia
  - If the fetus is Rh-positive
  - Oxygen level in fetal blood

Nursing Implications

- Determine if the patient
  - Signed a consent form
  - Has emptied her bladder
  - Can lie on her back
  - Is able to lie still

Understanding the Results

- The procedure takes less than 30 minutes. Results are known within 2 weeks.
- Normal test results indicate
  - Fetal blood is normal.
- Abnormal test results indicate
  - Fetal anemia.
  - The fetus is Rh-positive.
  - Abnormal oxygen level in the fetal blood.

Teach the Patient

- Explain
- Why the test is being performed.
- What the patient will experience during the test.
- That the patient will not feel any pain during the test, except a pinch when the local anesthetic is administered.
- That the patient should breathe slowly during the procedure to relax her abdominal muscle.
- That the patient may feel a cramp in the abdomen.
- That the patient must sign a consent form.
- That the patient must empty her bladder before the procedure.
- That the patient should avoid exercise for 24 hours following the test.
- That the patient should not have sexual intercourse for 24 hours following the test.
- That the patient should not douche or use tampons for 24 hours following the test.

NURSING ALERT

The patient should call her healthcare provider if she notices fluid or bloody discharge from the insertion site or if there is swelling and redness at the insertion site. She should also call her healthcare provider if she experience fever, pain, or cramping in her abdomen.

9. Cranial Ultrasound

A cranial ultrasound is performed on premature newborns to assess complications that might have arisen during the premature birth. During a cranial ultrasound, images of the newborn's brain are captured, displayed on a computer screen, and stored on a computer. The healthcare provider might order several cranial ultrasounds weeks apart. Some complications such as intraventricular hemorrhage (IVH) can be detected during the first week of birth while other complications such as periventricular leukomalacia (PVL) might occur 8 weeks after birth. PVL is damaged tissue around the ventricles.

> **NURSING ALERT**
>
> A cranial ultrasound is not performed after the child is 18 months of age because the cranium is fully formed and the fontanelle is closed.

What Is Being Examined?

- Assess the premature newborn's brain for complications resulting from the premature birth.

How Is the Procedure Performed?

- A conduction gel is placed on the newborn's head.
- A transducer is moved across the newborn's head, capturing images that appear on a computer monitor.

Rationale for the Test

- Assess
  - For hydrocephalus
  - For the risk of developing cerebral palsy
  - The cause of an enlarged head
  - For IVH
  - For PVL

Nursing Implications

- The mother can hold the newborn during the test.
- The newborn can be fed during the test.

Understanding the Results

- The procedure takes less than 30 minutes. Preliminary results are known immediately. Detailed results are known within a week.
- Normal test results indicate
  - No complications found
- Abnormal test results indicate
  - Complications found

Teach the Patient

- Explain
  - Why the test is being performed.
  - What the newborn will experience during the test.
  - That the newborn will not feel any pain during the test.
  - That the mother can hold and feed the newborn during the test.

10. Galactosemia Test

Newborns who have galactosemia may experience seizures, brain damage, and mental retardation if their body is unable to convert galactose, which is found in breast milk and formula, into glucose. This is because they lack three enzymes needed for this process. The galactosemia test determines if these enzymes are present in the newborn's blood.

NURSING ALERT

These enzymes can also be detected in a urine sample.

What Is Being Measured?

- Enzymes that convert galactose into glucose

How Is the Test Performed?

- A blood specimen is collected from the heel.

Rationale for the Test

- To screen for galactosemia

Nursing Implications

- Assess if the patient
  - Has had a blood transfusion
  - Has relief from galactosemia. Galactosemia is a genetic disorder.

Understanding the Results

- Test results are available within 2 days. The laboratory determines normal values based on calibration of testing equipment with a control test. Test results are reported as high, normal, or low based on the laboratory's control test.
- Normal (negative): The enzymes are present.
- Abnormal (positive): The enzymes are not present.

Teach the Patient

- Explain
  - Why blood sample is taken.
  - How the sample is taken.
  - That the newborn who has galactosemia must not ingest milk or milk by-products.

11. Karyotyping

Karyotyping is a test that determines the number and quality of chromosomes in a cell and is used to detect possible genetic disorders. Tissue samples for karyotyping are typically taken during chorionic villus sampling or amniocentesis.

What Is Being Examined?

- Chromosomes of fetal cells

How Is the Procedure Performed?

- The patient should undergo genetic counseling to understand the test and its results.
- The sample is taken using chorionic villus sampling or amniocentesis.
- Chromosomes are removed from cells and examined under a microscope.

Rationale for the Test

- To assess for fetal genetic disorder

Nursing Implications

- Determine if the patient has undergone genetic counseling

Understanding the Results

- The procedure takes less than 1 hour. Results are known within 2 weeks.
- Normal test results indicate
  - Normal number and quality of chromosomes.
- Abnormal test results indicate
  - Abnormal number and quality of chromosomes

Teach the Patient

- Explain
  - Why the test is being performed.
  - Why is it important to have genetic counseling to fully understand the test and its results.

12. Pap Smear

A Pap smear is a procedure that removes sample cells from the cervix to assess if there are any abnormal cells. The sample is sent to the laboratory for microscopic identification. Further examination is necessary if the sample is positive, indicating abnormal cells on the cervix.

> **NURSING ALERT**
>
> A negative Pap smear result does not mean that the patient is free from cervical cancer. It means that no abnormal cells were contained in the tissue sample. Abnormal cells might exist in areas of the cervix that was not tested.

What Is Being Examined?

- The cervix

How Is the Procedure Performed?

- The patient removes her clothing from below the waist.
- The patient lies on a table with her feet in stirrups.
- A speculum is placed into the vagina to spread the vaginal walls.
- The healthcare provider inserts a cytobrush to gather samples from several areas of the cervix and from the endocervical canal.
- The tissue sample is sent to the laboratory for identification.

Rationale for the Test

- To assess cervical tissue
- To identify abnormal tissue that might be cancerous

Nursing Implications

- Determine if the patient
  - Has been taking anticoagulant medication such as Plavix, Coumadin, heparin, or aspirin
  - Can lie on her back
  - Is pregnant
  - Is using birth control
  - Has undergone cervical surgery
  - Is not having her menstrual period
  - Is 8 to 12 days after her menstrual period
  - Has not used a tampon 24 hours prior to the procedure

- Has not douched 24 hours prior to the procedure
- Has not administered vaginal medications 24 hours prior to the procedure
- Did not have a pelvic, cervical, or vaginal infection within 6 weeks prior to the procedure

NURSING ALERT

Assess if the patient has been the victim of rape. If so, the patient may not feel comfortable having a pelvic examination or a Pap smear performed.

Understanding the Results

- The procedure takes less than 30 minutes. Results are available within 2 weeks.
- Normal test results indicate
  - Normal cervical tissue
- Abnormal test results indicate
  - Abnormal cervical tissue
- Inconclusive test results indicate
  - The same did not contain a sufficient amount of cells to make a determination if cells were normal.

Teach the Patient

- Explain
  - Why the procedure is being performed.
  - What the patient will experience during the procedure.
  - Not to use a tampon 24 hours prior to the procedure.
  - Not to douche 24 hours prior to the procedure.
  - Not to use vaginal medications 24 hours prior to the procedure.
  - That the patient cannot have the procedure performed during her menstrual period.
  - That the patient cannot have the procedure performed if she had a pelvic, cervical, or vaginal infection within 6 weeks prior to the procedure.
  - There may be a small amount of vaginal bleeding following the procedure.

13. Sperm Penetration Tests

Sperm penetration tests are performed, when a woman is having difficulty becoming pregnant, to determine if the sperm can move through the cervical mucus and into the fallopian tubes. The two types of sperm penetration tests are

- Sperm penetration assay: This test mixes sperm with hamster eggs to see if the sperm can penetrate the egg. The result is measured as a sperm capacitation index.
- Sperm mucus penetration: This test determines if sperm can move through the cervical mucus.

What Is Being Examined?

- Sperm penetration capability

How Is the Procedure Performed?

- The patient signs a consent form.
- Sperm penetration assay
- Ejaculation should not occur for 2 days before the semen sample is taken.
- Ejaculation should occur within 5 days before the semen sample is taken.
- Before the semen sample is taken, the patient should urinate.
- The patient's hands and penis should be washed.
- Do not use lubricants or condoms when collecting the sample.
- Do not collect a semen sample after withdrawal from intercourse.
- Place the semen sample in a sterile cup.
- Keep the sample at body temperature.
- Keep the sample from direct sunlight.
- Deliver the sample to the laboratory immediately.
- The laboratory will mix the semen with hamster eggs to determine the sperm capacitation index.

- Sperm mucus penetration test
  - The woman must be ovulating in order to perform this test.
  - Determine if she is ovulating by collecting a urine sample in the mid to late morning.
  - The woman should avoid drinking fluids before giving a urine sample.
  - The urine sample is analyzed for the presence of luteinizing hormone (LH). This hormone indicates that she is ovulating.
  - The woman is given a pelvic examination during which a sample of cervical mucus is collected.
  - The man provides a semen sample (see sperm penetration assay above).
  - The cervical mucus and the semen samples are combined at the laboratory to determine if sperm can move through the cervical mucus.

Rationale for the Test

- To determine the underlying cause of infertility

Nursing Implications

- Determine if the male patient
  - Has ejaculated for 2 days before the semen sample is taken
  - Has ejaculated within 5 days before the semen sample is taken
  - Has urinated before the semen sample was taken
  - Washed his hands and penis before the semen sample was taken
  - Used lubricants or condoms when collecting the semen sample
  - Collected a semen sample after withdrawal from intercourse
  - Placed the semen sample in a sterile cup
  - Kept the sample at body temperature
  - Kept the sample from direct sunlight
  - Delivered the sample to the laboratory immediately
  - Has signed a consent form
- Determine if the female patient
  - Was ovulating during the test

Understanding the Results

- The procedure takes less than 1 hour. Results are known within 2 days.
- Normal test results indicate
  - Sperm penetrated the hamster egg.
  - Sperm moved through the cervical mucus.
- Abnormal test results indicate
  - Sperm could not penetrate the hamster egg.
  - Sperm could not move through the cervical mucus.

Teach the Patient

- Explain
  - Why the procedure is being performed.
  - What the patient will experience during the procedure.
  - That the patient will not feel any pain during the procedure.
  - Must sign a consent form.
  - How to collect the semen sample.

14. Sweat Test

The sweat test is administered to a newborn between the ages of 2 days and 5 months to assess if the newborn might have cystic fibrosis. Children who have cystic fibrosis have increased sodium chloride in their sweat. The sweat test measures the amount of chloride in sweat in newborns.

What Is Being Examined?

- Chloride in sweat

How Is the Procedure Performed?

- The right arm or thigh is washed and dried.
- A small gauze pad is soaked with pilocarpine.
- Another small gauze pad is soaked with salt water.
- Both are placed on the skin.

- Electrodes are placed over the gauze pads.
- A mild current flows through the electrodes forcing the medication into the skin. The newborn may feel a slight tingling.
- The gauze pads are removed after 10 minutes.
- The skin under the gauze pad that contains pilocarpine is red.
- The skin is cleaned with water and dried.
- The reddened skin is covered with a dry gauze pad.
- The dry gauze pad is covered with plastic to prevent evaporation.
- The dry gauze pad remains in place for 30 minutes to soak up sweat.
- The dry gauze pad is removed and placed in a collection bottle, which is sealed and sent to the laboratory where the dry gauze is weighed to determine the amount of chloride and/or sodium that is on the gauze.
- The skin beneath the dry gauze pad is cleaned and dried.
- The skin remains reddened for less than 5 hours following the test.

NURSING ALERT

The healthcare provider may use the macroduct technique of collecting sweat, which uses a coil rather than gauze pads.

Rationale for the Test

- To assess for cystic fibrosis

Nursing Implications

- Determine if the patient
  - Is less than 4 weeks of age. Newborns less than 4 weeks of age usually do not produce enough sweat for the test.
  - Is dehydrated.
  - Is ill.
  - Is taking steroids.
  - Has a rash.

Understanding the Results

- The procedure takes less than 1 hour. Results are known within 2 days.
- Normal test results indicate
  - Normal amount of chloride
- Borderline test results indicate
  - A high level of chloride
- Abnormal test results indicate
  - A high level of chloride

> **NURSING ALERT**
>
> An abnormal result indicates that the newborn may have cystic fibrosis. Further testing is necessary to diagnose cystic fibrosis.

Teach the Patient

- Explain
- Why the test is being performed.
- What the newborn will experience during the test.
- That the newborn will not feel any pain during the test, except for a slight tingle when current is applied to the electrode.
- That any reddened skin will return to normal color within 5 hours of the test.

15. Vaginosis Tests

Vaginosis is inflammation of the vulva and vagina caused by an infection or a reaction to an irritant, resulting in a painful vaginal discharge and itching. The most common causes of vaginosis are

- *Candida albicans:* This is a yeast infection that causes lumpy white discharge and itching.
- *Trichomonas vaginalis:* This causes a foamy, yellow-green, odorous vaginal discharge.
- Bacterial vaginosis: This causes a milky thick vaginal discharge that gives off a fishy odor.

Vaginosis tests are performed by the healthcare provider taking a sample of the vaginal discharge and sending the sample to a laboratory for examination. The four vaginosis tests are

- Whiff test: Potassium hydroxide solution is dropped on the sample. If a fishy odor emanates, then the patient has bacterial vaginosis.
- KOH slide: The sample is mixed with potassium hydroxide solution. Only the yeast remains on the slide, indicating that the patient has a yeast infection.
- Wet mount: The sample is mixed with saline on one slide. The laboratory technician then identifies, through microscopic examination, the organism causing the infection.
- Vaginal pH: The pH level of the sample is tested. A pH level greater than 4.5 indicates bacterial vaginosis.

What Is Being Examined?

- The cause of vaginosis

How Is the Procedure Performed?

- The patient removes her clothing from below the waist.
- The patient lies on a table with her feet in stirrups.
- A speculum is placed into the vagina to spread the vaginal walls.
- The healthcare provider inserts a swab to gather a sample of the discharge.
- The sample is sent to the laboratory for identification.

Rationale for the Test

- To assess the cause of vaginal itching, inflammation, and discharge
- To identify the treatment of vaginosis

Nursing Implications

- Determine if the patient
  - Has taken anticoagulant medication such as Plavix, Coumadin, heparin, or aspirin
  - Can lie on her back
  - Is pregnant

- Is using birth control
- Has undergone cervical surgery
- Is 8 to 12 days after her menstrual period
- Has had sexual intercourse 24 hours before the procedure
- Has used a tampon 24 hours prior to the procedure
- Has douched 24 hours prior to the procedure
- Has administered vaginal medications 24 hours prior to the procedure
- Is having her menstrual period

NURSING ALERT

Assess if the patient has been the victim of rape. If so, the patient may not feel comfortable having a sample of the discharge taken.

Understanding the Results

- The procedure takes less than 30 minutes. Results are available within 2 days.
- Normal test results indicate
  - Normal vaginal discharge: No vaginosis
- Abnormal test results indicate
  - Presence of a microorganism that is causing vaginosis

Teach the Patient

- Explain
  - Why the procedure is being performed.
  - What the patient will experience during the procedure.
  - That the patient will have to sign a consent form.
  - Not to use a tampon 24 hours prior to the procedure.
  - Not to douche 24 hours prior to the procedure.
  - Not to use vaginal medications 24 hours prior to the procedure.
  - Cannot have the procedure performed during her menstrual period.
  - There will be a small amount of vaginal bleeding following the procedure.
  - Should not have sexual intercourse 24 hours before the procedure.

Summary

In this chapter you learned about commonly performed tests and procedures that assess a woman's breast and cervix for structural defects and disease. The tests involved visual examination of the patient's vulva, vagina, cervix, uterus, and fallopian tubes and looking through the skin using X-ray and ultrasound.

Any suspicious area of the breast or cervix is examined closely by taking a tissue sample or a biopsy of an abnormal growth to identify it. If the sample is cancerous, the healthcare provider will perform one of several procedures to remove either the affected area or affected organs.

In this chapter, you also learned of tests that assess the well-being of the fetus and of the newborn and procedures that prevent premature birth. In a high-risk pregnancy, a chorionic villus sampling or amniocentesis is performed to determine if the fetus has a genetic disorder or other health issues such as anemia. If the fetus is suspected of being anemic, a cordocentesis is likely performed in which a sample of blood is taken from the umbilical cord while in the womb.

A BPP test of the fetus is performed later in the pregnancy to assess the fetal heart rate, breathing and body movements, muscle tone, and the volume of amniotic fluid. During this time the mother undergoes a contraction stress test to determine if the fetus is healthy enough to survive the reduced oxygen levels that are common with natural childbirth.

In cases of incompetent cervix, which could result in the cervix opening prior to the 37th week of gestation causing a premature birth, the healthcare provider may perform a cervical cerclage, which temporarily closes the cervix until the mother enters labor. A premature birth can result in complications for the fetus. A cranial ultrasound might be performed to identify some complications.

QUIZ

1. **What is meant by a score of 7 on the biophysical profile (BPP) test?**
   A. Undetermined results. The test should be repeated.
   B. The fetus is normal.
   C. There are possible problems with the fetus.
   D. None of the above.

2. **Why is oxytocin administered during a contraction stress test?**

   A. To lower blood pressure of the fetus

   B. To stop contractions

   C. To induce contractions

   D. To keep the fetus from moving

3. **Why is a cranial ultrasound not performed after 18 months of age?**

   A. The fontanelle is closed.

   B. The fontanelle remains open.

   C. The test is too painful for the baby to undergo.

   D. Complications from a premature birth would have already manifested.

4. **Why is chorionic villus sampling preferred over amniocentesis?**

   A. Chorionic villus sampling can be performed earlier in the pregnancy than amniocentesis.

   B. Chorionic villus sampling can be performed later in the pregnancy than amniocentesis.

   C. Chorionic villus sampling is safer than amniocentesis.

   D. None of the above.

5. **What might an increase in bilirubin levels from an amniocentesis taken after the 20th week indicate?**

   A. The fetus is healthy.

   B. Fetal blood cells are attacking the mother's antibodies.

   C. Fetal blood cells are being attacked by the mother's antibodies.

   D. The fetus's lungs have matured.

6. **What does it mean if a woman's husband has the BRCA1 and BRCA2 genes?**

   A. He can pass these genes to the woman during sexual intercourse.

   B. The woman is at a high risk for cancer.

   C. The couple should refrain from unprotected sexual intercourse.

   D. The man might be at high risk for developing breast cancer and/or prostate cancer.

7. **A common yeast infection that causes vaginosis is**

   A. *Candida albicans*

   B. *Trichomonas vaginalis*

   C. Bacterial vaginosis

   D. None of the above

8. **What cause of vaginosis causes a fishy odor?**

   A. *Candida albicans*
   B. *Trichomonas vaginalis*
   C. Bacterial vaginosis
   D. None of the above

9. **What is the purpose of using pilocarpine during a sweat test?**

   A. Pilocarpine helps to draw sweat from the newborn.
   B. Pilocarpine prevents the newborn from sweating.
   C. Pilocarpine is not used in the sweat test.
   D. Pilocarpine protects the skin from electrodes that are placed on the skin during the test.

10. **How would you respond if the patient who is scheduled for a Pap smear today mentions that her menstrual period ended 7 days ago?**

    A. Prepare the patient for the test.
    B. Reschedule the test for the next day.
    C. Reschedule the test for the next week.
    D. Reschedule the test for 2 weeks.

ANSWERS

1. A. Undetermined results. The test should be repeated.
2. C. To induce contractions.
3. A. The fontanelle is closed.
4. A. Chorionic villus sampling can be performed earlier in the pregnancy than amniocentesis.
5. C. Fetal blood cells are being attacked by the mother's antibodies.
6. D. The man might be at high risk for developing breast cancer and/or prostate cancer.
7. A. *Candida albicans*.
8. C. Bacterial vaginosis.
9. A. Pilocarpine helps to draw sweat from the newborn.
10. B. Reschedule the test for the next day.

chapter 17

Tests for Males

KEY WORDS

Color duplex Doppler	Semen volume
Epididymis	Snap gauge
Fructose level	Sperm count
Intracavernosal injection	Sperm morphology
Liquefaction time	Sperm motility
Nocturnal penile tumescence (NPT)	Transillumination
Prostaglandin E1	Vas deferens

There are a number of medical tests and procedures that are specifically designed to diagnose and treat disorders that affect men. There are a group of tests and procedures focused on fertility.

When a man is unable to impregnate a woman, the healthcare provider orders tests to assess if there is an underlying problem with the man's reproductive organs. The initial test is a semen analysis that assesses the man's semen and sperm. Depending on the results, a testicular scan or testicular ultrasound is ordered to determine if there is a structural disorder. One such structural disorder is varicocele, which is a large vein that blocks blood flow to the testicles. This is relieved by performing a varicocele repair.

The healthcare provider may follow up with a testicular examination or an erectile dysfunction test. If the erectile dysfunction test returns positive results, the healthcare provider may perform a penile implant procedure where a device is inserted to cause an erection.

Some men desire to become infertile by having their vas deferens cut or blocked by a vasectomy. This prevents sperm from mixing with semen, resulting in no sperm in the ejaculate. A vasectomy in some instances can be reversed by performing a vasovasostomy.

Men are susceptible to developing an enlarged prostate gland, which could be caused by prostate cancer. Prostatic cancer cells are in part fueled by testosterone, which is produced by the testicles. The healthcare provider might perform an orchiectomy, which is the surgical removal of one or both testicles. This reduces the level of testosterone in the patient's body.

Alternatively, the healthcare provider may perform a prostatectomy, which is the removal of the prostate gland. However, this procedure may leave the patient with erectile dysfunction and urinary incontinence.

In this chapter, you will learn about these tests and procedures.

1. Erectile Dysfunction Tests

Erectile dysfunction is commonly caused by psychological, blood vessel, and nerve disorders. There are three tests that are commonly ordered to assess erectile dysfunction. These are

- Color duplex Doppler: This test assesses blood flow through the penis using an ultrasound.
- Nocturnal penile tumescence (NPT): This test assesses if the patient has erections during sleep.
- Intracavernosal injection: This test injects prostaglandin E1 into the base of the penis to cause an erection.

What Is Being Examined?

- Penile erection

How Is the Procedure Performed?

- The patient signs a consent form.
- The patient removes clothing below the waist.
- The patient lies on a table.
- Color duplex Doppler.
  - Conductive gel is placed on the penis.
  - The Doppler ultrasound transducer is moved across the penis.
  - An image on a video screen shows the direction and velocity of blood flowing through the penis.
- NPT
  - A snap gauge is placed around the penis when the patient goes to sleep.
  - An erection during sleep will snap the film, indicating that the patient had an erection while sleeping.
  - Alternatively, a transducer is placed on the penis when the patient goes to sleep and it records the number of erections, the length of time of the erection, and how rigid the erection was during sleep.
- Intracavernosal injection
  - Prostaglandin E1 is injected into the base of the penis causing an erection.
  - A measurement is taken of the duration and how rigid the erection is.

Rationale for the Test

- To assess the underlying cause of erectile dysfunction

Nursing Implications

- Determine if the patient
  - Has signed a consent form
  - Is stressed or depressed
  - Has not taken Cialis, Levitra, or Viagra prior to the test
  - Has any allergies
  - Has not taken sleeping pills 2 days before the test, if the patient is undergoing the NPT test
  - Has not ingested alcohol 2 days before the test, if the patient is undergoing the NPT test
  - Has not had an erection lasting more than 4 hours
  - Has not ingested nicotine within 2 hours of the test
  - Has not been taking anticoagulant medication such as Plavix, Coumadin, heparin, or aspirin
  - Can lie still

Understanding the Results

- The procedure takes less than 1 hour except for the NPT test, which is performed overnight. Results are immediate.
- Normal test results indicate
  - Normal blood flow in the penis
  - Normal erection immediately and overnight
- Abnormal test results indicate
  - Abnormal blood flow in the penis
  - Abnormal or no erection

Teach the Patient

- Explain
  - Why the procedure is being performed.

- What the patient will experience during the procedure.
- That the patient will not feel any pain during the procedure except for a pinch from the needle if intracavernosal injection is performed,
- That the patient will have to sign a consent form.
- That the patient must not take Cialis, Levitra, or Viagra prior to the test.
- That the patient must not have taken sleeping pills 2 days before the test, if the patient is undergoing the NPT test.
- That the patient must not ingest alcohol 2 days before the test, if the patient is undergoing the NPT test.
- That the patient must not ingest nicotine within 2 hours of the test.
- That the patient must stop taking anticoagulant medication such as Plavix, Coumadin, heparin, or aspirin until after the test is completed.

2. Semen Analysis

Semen analysis is performed to assess the volume of semen and number of quality sperm that is produced in an ejaculation to determine the underlying cause of infertility. There are eight factors that are analyzed. These are

- Semen volume: This is the amount of semen in an ejaculation.
- Liquefaction time: This is the time it takes for the semen to liquefy.
- Sperm morphology: This is the number of normally shaped sperm.
- Sperm motility: This is the percentage of sperm that shows forward movement.
- Sperm count: This is the number of sperm in a milliliter of semen in one ejaculation.
- Fructose level: This is the amount of fructose in semen to provide energy for sperm.
- pH: This measures the pH level of the semen.
- White blood cell count: This measures the number of white blood cells in semen, which is normally zero.

What Is Being Examined?

- Semen and sperm

How Is the Procedure Performed?

- The patient signs a consent form.
- Ejaculation should not occur for 2 days before the semen sample is taken.
- Ejaculation should occur within 5 days before the semen sample is taken.
- Before the semen sample is taken, the patient should urinate.
- The patient's hands and penis should be washed.
- The patient should not use lubricants or condoms when collecting the sample.
- The patient should not collect a semen sample after withdrawing from intercourse.
- The patient should place the semen sample in a sterile cup.
- The patient should keep the sample at body temperature.
- The patient should keep the sample away from direct sunlight.
- The patient should deliver the sample to the laboratory immediately.

Rationale for the Test

- To determine the underlying cause of infertility
- To assess the vasectomy
- To assess the vasovasostomy

Nursing Implications

- Determine if the patient
  - Has not taken tegument, sulfasalazine, testosterone, estrogen, or nitrofurantoin
  - Has not taken Echinacea, St. John's wort, caffeine, cocaine, alcohol, marijuana, or tobacco
  - Has not ejaculated for 2 days before the semen sample is taken
  - Has ejaculated within 5 days before the semen sample is taken
  - Has urinated before the semen sample was taken
  - Had washed his hands and penis before the semen sample was taken
  - Did not use lubricants or condoms when collecting the semen sample
  - Did not collect a semen sample after withdrawing from intercourse

- Placed the semen sample in a sterile cup
- Kept the sample at body temperature
- Kept the sample away from direct sunlight
- Deliver the sample to the laboratory immediately
- Has signed a consent form

Understanding the Results

- The procedure takes less than 1 hour. Results are known within 2 days.
- Normal test results indicate
  - Normal semen volume.
  - Liquefaction time is less than 60 minutes.
  - 70% of sperm have normal shape.
  - 70% of sperm show forward mobility.
  - Sperm count is more than 20 million sperm per milliliter of semen or zero if a vasectomy was performed.
  - Semen pH is between 7.1 and 8.0.
  - 300 mg of fructose in 100 mL of semen.
  - No white blood cells in the semen.
- Abnormal test results indicate
  - Low semen volume.
  - Liquefaction time is 60 minutes or greater.
  - Less than 70% of sperm have normal shape.
  - Less than 70% of sperm show forward mobility.
  - Sperm count is less than 20 million sperm per milliliter of semen or greater than zero if a vasectomy was performed.
  - Semen pH is less than 7.1 or greater than 8.0.
  - Less than 300 mg of fructose in 100 mL of semen.
  - White blood cells present in the semen.

Teach the Patient

- Explain
  - That the patient will not feel any pain during the procedure.
  - Why the procedure is being performed.

- What the patient will experience during the procedure.
- That the patient must sign a consent form.
- How to collect the semen sample.
- That the patient must not take tegument, sulfasalazine, testosterone, estrogen, or nitrofurantoin.
- That the patient must not take Echinacea, St. John's wort, caffeine, cocaine, alcohol, marijuana, or tobacco.

3. Testicular Examination

A testicular examination is performed to assess the patient's testicles, scrotum, and penis for testicular atrophy, growths, and abnormalities.

What Is Being Examined?

- The testicles, scrotum, and penis

How Is the Procedure Performed?

- The patient empties his bladder prior to the examination.
- The patient removes clothing below the waist.
- The patient lies on a table and then stands during the examination.
- The scrotum and testicles are palpated.
- Transillumination is performed to highlight any growth found during palpation. This is where a light is placed behind the testicles, making the outline of the growth visible.
- The healthcare provider assesses the testicles for consistency, weight, size, and texture.
- Lymph nodes in the groin and thigh are palpated.

Rationale for the Test

- To assess the testicles, scrotum, and penis

Nursing Implications

- Determine if the patient
  - Can lie still
  - Can stand

Understanding the Results

- The procedure takes less than 1 hour. Results are known immediately.
- Normal test results indicate
  - Normal shape and size of the testicles, scrotum, and penis
  - Normal shape and size of the lymph nodes
- Abnormal test results indicate
  - Abnormal shape and size of the testicles, scrotum, and penis
  - Abnormal shape and size of the lymph nodes

Teach the Patient

- Explain
  - Why the examination is being performed.
  - What the patient will experience during the examination.
  - That the patient will not feel any pain during the examination.
  - That the patient should empty his bladder before the examination.

4. Testicular Scan

A testicular scan assesses the function of the testicles and is used to identify blockages. A radioactive tracer is injected in the patient's vein. The tracer flows into the testicles. A camera takes an image of the tracer as the tracer flows through the testicles.

What Is Being Examined?

- The testicles

How Is the Procedure Performed?

- The patient signs a consent form.
- The patient removes clothing below the waist.
- The patient lies on a table.
- The penis is taped to the abdomen.
- The testicles are supported by a towel.
- The injection site is cleaned.

- The patient is injected with the radioactive tracer.
- The camera is moved into position.
- Two images are taken, one every 15 minutes.

Rationale for the Test

- To assess the testicles

Nursing Implications

- Determine if the patient
  - Has signed a consent form
  - Has allergies
  - Has had a barium test performed 4 days prior to the test
  - Has taken aspirin

Understanding the Results

- The procedure takes less than 1 hour. Results are known within 2 days.
- Normal test results indicate
  - No blockages in the testicles
  - Normal shape and size of the testicles
- Abnormal test results indicate
  - Abnormal shape and size of the testicles.
  - Testicles are inflamed or blocked.

Teach the Patient

- Explain
  - Why the procedure is being performed.
  - What the patient will experience during the procedure.
  - That the patient will not feel any pain during the procedure except for a pinch when the tracer is injected into his vein.
  - That the patient must sign a consent form.
  - That the patient should not take anticoagulant medication such as Plavix, Coumadin, heparin, or aspirin for 2 weeks prior to the test.

- That the patient must drink lots of fluids to flush the tracer following the test.
- That the patient should flush the toilet immediately after urinating and defecating.
- That the patient should wash hands thoroughly after urinating and defecating.
- That the patient should apply a warm compress to the injection site if there is swelling.

5. Testicular Ultrasound

A testicular ultrasound is a procedure used to produce an image of the testicles, scrotum, epididymis, and vas deferens to detect if there is any structural dysfunction.

What Is Being Examined?

- Testicles, scrotum, epididymis, and vas deferens

How Is the Procedure Performed?

- The patient removes clothing below the waist.
- The patient lies on a table.
- Conductive gel is placed on the scrotum.
- A transducer is moved across the scrotum.
- An image of the testicles, scrotum, epididymis, and vas deferens is seen on a video screen.

Rationale for the Test

- To assess a mass on the testicles
- To identify the underlying cause of pain in the scrotum
- To assess structures within the scrotum

Nursing Implications

- Determine if the patient can lie still.

Understanding the Results

- The procedure takes 1 hour. Results are known within 2 days.
- Normal test results indicate
  - Normal structures in the scrotum
- Abnormal test results indicate
  - Inflammation.
  - Twisted spermatic cord.
  - Growth.
  - Pyocele, spermatocele, or hematocele in the scrotum.
  - Hernia is present.

Teach the Patient

- Explain
  - Why the procedure is being performed.
  - What the patient will experience during the procedure.
  - That the patient will not feel any pain during the procedure.

Summary

In this chapter you learned about tests and procedures specifically designed to diagnose and treat disorders that affect men.

You saw how semen analysis determines the quality of semen and sperm and how a testicular scan or testicular ultrasound gives the healthcare provider a view inside the structural defects of the patient's testicles, which do not show up on a testicular examination. The healthcare provider can remove structural disorders by performing procedures such as varicoceles repair.

Erectile dysfunction is a problem that affects some patients. You learned about the various erectile dysfunction tests that are used to diagnose this condition and about the penile implant procedure that restores the erection.

The healthcare provider can perform a vasectomy to cut or block the vas deferens, preventing sperm from mixing with semen resulting in no sperm in the ejaculate. A vasectomy in some instances can be reversed by performing a vasovasostomy.

An enlarged prostate gland could be caused by prostate cancer. An orchiectomy can be performed to remove one or both testicles resulting in a reduction of testosterone, which fuels prostate cancer cells. If this fails to reduce the prostate gland, then the healthcare provider may perform a prostatectomy—the removal of the prostate gland.

QUIZ

1. **What test measures if the patient has erections during sleep?**

    A. Intracavernosal injection

    B. NPT

    C. Color duplex Doppler

    D. Liquefaction time

2. **What is sperm morphology?**

    A. Liquefaction time

    B. Semen volume

    C. The number of normally shaped sperm

    D. Fructose level

3. **How does the snap gauge work?**

    A. It measures the size of an erection.

    B. The snap gauge consisting of a film is placed around the penis. The film snaps when the patient has erection.

    C. It measures the length of time of an erection.

    D. All of the above.

4. **Why is transillumination performed?**

    A. To highlight growths found during a testicular examination

    B. To visualize the prostate gland through the urethra

    C. To scan the prostate gland

    D. To scan the bladder

5. **What is liquefaction time?**

    A. The time necessary for semen to liquefy

    B. The time necessary for semen to dehydrate

    C. The time necessary for sperm to liquefy

    D. The time necessary for sperm to dehydrate

6. **What might cause low sperm motility?**

    A. Sample not kept at body temperature

    B. Delay in delivering the sample to the laboratory

    C. Sample not kept away from direct sunlight

    D. All of the above

7. **What might cause a low sperm count?**

    A. The sample was taken within 2 days of the last ejaculation.

    B. Having sexual intercourse 10 days before the sample is taken.

    C. Unable to have an erection.

    D. Unable to have an erection while sleeping.

8. **Why is the fructose level in semen measured?**

    A. Fructose prevents sperm motility.

    B. Fructose provides energy for sperm.

    C. Fructose reduces sperm count.

    D. Fructose increases semen volume.

9. **What is the purpose of the Color duplex Doppler test?**

    A. To assess the velocity and direction of blood flowing through the penis

    B. To assess size of an erection

    C. To assess if the patient had an erection during sleep

    D. To assess if the patient has urine in his bladder

10. **What is the purpose of an intracavernosal injection?**

    A. To increase sperm count

    B. To prevent an erection

    C. To cause an erection

    D. None of the above

ANSWERS

1. B. NPT.
2. C. The number of normally shaped sperm.
3. B. The snap gauge consisting of a film is placed around the penis. The film snaps when the patient has erection.
4. A. To highlight growths found during a testicular examination.
5. A. The time necessary for semen to liquefy.
6. D. All of the above.
7. A. The sample was taken within 2 days of the last ejaculation.
8. B. Fructose provides energy for sperm.
9. A. To assess the velocity and direction of blood flowing through the penis.
10. C. To cause an erection.

chapter 18

Lung, Chest, Abdominal, Urinary Tract Tests and Procedures

LEARNING OBJECTIVES

1. D-xylose Absorption Test
2. Enterotest (Giardiasis String Test)
3. Esophagus Test Series
4. Fecal Occult Blood Test (FOBT)
5. Gallbladder Scan
6. Kidney Scan
7. Liver and Spleen Scan
8. Lung Scan

⑨ Overnight Dexamethasone Suppression Test

⑩ Pulmonary Function Tests

⑪ Renin Assay Test

⑫ Salivary Gland Scan

⑬ Stool Analysis

⑭ Stool Culture

⑮ Thyroid and Parathyroid Ultrasound

⑯ Thyroid Hormone Tests

⑰ Thyroid Scan

⑱ Thyroid Surgery

⑲ Thyroid-Stimulating Hormone (TSH) Test

⑳ Upper Gastrointestinal (UGI) Series

㉑ Urinalysis

㉒ Urine Culture and Sensitivity Test

KEY WORDS

Bladder scan
Body plethysmograph test
Bravo wireless
Carbon monoxide diffusing capacity
Cholecystokinin
Esophageal acidity test
Esophageal manometry
Exercise stress tests
Expiratory reserve volume (ERV)
Forced expiratory volume (FEV)
Forced vital capacity (FVC)
Free thyroxine (FT4)
Function study
Functional residual capacity (FRC)
Gas diffusion tests
Inhalation challenge test
Lobectomy
Malabsorption syndrome

Maximum voluntary ventilation (MVV)
Near-total thyroidectomy
Peak expiratory flow (PEF)
Perfusion scan
Perfusion study
Pneumonectomy
Pulmonary emboli
Radioactive iodine uptake (RAIU) test
Slow vital capacity (SVC)
Spirometry test
Total lung capacity (TLC)
Total thyroidectomy
Total thyroxine (T4)
Triiodothyronine (T3)
V/Q scan
Ventilation scan
Whole-body thyroid scan

When there are suspected disorders of the upper gastrointestinal tract, the thyroid gland, the liver, gallbladder, kidneys, spleen, the urinary tract, and other organs in the upper part of the body, the healthcare provider is likely to order a number of tests to uncover the underlying problem.

Some tests enable the healthcare provider to look down the esophagus to examine the stomach, duodenum, and the bile and pancreatic ducts and to take a biopsy or, in some cases, remove an obstruction.

Other tests enable the healthcare provider to scan the liver, spleen, gallbladder, and kidneys by using contrast material to highlight the structure of the organ. Images of the organ are captured with a camera and studied to uncover diseases and disorders.

There are also procedures that the healthcare provider can perform to temporarily or permanently repair a problem. It can be to remove a cancerous thyroid gland, remove a tumor from the bladder, or fix urinary incontinence.

The lungs exchange carbon dioxide and oxygen in the hemoglobin in red blood cells. In order to do so effectively, the lungs must be able to expand and retract and blood must flow freely to the lungs. When the patient experiences signs and symptoms of lung disorder and disease, the healthcare provider tests the lungs and orders procedures to evaluate the respiratory system.

The healthcare provider can examine the respiratory tract using bronchoscopy and removes samples of suspicious tissue for microscopic examination. The capacity and function of the lungs are measured using several pulmonary function tests. Blood flow to the lungs is monitored by a lung scan and by performing a pulmonary angiogram to identify restriction or blockage of blood flow to the lungs. This is also performed using CT imaging.

The patient may experience difficulty breathing when excess fluid builds in the plural space, inhibiting the expansion of the lung. A thoracentesis is sometimes performed, which removes the excess fluid.

Diseases such as lung cancer can destroy part of or the entire lung, requiring the healthcare provider to surgically remove a portion (wedge resection), lobes of the lung (lobectomy), or the entire lung (pneumonectomy).

You will learn about these and other tests and procedures in this chapter.

1. D-xylose Absorption Test

Patients with malabsorption syndrome are unable to absorb certain nutrients into their blood from the intestinal tract. This can result in malnutrition and chronic diarrhea. The D-xylose absorption test assesses whether or not these signs are a result of malabsorption syndrome by asking the patient to drink a solution of D-xylose and then measuring the amount of D-xylose in the patient's blood and urine.

What Is Being Measured?

- Absorption of D-xylose

How Is the Test Performed?

- A sample of urine and blood is taken.
- The patient drinks a solution containing D-xylose.
- A blood sample is taken 2 hours after the patient drinks the solution.
- A 24-hour urine sample is collected once the patient drinks the solution.
- Urine and blood samples are then sent to the laboratory for analysis.

Rationale for the Test

- Assess the intestine's ability to absorb D-xylose.

Nursing Implications

- Determine if the patient
  - Has eaten fruits, jellies, pastries, or other foods high in pentose for 24 hours prior to the test
  - Has taken aspirin, indomethacin, cardiac medication, or antibiotics
  - Has eaten or drunk, except for water, for 12 hours prior to the test
  - Has emptied the bladder prior to the test
  - Has an infection
  - Has rested prior to and during the test
  - Has a digestive disorder that reduces the time it takes the stomach to empty

Understanding the Results

- The results are available quickly. The laboratory determines normal values based on calibration of testing equipment with a control test. Test results are reported as high, normal, or low based on the laboratory's control test.

- Normal test results indicate
  - The patient's intestines absorb D-xylose without a problem.
- Low value test results indicate
  - Malabsorption syndrome
  - Celiac disease
  - Whipple disease
  - Crohn disease
- High value results indicate
  - Hodgkin disease
  - Scleroderma

Teach the Patient

- Explain
  - Why the test is administered.
  - How the test is performed.
  - How to collect a 24-hour urine sample.
  - That the patient will not feel pain except a pinch when blood samples are taken.
  - Should not eat fruits, jellies, pastries, or other foods high in pentose for 24 hours prior to the test.
  - Should not take aspirin, indomethacin, cardiac medication, or antibiotics.
  - Should not eat or drink, except for water, 12 hours prior the test.
  - Should empty his bladder prior to the test.
  - Should rest prior to and during the test.

2. Enterotest (Giardiasis String Test)

A patient who has severe diarrhea might have giardiasis. Giardiasis is caused by an intestinal parasite called *Giardia intestinalis,* which is found in water, food, or soil that are contaminated with feces. The enterotest determines if the patient has giardiasis by sampling fluid in the duodenum. The patient swallows a gelatin capsule that is attached to a string. The string is taped to the outside of the patient's mouth while the capsule dissolves in the stomach and the duodenum. The string is then removed and examined under a microscope.

What Is Being Measured?

- Fluid in the duodenum

How Is the Test Performed?

- The patient swallows a gelatin capsule that is attached to a string.
- The string is taped to the outside of the patient's cheek.
- The patient waits 6 hours.
- The string is removed and sent to the laboratory for microscopic analysis to determine the presence of *G intestinalis*.

Rationale for the Test

- Assess for the presence of *G intestinalis*.

Nursing Implications

- Determine if the patient
  - Can swallow
  - Is able to have the string attached to the outside of his/her mouth

Understanding the Results

- The result is available within 3 days.
- Normal test results indicate
  - No *G intestinalis* is present.
- Abnormal test results indicate
  - *Giardia intestinalis* is present.

Teach the Patient

- Explain
  - Why the test is administered.
  - How the test is performed.
  - How to collect the stool sample.

- The patient should not take antibiotics or medication to treat an infection.
- That the patient will not feel pain although the string might feel uncomfortable.

3. Esophagus Test Series

The esophagus test series consists of two tests that assess the esophagus and esophageal sphincters. These tests are
- Esophageal manometry: Measures esophageal muscle contractions
- Esophageal acidity test: Measures the pH of the esophagus

What Is Being Examined?

- The esophagus

How Is the Procedure Performed?

- The patient signs a consent form.
- The patient removes clothing.
- The patient lies on a table with head slightly raised.
- Esophageal manometry
  - The patient swallows a transducer that is attached to a tube.
  - The tube contains pressure-sensing holes.
  - The patient is asked to swallow several times during the test. Pressure in the esophagus is measured with each swallow.
  - A graph depicting the pressure is recorded and assessed by the health-care provider.
- Esophageal acidity test (bravo wireless)
  - The patient swallows a capsule that contains a transmitter. The transmitter measures the acidity of his/her stomach and transmits it to a receiver carried by him/her.
  - The patient keeps a diary of his/her activities.
  - The patient is asked to press a button on the pager when he/she experiences a symptom.
  - The transmitter passes through bowel movement within 1 week.

- Esophageal acidity test (nonwireless)
  - An anesthetic is sprayed in the back of patient's throat and in his/her nose.
  - A tube containing a probe that measures acidity is passed through the patient's nose and down the esophagus.
  - The probe remains in place for 24 hours as it records the acidity level in the esophagus while patient goes about normal daily activities.
  - The patient keeps a diary of his/her activities and symptoms.
  - The patient must avoid activities that may cause the monitor to become wet.
  - The probe is removed after 24 hours and the results are analyzed by the healthcare provider.

Rationale for the Test

- To assess the cause of gastroesophageal reflux disease (GERD)
- To assess the cause of chest pain

Nursing Implications

- Determine that the patient
  - Has signed a consent form
  - Has not eaten or drunk for 12 hours before the test
  - Has not smoked or ingested alcohol 24 hours before the test
  - Does not have esophageal varices
  - Does not have heart failure
  - Has been taking anticoagulant medications such as Plavix, Coumadin, heparin, or aspirin
  - Can lie on the back
  - Can swallow
  - Has not taken Prevacid, Prilosec, Protonix, Nexium, Aciphex, Zantac, Pepcid, Axid, Tagamet, or antacids prior to and during the test
  - Has not taken corticosteroids
  - Has not taken blood pressure medication
  - Has not taken medication to treat bladder and intestinal muscle spasms
  - Has not taken medication for Parkinson disease
  - Has not taken theophylline

Understanding the Results

- The procedure takes less than 1 hour. The esophageal acidity test takes 24 hours. Results are known within 2 weeks of the test.
- Normal test results indicate
  - Normal structure and function of the esophagus or normal pH level
- Abnormal test results indicate
  - Abnormal structure or function of the esophagus or acidic pH level

Teach the Patient

- Explain
  - Why the procedure is being performed.
  - What the patient will experience during the procedure.
  - That the patient will not feel any pain during the procedure.
  - That the patient should not eat or drink for 12 hours before the test.
  - Should not have smoked or ingested alcohol 24 hours before the test.
  - Should not take Prevacid, Prilosec, Protonix, Nexium, Aciphex, Zantac, Pepcid, Axid, Tagamet, or antacids prior to and during the test.

4. Fecal Occult Blood Test

Blood in the stool is not always visible. The fecal occult blood test (FOBT) examines the stool for blood that is not visible to the naked eye. This is referred to as occult blood. Although the presence of occult blood is linked to colon cancer, there are many other causes of occult blood in the stool.

What Is Being Measured?

- Occult blood in the stool

How Is the Test Performed?

- Urinate prior to defecating.
- Do not mix urine and stool.
- The patient is asked to defecate in a basin in the toilet or bedpan. Do not defecate in the toilet, since this might contaminate the sample.

- Place on clean gloves.
- A sample of stool is placed on a card that is chemically treated. It is critical that the stool sample is not contaminated with hair, toilet paper, and other elements that might produce a false-positive test result.
- A reaction agent is placed on the stool sample. If the sample turns blue, then there is blood in the stool sample.
- Wash hands immediately.

> **NURSING ALERT**
>
> The healthcare provider may collect a stool sample during a digital rectum examination rather than ask the patient to defecate.

Rationale for the Test

- Assess for blood in the stool.

Nursing Implications

- Determine if the patient
  - Has her menstrual period
  - Has contaminated the stool sample
  - Has been taking anticoagulant medications such as Plavix, Coumadin, aspirin, or heparin.

Understanding the Results

- The results are available immediately.
- Normal test results indicate
  - No blood in the stool sample
- Abnormal test results indicate
  - Anal fissures
  - Peptic ulcer
  - Polyps
  - Hemorrhoids
  - Gastroesophageal reflux disease

- Ulcerative colitis
- Use of anticoagulation medication
- Crohn disease

Teach the Patient

- Explain
- Why the test is administered.
- How the test is performed.
- How to collect the stool sample.
- Not to take the sample during her menstrual period.
- Stop taking anticoagulant medications such as Plavix, Coumadin, aspirin, or heparin.
- The patient will not feel pain.

5. Gallbladder Scan

A gallbladder scan assesses the function of the gallbladder and is used to identify blockages in the bile ducts. A radioactive tracer is injected into the patient's vein. The tracer is removed from the blood by the liver, which places and adds the tracer to bile that flows into the gallbladder and into the duodenum. A camera takes an image of the tracer as the tracer flows through the liver to the duodenum.

What Is Being Examined?

- The gallbladder

How Is the Procedure Performed?

- The patient signs a consent form.
- The patient removes clothing.
- The patient lies on a table.
- The injection site is cleaned.
- The patient is injected with the radioactive tracer.
- The camera is moved into position.
- Images are taken immediately, then every 10 minutes for 90 minutes.

- The patient is administered cholecystokinin to stimulate the gallbladder.
- The patient may be administered morphine sulfate to diagnose gallbladder inflammation.
- The patient should drink lots of fluid to flush the tracer from his/her body.
- The patient should flush the toilet quickly after urinating and defecating, since the tracer is excreted in urine and feces for 2 days following the test.

Rationale for the Test

- To assess the gallbladder
- To assess the cause of upper right abdominal pain

Nursing Implications

- Determine if the patient
  - Has signed a consent form
  - Has not eaten or drunk for 12 hours before the test
  - Has allergies
  - Is pregnant
  - Has recently had a barium test performed within 4 days prior to the test
  - Has been taking anticoagulant medications such as Plavix, Coumadin, heparin, or aspirin
  - Has taken Pepto-Bismol

Understanding the Results

- The procedure takes less than 2 hours and results are known within 2 days.
- Normal test results indicate
  - Gallbladder is functioning normally.
  - Normal shape and size of the gallbladder.
- Abnormal test results indicate
  - Possible liver disease if the tracer does not flow into the gallbladder.
  - Gallbladder is inflamed or blocked.
  - The bile duct is narrowed or blocked.

Teach the Patient

- Explain
- Why the procedure is being performed.
- What the patient will experience during the procedure.
- That the patient will not feel any pain during the procedure except for a pinch when the tracer is injected into the vein.
- That the patient must sign a consent form.
- That the patient must not eat or drink for 12 hours before the test.
- That the patient should not take anticoagulant medications such as Plavix, Coumadin, heparin, or aspirin for 2 weeks prior to the test.
- That the patient should not take Pepto-Bismol for 48 hours before the test.
- That the patient should drink lots of fluids to flush the tracer following the test.
- That the patient should flush the toilet immediately after urinating or defecating.
- That the patient should wash hands thoroughly after urinating or defecating.
- That the patient should apply a warm compress to the injection site if there is swelling.
- If the patient is breast-feeding, breast milk must be discarded for 2 days after the scan.

6. Kidney Scan

A kidney scan assesses the function of the kidneys. A radioactive tracer is injected in the patient's vein. The tracer moves through the blood vessels in the kidneys. A camera takes images of the tracer as the tracer flows through the kidney, illustrating where blood flows unobstructed and where blood flow is blocked. There are two types of kidney scans. These are

- Function study: This measures the time that the tracer takes to pass through the kidneys and enter the bladder as part of urine.
- Perfusion study: This assesses blood flow through the kidneys.

NURSING ALERT

A kidney scan is an alternative to the intravenous pyelogram (IVP) test.

What Is Being Examined?

- The kidneys

How Is the Procedure Performed?

- The patient signs a consent form.
- The patient removes clothing.
- The patient lies on a table, although he/she may be asked to sit or stand during the test.
- The injection site is cleaned.
- The patient is injected with the radioactive tracer.
- The camera is moved into position.
- Function study
  - Images are taken every 3 minutes for 30 minutes.
  - The patient may be administered a diuretic to increase kidney function.
- Perfusion study
  - Movement of the tracer through the kidneys is recorded on a renogram.
- The patient should drink lots of fluid to flush the tracer from body.
- The patient should flush the toilet quickly after urinating or defecating, since the tracer is excreted in urine and feces for 2 days following the test.

Rationale for the Test

- To assess blood flow through the kidneys
- To assess the function of the kidneys

Nursing Implications

- Determine if the patient
  - Has signed a consent form.
  - Has drunk 3 glasses of water before the test.

- Can lie still.
- Has allergies.
- Is pregnant.
- Has recently had a barium test performed within 4 days prior to the test.
- Has been taken anticoagulant medications such as Plavix, Coumadin, heparin, or aspirin.
- Has taken Pepto-Bismol.
- Has taken antihypertensives.
- If the patient is breast-feeding, breast milk must be discarded for 2 days after the scan.

Understanding the Results

- The procedure takes less than 2 hours. Preliminary results are known within 2 days.
- Normal test results indicate
  - Kidney is functioning normally.
  - Normal kidney size and shape.
- Abnormal test results indicate
  - Abnormal kidney function.
  - Abnormal kidney size and shape.
  - There is narrowing or blockage of blood vessels.

Teach the Patient

- Explain
- Why the procedure is being performed.
- What the patient will experience during the procedure.
- That the patient will not feel any pain during the procedure except for a pinch when the tracer is injected into his vein.
- That the patient must sign a consent form.
- That the patient must drink 3 glasses of water before the test.
- That the patient should not take anticoagulant medications such as Plavix, Coumadin, heparin, or aspirin for 2 weeks prior to the test.

- That the patient should not take Pepto-Bismol for 48 hours before the test.
- That the patient should drink lots of fluids to flush the tracer following the test.
- That the patient flushes the toilet immediately after urinating or defecating.
- That the patient should wash hands thoroughly after urinating or defecating.
- That the patient should apply a warm compress to the injection site if there is swelling.
- If the patient is breast-feeding, breast milk must be discarded for 2 days after the scan.

7. Liver and Spleen Scan

A liver and spleen scan assesses the function of the liver and spleen. A radioactive tracer is injected into the patient's vein. The tracer moves through the blood vessels in the liver and spleen. A camera takes an image of the tracer as it flows through the liver and spleen, illustrating where blood flows unobstructed and where blood flow is blocked.

What Is Being Examined?

- The liver and spleen

How Is the Procedure Performed?

- The patient signs a consent form.
- The patient will empty the bladder.
- The patient removes clothing.
- The patient lies on a table.
- The injection site is cleaned.
- The patient is injected with the radioactive tracer.
- The camera is moved into position.
- Several images are taken.
- The patient should drink lots of fluid to flush the tracer from body.

- The patient should flush the toilet quickly after urinating or defecating, since the tracer is excreted in urine and feces for 2 days following the test.

Rationale for the Test

- To assess blood flow through the liver and spleen
- To assess if cancer metastasized to the liver
- To assess the spleen after an injury
- To assess treatment for cancer

Nursing Implications

- Determine if the patient
  - Has signed a consent form.
  - Can lie still.
  - Has allergies.
  - Is pregnant.
  - Has recently had a barium test performed within 4 days prior to the test.
  - Has been taking anticoagulant medication such as Plavix, Coumadin, heparin, or aspirin.
  - Has taken Pepto-Bismol.
  - Has emptied the bladder.
  - If the patient is breast-feeding, breast milk must be discarded for 2 days after the scan.

Understanding the Results

- The procedure takes less than 2 hours. Results are known within 2 days.
- Normal test results indicate
  - Liver and spleen are functioning normally.
  - Normal size and shape of the liver and spleen.
- Abnormal test results indicate
  - Abnormal liver function
  - Abnormal spleen function
  - Abnormal size and shape of the spleen
  - Abnormal size and shape of the liver

Teach the Patient

- Explain
- Why the procedure is being performed.
- What the patient will experience during the procedure.
- That the patient will not feel any pain during the procedure except for a pinch when the tracer is injected into the vein.
- That the patient must sign a consent form.
- That the patient must have an empty bladder.
- That the patient should not take anticoagulant medications such as Plavix, Coumadin, heparin, or aspirin for 2 weeks prior to the test.
- That the patient should not take Pepto-Bismol for 48 hours before the test.
- That the patient should drink lots of fluids to flush the tracer following the test.
- That the patient should flush the toilet immediately after urinating or defecating.
- That the patient should wash hands thoroughly after urinating or defecating.
- That the patient should apply a warm compress to the injection site if there is swelling.
- If the patient is breast-feeding, breast milk must be discarded for 2 days after the scan.

8. Lung Scan

A lung scan is performed to detect pulmonary emboli that imbed blood flow in the lungs. Following are the three types of lung scans:

- Perfusion: In a perfusion scan, a radioactive tracer is injected into a blood vessel of the patient. An image is taken of the lungs as the tracer circulates in the lungs. A pulmonary embolus is suspected in areas of the lung where the tracer is not seen.
- Ventilation: In a ventilation scan, the patient inhales gas that contains a radioactive tracer. An image is taken of the lungs. A pulmonary embolus is suspected in areas of the lung that are not receiving the tracer.

- V/Q: A V/Q scan consists of both the perfusion scan and the ventilation scan. The ventilation scan is performed first. This is the most commonly performed lung scan.

What Is Being Examined?

- The presence of the pulmonary emboli

How Is the Test Performed?

- The patient removes his/her clothing.
- The patient lies on a table.
- Perfusion scan
  - The radioactive trace is injected into the patient's arm.
- Ventilation scan
  - A mask is placed over the patient's mouth and nose.
  - The patient is asked to take a deep breath to inhale a mixture of oxygen and tracer gas and hold it for 10 seconds as the image is taken.
- The scanning camera is placed over the patient's chest.
- The patient must remain still when each image is taken.
- The scanning camera may be repositioned during the procedure.
- The patient may be repositioned during the procedure.

Rationale for the Test

- Assess blood flow to the lungs.

Nursing Implications

- Determine if the patient
  - Has signed a consent form
  - Takes anticoagulants such as Coumadin, aspirin, heparin, or Plavix
  - Is pregnant
  - Can lie still on the back
  - Has pulmonary disease
  - Has cardiac disease

- Can hold the breath for 10 seconds, if the ventilation scan is performed
- Has taken Pepto-Bismol or barium prior to the procedure

Understanding the Results

- The lung scan takes about 30 minutes to perform. The results are usually known immediately.
- Normal test results indicate
  - Normal blood flow throughout the lungs
- Abnormal test results indicate
  - Obstructed blood flow in a portion of the lungs
  - Pulmonary emboli identified

Teach the Patient

- Explain
- Why the procedure is being performed.
- That the patient will need to sign a consent form.
- What the patient will experience during the procedure.
- That the patient will not feel any pain during the procedure except for a pinch from the needle used to administer the tracer, if the perfusion scan is performed.
- That the patient must tell the healthcare provider if he/she is taking anticoagulants.
- That the patient may be asked to change positions during the procedure.
- That the patient might have swelling at the injection site that is relieved by placing warm compresses on the site.
- After using the toilet following the procedure, the patient should promptly flush the toilet and wash hands thoroughly with soap and water since the tracer exits the body through urine and stool.
- If the patient is breast-feeding, any breast milk produced up to 2 days following the procedure should be discarded.

9. Overnight Dexamethasone Suppression Test

The overnight dexamethasone suppression test is used to assess if the patient has Cushing syndrome. The pituitary gland secretes adrenocorticotropic hormone (ACTH) based on the amount of cortisol in the patient's blood.

ACTH signals the adrenal glands to secrete cortisol. In Cushing syndrome, cortisol is secreted regardless of the secretion of the ACTH level. The overnight dexamethasone suppression test requires the patient to take dexamethasone, which is a corticosteroid. This increases the cortisol level in the patient's blood and, therefore, signals the pituitary gland not to secrete ACTH. As a result, the adrenal glands should not secrete cortisol. In the morning, the patient's cortisol level should be relatively low. If not, then the patient might have Cushing syndrome.

What Is Being Measured?

- Cortisol level in blood

How Is the Test Performed?

- At 11.00 PM, the patient is administered dexamethasone by mouth with milk or antacid.
- A blood sample is taken at 8.00 AM.
- The level of cortisol in the blood sample is measured.

Rationale for the Test

- Assess
  - For Cushing syndrome

Nursing Implications

- Determine if the patient
  - Has eaten or drunk 12 hours prior to drawing the blood sample
  - Has taken methadone, aspirin, MAOIs, lithium, diuretics, 48 hours before the blood sample is drawn

Understanding the Results

- The results are available quickly. The laboratory determines normal values based on calibration of testing equipment with a control test. Test results are reported as high, normal, or low based on the laboratory's control test.
- Normal value results indicate
  - A relatively low level of cortisol in the blood sample

- High value results indicate
  - Cushing syndrome
  - Cancer
  - Diabetes
  - Hyperthyroidism

Teach the Patient

- Explain
- Why the test is administered.
- How the test is performed.
- Do not eat or drink 12 hours prior to drawing the blood sample.
- Do not take methadone, aspirin, MAOIs, lithium, diuretics, 48 hours before the blood sample is drawn.

10. Pulmonary Function Tests

There are a number of pulmonary function tests used to assess how well the patient's lungs perform. They are as follows:

- Gas diffusion: Measures the amount of gasses that cross the alveoli per minute. These include arterial blood gases and the carbon monoxide diffusing capacity.
- Spirometry: Measures the volume and capacity of the lungs.
- Exercise stress: Measures the effect the exercise has on the lungs.
- Body plethysmograph: Measures the volume and capacity of the lungs.
- Inhalation challenge: Assesses the patient's airway responses to allergens.

What Is Being Examined?

- Function of the lungs

How Is the Test Performed?

- A nose clip may be placed on the patient's nose to prevent the patient from breathing through the nose, depending on the test that is being performed.

- A mouthpiece connected to the measuring device is placed in the patient's mouth.
- Gas diffusion tests
  - Arterial blood gases
  - A needle is inserted into an artery in the patient's arm.
  - A sample of blood is removed from an artery.
  - Pressure is placed on the site for approximately 5 minutes to stop any bleeding.
  - A bandage is then placed over the site.
- Carbon monoxide diffusing capacity
  - A mask is connected to a container of a mixture of air and a small amount of carbon monoxide.
  - The patient breathes the gas mixture.
  - A mouthpiece connected to the measuring device is placed in the patient's mouth.
  - The patient exhales. The amount of carbon monoxide in the patient's breath is measured by the device. This is referred to as the diffusing capacity of the patient's lungs.
- Spirometry test
  - A nose clip is placed on the patient's nose to prevent breathing through the nose.
  - A mouthpiece connected to the spirometer is placed in the patient's mouth.
  - The patient inhales, and then exhales with force to measure the forced vital capacity (FVC). The exhaled air flow is also measured halfway through exhalation to measure the forced expiratory flow 25% to 75%. The peak exhale flow is also measured, which is referred to as the peak expiratory flow (PEF).
  - The patient inhales, then exhales with force. The amount of air exhaled is measured each second for 3 seconds to determine the forced expiratory volume (FEV).
  - The patient is asked to take a deep breath and then exhale to measure the maximum voluntary ventilation (MVV).
  - The patient is asked to take a deep breath and then slowly exhale to measure the slow vital capacity (SVC) and the total lung capacity (TLC).

- The patient is asked to take a normal breath and exhale to measure the functional residual capacity (FRC).
- The patient is asked to inhale normally and then exhale with force (RV). The amount exhaled is subtracted from the FRC to calculate the expiratory reserve volume (ERV).
- The patient's ERV is calculated by subtracting the reserve volume (RV) from the FRC.
- The radioactive trace is injected into the patient's arm.
- Exercise stress test
  - The patient undergoes a spirometry test.
  - The patient exercises.
  - The patient undergoes another spirometry test.
  - Results of both spirometry tests are compared to assess the patient's lung function before and after exercising.
- Inhalation challenge test
  - The patient undergoes a spirometry test.
  - The patient places a face mask over nose and mouth.
  - The face mask is attached to a nebulizer.
  - An allergen is gradually added to the mixture in the nebulizer.
  - The patient inhales a fine mist that contains the allergen from the nebulizer.
  - The patient is monitored for bronchospasm that may be triggered by the allergen.
  - The patient undergoes another spirometry test.
  - The results of both spirometry tests are compared to determine the effect that the antigen had on the patient.
- Body plethysmography test
  - The patient sits inside an airtight plethysmograph booth.
  - The booth is filled with a mixture of oxygen and helium or 100% oxygen.
  - Instruments attached to the booth measure pressure changes within the booth as the patient breathes.

Rationale for the Test

- Assess the function of the patient's lungs.
- Monitor the progress of lung therapy.

Nursing Implications

- Determine if the patient
  - Has eaten a heavy meal 8 hours before the test
  - Is able to have nose pinched
  - Is able to breathe through a mouthpiece
  - Is able to breathe normally
  - Is able to follow directions during the test
  - Has removed dentures if they prevent a tight seal around the patient's mouth
  - Has smoked 6 hours before the test
  - Has ingested caffeine 6 hours before the test
  - Has exercised 6 hours before the test
  - Is wearing comfortable clothes if the patient is taking the exercise stress test
  - Has taken medication that affects the respiratory tract
  - Has taken a sedative before the test
  - Has cardiovascular disease
  - Has allergies
  - Is pregnant

Understanding the Results

- The lung scan takes about 30 minutes to perform. The results are usually known immediately.
- Normal test results indicate
  - Normal for age, height, sex, weight, and race
- Abnormal test results indicate
  - Decreased pulmonary function based on the patient's age, height, sex, weight, and race

Teach the Patient

- Explain
  - Why the procedure is being performed.
  - What the patient will experience during the procedure.

- That the patient will not feel any pain during the test except if undergoing the arterial blood gas test, during which he/she will feel a pinch when the needle is inserted into the his/her arm.
- That the patient should avoid taking a sedative prior to the test.
- That the patient may be asked to stop taking respiratory medication 24 hours before the test. Taking medication may be resumed after the test.
- That the patient may be given instructions during the test.
- That the patient should not eat a big meal 8 hours before the test.
- That the patient should wear comfortable clothes the day of the test, especially undergoing an exercise stress test.
- After using the toilet following the procedure, the patient should promptly flush the toilet and wash hands thoroughly with soap and water since the tracer exits the body through urine and stool.
- If the patient is breast-feeding, any breast milk produced up to 2 days following the procedure should be discarded.
- That the patient should tell the healthcare provider if feeling light-headed when breathing rapidly during the test. The patient will be given time to adjust his/her breathing, which normally relieves the lightheadedness.

11. Renin Assay Test

The renin assay test is performed along with the aldosterone test to determine the underlying cause of hypertension. Renin is an enzyme produced by the kidneys. Aldosterone is a hormone produced by the adrenal glands. Together these work to balance the sodium and potassium levels within the patient. A high renin level might indicate a kidney disorder. A low renin level might indicate Conn syndrome. A low renin level and a high aldosterone level might indicate an adrenal gland tumor.

What Is Being Examined?

- Renin level in blood

How Is the Procedure Performed?

- See "How to Collect Blood Specimen From a Vein" in Appendix A.

Rationale for the Test

- To assess the underlying cause of hypertension

Nursing Implications

- Determine that the patient
  - Has not taken β-blockers, ACE inhibitors, diuretics, aspirin, corticosteroids, and estrogen 4 weeks prior to the test
  - Has not eaten natural black licorice for 2 weeks prior to the test
  - Has not ingested caffeine 24 hours prior to the test
  - Has eaten a low-sodium diet 3 days prior to the test
  - Has not eaten or drunk 8 hours prior to the test
  - Is not pregnant

Understanding the Results

- Test results are available quickly. The laboratory determines normal values based on calibration of testing equipment with a control test. Test results are reported as high, normal, or low based on the laboratory's control test.
- Normal test results indicate
  - Normal levels of renin and aldosterone
- Abnormal test results indicate
  - High renin levels might indicate a kidney disorder.
  - Low renin levels might indicate Conn syndrome.
  - Low renin levels and high aldosterone levels might indicate an adrenal gland tumor.

Teach the Patient

- Explain
- Why the test is being performed.
- What the patient will experience during the test.
- That the patient will not feel any pain during the test except a pinch when the blood sample is taken.
- That the patient should not take β-blockers, ACE inhibitors, diuretics, aspirin, corticosteroids, and estrogen 4 weeks prior to the test.

- That the patient should not eat natural black licorice for 2 weeks prior to the test.
- That the patient should not ingest caffeine 24 hours prior to the test.
- That the patient should eat a low-sodium diet 3 days prior to the test.
- That the patient should not eat or drink 8 hours prior to the test.

12. Salivary Gland Scan

A salivary gland scan assesses the function of the salivary glands to determine the underlying cause of xerostomia (dry mouth) or swelling.

What Is Being Examined?

- The salivary glands

How Is the Procedure Performed?

- The patient signs a consent form.
- The patient removes clothing above the waist.
- The patient removes dentures.
- The patient removes jewelry from the upper part of the body.
- A radioactive tracer is injected into the patient's vein.
- The patient lies on a table.
- The table is tipped backward.
- The gamma scintillation camera takes images of the salivary glands.
- The patient sucks a lemon, which normally causes the glands to release more saliva.
- The patient should drink lots of fluid to flush the tracer from the body.
- The patient should discard breast milk for 2 days following the test if she is breast-feeding.
- The patient should flush the toilet quickly after urinating or defecating, since the tracer is excreted in urine and feces for 2 days following the test.

Rationale for the Test

- To assess the salivary glands function
- To assess the underlying cause of swollen salivary glands
- To assess the underlying cause of dry mouth

Nursing Implications

- Determine if the patient
- Has signed a consent form
- Has allergies
- Is pregnant
- Is breast-feeding
- Has recently had a radioactive iodine test performed within 4 weeks prior to the test
- Has been taking anticoagulant medications such as Plavix, Coumadin, heparin, or aspirin

Understanding the Results

- The procedure takes less than 1 hour. Results are known within a week.
- Normal test results indicate
- Salivary glands are functioning normal.
- Abnormal test results indicate
- Abnormal shape or size of the salivary glands.
- Nodules are found on the salivary glands.
- Blockage is found on the salivary glands.

Teach the Patient

- Explain
- Why the test is being performed.
- What the patient will experience during the test.
- That the patient will not feel any pain during the procedure except for a pinch when the tracer is injected into the vein.
- The patient may feel flushed when tracer is injected.
- The patient must sign a consent form.
- The patient should not take anticoagulant medications such as Plavix, Coumadin, heparin, or aspirin for 2 weeks prior to the test.
- The patient should drink lots of fluids to flush the tracer following the test.
- The patient should flush the toilet immediately after urinating or defecating.

- The patient should wash hands thoroughly after urinating and defecating.
- If the patient is breast-feeding, breast milk must be discarded for 2 days after the scan.

13. Stool Analysis

Stool analysis is the examination of the patient's feces to identify digestive tract disorders. The patient's stool sample is examined for color, volume, consistency, odor, and the presence of blood, fat, mucus, fiber, bile, and glucose.

What Is Being Measured?

- Stool sample

How Is the Test Performed?

- Urinate prior to defecating.
- Do not mix urine and stool.
- The patient is asked to defecate in a basin in the toilet or bedpan. Do not defecate in the toilet, since this might contaminate the sample.
- Place on clean gloves.
- A sample of stool is placed in a clean container. It is critical that the stool sample isn't contaminated with hair, toilet paper, and other elements that might produce a false-positive test result.
- Cap and label the container.
- Wash hands immediately to prevent the spread of the microorganism.
- The container is immediately sent to the laboratory.

Rationale for the Test

- Assess
  - Digestive tract disorder
  - Liver disorder
  - Pancreatic disorder
  - Colon cancer
  - Absorption disorder

Nursing Implications

- Determine if the patient
  - Has her menstrual period
  - Has taken aspirin, Aleve, ibuprofen, antacids, NSAIDs, laxatives, antid-iarrheal medication, antibiotics, or medication to treat an infection for 2 weeks prior to the test
  - Has had a test that used contrast material within 10 days of the test
  - Has contaminated the stool sample
  - Has eaten cauliflower, bananas, red meat, cantaloupe, parsnips, turnips, or beets prior to the test
  - Has taken vitamin C prior to the test
  - Has drunk alcohol prior to the test
  - Has had an enema prior to the test

Understanding the Results

- The results are available within 3 days.
- Normal test results indicate
  - Stool is well-formed, soft, and brown
  - No mucus or blood in the stool
  - Minimum amount of glucose
- Abnormal test results indicate
  - Stool is loose, hard, or a color other than brown
  - Mucus or blood in the stool
  - Significant amount of glucose, fat, trypsin, or elastase in stool

Teach the Patient

- Explain
  - Why the test is administered.
  - How the test is performed.
  - How to collect the stool sample.
  - Not to take the sample during her menstrual period.

- Not to take aspirin, Aleve, ibuprofen, antacids, NSAIDs, laxatives, antidiarrheal medication, antibiotics, or medication to treat an infection for 2 weeks prior to the test.
- Not to eat cauliflower, bananas, red meat, cantaloupe, parsnips, turnips, or beets prior to the test.
- Not to take vitamin C prior to the test.
- Not to drink alcohol prior to the test.
- Not to have an enema prior to the test.
- The patient will not feel pain.

14. Stool Culture

A patient may exhibit diarrhea and other signs of an infection. The healthcare provider orders a stool culture to determine if the underlying cause is a microorganism. A sample of the patient's stool is sent to the laboratory where it is placed in an environment that encourages microorganisms to grow. After 3 days, laboratory technicians determine if a microorganism is present and if so, which microorganism.

> **NURSING ALERT**
>
> The healthcare provider typically orders a sensitivity test of the sample along with the stool culture. The sensitivity test determines the medication that kills the microorganism.

What Is Being Measured?

- Microorganism in a stool sample

How Is the Test Performed?

- Urinate prior to defecating.
- Do not mix urine and stool.
- The patient is asked to defecate in a basin in the toilet or bedpan. Do not defecate in the toilet, since this might contaminate the sample.
- Place on clean gloves.

- A sample of stool is placed in a clean container. It is critical that the stool sample is not contaminated with hair, toilet paper, and other elements that might produce a false-positive test result.
- Cap and label the container.
- Wash hands immediately to prevent the spread of the microorganism.
- The container is immediately sent to the laboratory.

Rationale for the Test

- Assess if there is a microorganism in the stool sample.
  - Identify the microorganism in the stool sample.

Nursing Implications

- Determine if the patient
  - Has her menstrual period
  - Has taken antibiotics or medication to treat an infection
  - Has had a test that used contrast material within 10 days of the test
  - Has contaminated the stool sample

Understanding the Results

- The results are available within 3 days.
- Normal test results indicate
  - No disease causing microorganism
- Abnormal test results indicate
  - Disease causing microorganism identified
- Indeterminate
  - Insufficient sample size
  - Contaminated sample

Teach the Patient

- Explain
  - Why the test is administered.
  - How the test is performed.

- How to collect the stool sample.
- Not to take the sample during her menstrual period.
- Not to take antibiotics or medication to treat an infection.
- The patient will not feel pain.

15. Thyroid and Parathyroid Ultrasound

The thyroid and parathyroid ultrasound is used to assess the size and shape of the thyroid gland and the parathyroid glands, which are located behind the thyroid gland.

> **NURSING ALERT**
>
> This test is not used to assess the function of these glands.

What Is Being Examined?

- The thyroid and parathyroid glands

How Is the Procedure Performed?

- The patient signs a consent form.
- The patient removes clothing above the waist.
- The patient lies on a table with neck stretched.
- Conductive gel is placed on the patient's neck.
- A transducer is moved over the thyroid gland.
- Images are displayed on a computer screen and saved in a computer.
- The gel is wiped from the patient's neck.

Rationale for the Test

- To assess the size and shape of the thyroid and parathyroid glands.

Nursing Implications

- Determine if the patient
  - Has signed a consent form

- Removed jewelry from the neck
- Removed his/her clothing above the waist
- Is able to lie still

Understanding the Results

- The procedure takes less than 1 hour. Results are known within a week.
- Normal test results indicate
  - Normal shape and size of the thyroid
  - Normal shape and size of the parathyroid glands
- Abnormal test results indicate
  - Abnormal shape or size of the thyroid
  - Abnormal shape or size of the parathyroid glands

Teach the Patient

- Explain
  - Why the test is being performed.
  - What the patient will experience during the test.
  - That the patient will not feel any pain during the test.
  - That the patient must sign a consent form.

16. Thyroid Hormone Tests

The thyroid gland produces two hormones. These are thyroxine (T4) and triiodothyronine (T3). The thyroid hormone tests measure the level of thyroid hormones in the patient's blood. There are three thyroid hormone tests. These are

- Free T4: This test determines the amount of thyroxine that is not bound to globulin.
- Total T4: This test determines the total amount of thyroxine that is attached to globulin and that is not bound to globulin.
- T3: This test determines the total amount of triiodothyronine that is attached to globulin and not bound to globulin.

What Is Being Examined?

- The thyroid hormone level in blood

How Is the Procedure Performed?

- See "How to Collect Blood Specimen From a Vein" in Appendix A.

Rationale for the Test

- To assess for hyperthyroidism and hypothyroidism
- To assess for the cause of abnormal thyroid-stimulating hormone (TSH) test results
- To assess for treatment of hyperthyroidism and hypothyroidism

Nursing Implications

- Determine that the patient
  - Has not taken birth control pills, corticosteroids, estrogen, Dilantin, Tegretol, amiodarone, propranolol, or lithium 4 weeks prior to the test
  - Has not been taking anticoagulant medications such as Plavix, Coumadin, heparin, or aspirin
  - Is not pregnant
  - Has not undergone a test that used contrast material 4 weeks prior to the test

Understanding the Results

- Test results are available quickly. The laboratory determines normal values based on calibration of testing equipment with a control test. Test results are reported as high, normal, or low based on the laboratory's control test.
- Normal test results indicate
  - Normal level of T4 and T3
- Abnormal test results indicate
  - High levels might indicate hyperthyroidism, Graves disease, goiter, thyroiditis, excess intake of thyroid medication.
  - Low levels might indicate hypothyroidism, pituitary gland disorder, thyroiditis.

Teach the Patient

- Explain
  - Why the test is being performed.

- What the patient will experience during the test.
- That the patient will not feel any pain during the test except a pinch when the blood sample is taken.
- That the patient should not take birth control pills, corticosteroids, estrogen, Dilantin, Tegretol, amiodarone, propranolol, lithium, or anti-coagulant medications such as Plavix, Coumadin, heparin, or aspirin 4 weeks prior to the test.

17. Thyroid Scan

A thyroid scan assesses the function of the thyroid gland. There are two types of thyroid scans. These are

- Radioactive iodine uptake (RAIU) test: This assesses the absorption of a radioactive tracer by the thyroid gland.
- Whole-body thyroid scan: This test assesses whether or not thyroid cancer has metastasized.

What Is Being Examined?

- The thyroid

How Is the Procedure Performed?

- A blood sample is taken to measure the amount of thyroid hormones in the blood.
- The patient signs a consent form.
- The patient removes clothing above the waist.
- The patient removes dentures.
- The patient removes jewelry from the upper part of the body.
- The patient either swallows the radioactive tracer 24 hours before the test or is administered technetium 2 hours prior to the test.
- The patient lies on a table.
- The table is tipped backward.
- The gamma scintillation camera takes images of the thyroid gland.
- Images are also taken again 24 hours after the initial images were taken.
- The patient should drink lots of fluid to flush the tracer from body.

- The patient should discard breast milk for 2 days following the test if she is breast-feeding.
- The patient should flush the toilet quickly after urinating or defecating, since the tracer is excreted through urine and feces for 2 days following the test.

Rationale for the Test

- To assess the thyroid function
- To assess the treatment for thyroid disease

Nursing Implications

- Determine that the patient
  - Has signed a consent form
  - Has not eaten or drunk 2 hours before the test
  - Has not taken antithyroid medication, thyroid hormones, Cordarone, Pacerone, iodine, or kelp a week before the test
  - Has eaten a low-iodine diet
  - Has allergies
  - Is not pregnant
  - Is breast-feeding
  - Has recently had a radioactive iodine test performed within 4 weeks prior to the test
  - Has been taking anticoagulant medications such as Plavix, Coumadin, heparin, or aspirin

Understanding the Results

- The procedure takes less than 1 hour. Results are known within 1 week.
- Normal test results indicate
  - Thyroid is functioning normally.
  - Normal shape and size of the thyroid.
- Abnormal test results indicate
  - Abnormal shape or size of the thyroid.
  - Nodules are found on the thyroid.
  - Iodine is in other tissues indicating that thyroid cancer may have metastasized.

Teach the Patient

- Explain
  - Why the test is being performed.
  - What the patient will experience during the test.
  - That the patient will not feel any pain during the procedure except for a pinch when the tracer is injected into the vein.
  - That the patient may feel flushed when technetium is injected, if it is administered.
  - The patient swallows the capsule with water that contains the tracer if the capsule is used.
  - Must sign a consent form.
  - Must not eat or drink for 2 hours before the test.
  - Should not take anticoagulant medications such as Plavix, Coumadin, heparin, or aspirin for 2 weeks prior to the test.
  - Drink lots of fluids to flush the tracer following the test.
  - Flush the toilet immediately after urinating or defecating.
  - Wash hands thoroughly after urinating or defecating.
  - If the patient is breast-feeding, breast milk must be discarded for 2 days after the scan.
  - Should not take antithyroid medication, thyroid hormones, Cordarone, Pacerone, iodine, or kelp a week before the test.
  - Should eat a low-iodine diet.

18. Thyroid Surgery

Thyroid surgery is performed to remove a portion or all of the thyroid gland to treat thyroid cancer or to remove a benign nodule that is interfering with the patient's swallowing or breathing. There are three types of thyroid surgical procedures. These are

- Near-total thyroidectomy: One lobe, the isthmus, and part of the other lobe of the thyroid gland are removed to treat Graves disease.
- Total thyroidectomy: The whole thyroid gland is removed in addition to neighboring lymph nodes to treat thyroid cancer.
- Thyroid lobectomy: A lobe of the thyroid gland is removed. The healthcare provider may or may not remove the isthmus that connects the lobes of the thyroid gland. This is commonly performed to assess the lobe for cancer.

What Is Being Examined?

- Surgical removal of part or all of the thyroid gland

How Is the Procedure Performed?

- The patient signs a consent form.
- The patient removes clothing.
- The patient will lie on a table with head tipped backward.
- An intravenous line is inserted into the patient's arm.
- The patient is administered a general anesthetic.
- A breathing tube is placed down the patient's throat.
- The patient is connected to an ECG during the procedure.
- The patient is connected to a pulse oximeter.
- The insertion site is cleaned with an anesthetic.
- An incision is made in the skin above the thyroid gland.
- Part or the entire thyroid is removed.
- A drain might be inserted into the neck and connected to a collection device. The drain is emptied frequently and removed once drainage has stopped.
- The incision is closed with stitches and the site is covered with colloidin, which is a clear protective waterproof glue.

Rationale for the Test

- To assess for cancerous tissues
- To remove a cancerous thyroid gland
- To treat Graves disease

Nursing Implications

- Determine if the patient
  - Has signed a consent form
  - Removed dentures
  - Has any allergies
  - Has been taking anticoagulant medication such as Plavix, Coumadin, heparin, or aspirin

- Is pregnant
- Has recently had a radioactive iodine test performed within 4 weeks prior to the surgery
- Can lie on the back
- Is able to lie still
- Has eaten or drunk 12 hours before the surgery

Understanding the Results

- The procedure takes less than 1 hour. Results are ready within 2 weeks of the procedure.
- Normal test results indicate
  - Thyroid is removed.
- Abnormal test results indicate
  - Thyroid tissue was cancerous.

> **NURSING ALERT**
>
> A normal result does not mean that the patient is cancer free. It means that no cancerous cells were found in the tissue sample.

Teach the Patient

- Explain
  - Why the procedure is being performed.
  - What the patient will experience during the procedure.
  - That the patient will not feel any pain during the procedure except for a pinch from the needle used to the insert the intravenous saline lock.
  - That the patient cannot eat 12 hours before the surgery.
  - The incision site may be sore for 3 days following the surgery.
  - A bruise may develop around the site.
  - That the patient should avoid any stretching or pulling of neck muscles for 24 hours after the procedure.

- The patient should gargle with warm salt water to ease a sore throat that follows the surgery.
- The patient's neck will feel tender, stiff, and swollen following the procedure. Tenderness resolves in 1 week. The swelling resolves in 8 weeks.
- The patient might have a small scar on the neck.
- The patient must sign a consent form.
- The patient must remove dentures.
- The patient must stop taking anticoagulant medication such as Plavix, Coumadin, heparin, or aspirin.
- The patient might be required to undergo lifetime thyroid hormone replacement therapy and calcium replacement therapy, depending on the surgical procedure.
- Support the back of patient's neck when raising the head.

NURSING ALERT

The patient should call the healthcare provider if he/she has fever, experiences redness and drainage from the incision site after the drain has been removed, or has pain a week or more following the procedure. The patient should also call the healthcare provider if experiencing muscle cramps, hoarseness, tingling around the lips, hands, and feet, which are signs of hypocalcemia.

19. Thyroid-Stimulating Hormone Test

The hypothalamus produces thyrotropin-releasing hormone (TRH), which causes the pituitary gland to produce the TSH, causing the thyroid to produce thyroid hormones. The TSH test determines the underlying cause of thyroid disorder.

What Is Being Examined?

- The TSH level in blood

How Is the Procedure Performed?

- See "How to Collect Blood Specimen From a Vein" in Appendix A.

Rationale for the Test

- Assess the underlying cause of hyperthyroidism and hypothyroidism.

Nursing Implications

- Determine that the patient
  - Has not taken lithium, Tapazole, propylthiouracil, or corticosteroids 4 weeks prior to the test
  - Has not taken anticoagulant medication such as Plavix, Coumadin, heparin, or aspirin
  - Is not pregnant
  - Has not undergone a test that used contrast material 4 weeks prior to the test

Understanding the Results

- Test results are available quickly. The laboratory determines normal values based on calibration of testing equipment with a control test. Test results are reported as high, normal, or low based on the laboratory's control test.
- Normal test results indicate
  - Normal level TSH
- Abnormal test results indicate
  - High levels might indicate hypothyroidism, Hashimoto thyroiditis, pituitary gland tumor, insufficient dose of thyroid hormone.
  - Low levels might indicate hyperthyroidism, Graves disease, goiter, pituitary gland disorder, excess dose of thyroid hormone.

Teach the Patient

- Explain
  - Why the test is being performed.
  - What the patient will experience during the test.
  - That the patient will not feel any pain during the test except a pinch when the blood sample is taken.
  - That the patient should not take lithium, Tapazole, propylthiouracil, or corticosteroids 4 weeks prior to the test.

20. Upper Gastrointestinal Series

The upper gastrointestinal (UGI) series consists of a group of tests that assess the esophagus, stomach, and the duodenum. Prior to the series, the patient ingests barium contrast material and water. X-ray images of the esophagus, stomach, and duodenum are taken using a fluoroscope as the barium moves through the UGI tract. Images are displayed on a computer screen and stored for further review. If the healthcare provider sees anything suspicious, he might perform an endoscopy where an endoscope is inserted down the esophagus and into the stomach and duodenum to directly view the UGI tract.

> ### NURSING ALERT
>
> The UGI series is also performed during a full gastrointestinal series, which also involves examination of the lower gastrointestinal tract.

What Is Being Examined?

- The esophagus, stomach, and duodenum

How Is the Procedure Performed?

- Twelve hours before the test, the patient is administered a laxative.
- The patient signs a consent form.
- The patient removes clothing.
- The patient lies on the back.
- An X-ray of the UGI tract is taken.
- The patient is sitting when drinking the barium contrast material.
- A series of X-rays are taken.
- The patient may be asked to drink additional amounts of barium contrast material during the test. After each swallow, additional X-rays are taken.

Rationale for the Test

- To assess the cause of stomach pain and indigestion
- To assess the cause of malabsorption syndrome

Nursing Implications

- Determine if the patient
  - Has signed a consent form
  - Has any allergies
  - Has been taking anticoagulant medications such as Plavix, Coumadin, heparin, or aspirin
  - Can lie on the back or stomach
  - Is able to lie still
  - Is able to follow instructions
  - Has eaten a low-fiber diet for 3 days before the test
  - Has not eaten or drunk 12 hours before the test
  - Has taken a laxative 12 hours before the test
  - Has removed dentures before the test
  - Is able to swallow the barium contrast material

Understanding the Results

- The procedure takes less than 1 hour. Preliminary results are known immediately. Comprehensive results are ready within 2 weeks of the procedure.
- Normal test results indicate
  - Normal structure of the UGI tract
- Abnormal test results indicate
  - Abnormal structure of the UGI tract

Teach the Patient

- Explain
  - Why the procedure is being performed.
  - What the patient will experience during the procedure.
  - That the patient will not feel any pain during the procedure.
  - Should eat a low-fiber diet for 3 days before the test.
  - Must not eat or drink 12 hours before the test.
  - Should take a laxative 12 hours before the test.

- Will be swallowing the barium contrast material several times during the test. Barium contrast material is sweet flavored.
- The patient might feel bloated following the test.
- The patient might feel nausea following the test.
- Feces will appear white for 3 days following the test.
- The healthcare provider may administer a stool softener following the test to prevent constipation from the barium contrast material.

> **NURSING ALERT**
>
> The patient should call the healthcare provider if he/she has not had a bowel movement within 3 days following the test.

21. Urinalysis

Waste material carried by blood is filtered by kidneys and excreted as urine. A urinalysis is performed to determine the characteristics of the urine and to determine the existence and amount of substances in the urine. Urine characteristics:

- Clarity: How clear is the urine?
- Color: What is the color of the urine?
- Specific gravity: The balance between water and substances in the urine.
- Odor: The aroma of urine.
- pH: How acidic or alkaline is the urine?

There are several methods used to capture the urine sample. These are

- Clean-catch, midstream, one-time urine collection: Urine is collected after the patient begins to urinate.
- Double-voided urine collection: Urine is collected the second time that the patient voids.
- 24-hour urine collection: Urine is collected over a 24-hour period.

What Is Being Examined?

- Urine

How Is the Procedure Performed?

- The patient washes hands.
- The patient opens the collection cup without touching the inside of the cup.
- Clean the urethral area with an antiseptic.
- Do not touch the cup to the urethra or any skin when collecting the sample.
- Do not contaminate the urine sample with feces, pubic hair, or other substances.
- If the sample becomes contaminated, then begin again with a new collection cup.
- Double-voided urine collection.
  - The patient urinates.
  - The patient drinks a lot of water.
  - The patient waits until he/she has the feeling to urinate.
- Urinate for 5 seconds making sure no skin aside from the urethra touches the urine.
- Move the collection cup into the urine stream.
- Do not touch the collection cup to the urethra or any skin.
- Remove the collection cup and continue urinating.
- Place the lid on the collection cup.
- Refrigerate the collection cup until the sample is sent to the laboratory.
- 24-hour urine collection
  - The patient empties bladder the first thing in the morning.
  - The patient collects urine the next and subsequent times that he/she urinates for the 24-hour period.
  - The patient must note the time when urinates. This begins the 24-hour period.
  - Urine is kept in a gallon container that must be refrigerated between collections.
  - The patient must note the last time when urinated at the end of the 24-hour period.
  - If patients urinate within the 24-hour period and do not collect the urine, then they must begin the 24-hour urine collection again.

Rationale for the Test

- To assess for kidney and other disorders

Nursing Implications

- Determine if the patient
  - Has collected the urine properly
  - Has exercised prior to the test
  - Is menstruating
  - Has eaten blackberries, beets, or foods that might color urine
  - Has been exposed to sun
  - Is on extended bed rest
  - Has recently undergone a test that used contrast material
  - Has ingested nicotine or caffeine
  - Has had a recent illness or is under stress
  - Keeps warm during testing if testing catecholamine levels
  - Is pregnant
  - Has had severe vomiting
  - Has taken Dilantin, Pyridium, vitamin B, diuretics, rifampin, Trimpex, ascorbic acid, Probalan, Benemid, allopurinol, insulin, lithium, laxatives, steroids, antacids, NSAIDs, antibiotics, potassium supplements, growth hormones or parathyroid hormone, aspirin, antidepressants (including tricyclic), nitroglycerin, tetracycline, theophylline, cold and sinus medication
  - Has recently taken sodium-based medication

Understanding the Results

- The collection takes a few seconds except for the 24-hour collection. Results are known within 2 days.
- The laboratory determines normal values based on calibration of testing equipment with a control test. Test results are reported as high, normal, or low based on the laboratory's control test.
- Normal
  - Color: pale to dark amber

- Clarity: clear
- Odor: Nutty
- Specific gravity: 1.005 to 1.030
- pH: 4.6 to 8.0
- Protein: None
- Glucose: None
- Ketones: None
- Leukocytes: None
- Erythrocytes: None
- Casts: None
- Microorganism: None
- Crystals: Slight
- Squamous cells: None
- Uric acid: 250 to 800 mg (24-hour urine collection)
- Calcium: 100 to 250 mg (24-hour urine collection)
- Catecholamines: < 100 mcg (24-hour urine collection)
- Epinephrine: < 20 mcg (24-hour urine collection)
- Norepinephrine: < 100 mcg (24-hour urine collection)
- Dopamine: 65 to 400 mcg (24-hour urine collection)
- Normetanephrine: 10 to 80 mcg (24-hour urine collection)
- Metanephrine: < 1.3 mg (24-hour urine collection)
- Vanillylmandelic acid: < 6.8 mg (24-hour urine collection)
- Cortisol: < 100 mcg (24-hour urine collection)
- Phosphate: 0.9 to 1.3 g (24-hour urine collection)
- Potassium: 25 to 100 mEq/L (24-hour urine collection)
- Sodium: 40 to 220 mEq (24-hour urine collection)
- Microalbumin: < 30 mg (24-hour urine collection)
- Abnormal
  - Color: Clear (chronic kidney disease, diabetes), dark (dehydration), or red (blood)
  - Clarity: Cloudy (microorganism)
  - Odor: Fruity (diabetes), foul (urinary tract infection), maple syrup (maple syrup urine disease)

- Specific gravity: < 1.005 (overhydration, kidney disease, diuretics) or > 1.030 (dehydration, hyperglycemia, vomiting, diarrhea)
- pH: < 4.6 (diabetes, dehydration, excess alcohol, aspirin overdose) or > 8.0 (vomiting, urinary tract infection, kidney disease)
- Protein: Present (infection, high blood pressure, kidney disorder, glomerulonephritis)
- Glucose: Present (diabetes, liver disease, kidney disorder, adrenal gland disorder)
- Ketones: Present (diabetes, starvation, anorexia, bulimia, alcoholism)
- Leukocytes: Present (urinary tract infection, glomerulonephritis, kidney stones, kidney disorder)
- Erythrocytes: Present (urinary tract infection, glomerulonephritis, kidney stones, kidney disorder)
- Casts: Present (inflammation, kidney disorder, lead poisoning, heart failure)
- Microorganism: Present (urinary tract infection)
- Crystals: Large amount (kidney stone, kidney disorder)
- Squamous cells: Present (contaminated urine sample)
- Uric acid: < 250 or > 800 mg (24-hour urine collection) (kidney stones, gout)
- Calcium: < 100 or > 250 mg (24-hour urine collection) (hyperparathyroidism, osteoporosis, excess vitamin D, excess dietary calcium, dehydration)
- Catecholamines: > 100 mcg (24-hour urine collection) (pheochromocytoma)
- Epinephrine: > 20 mcg (24-hour urine collection) (infection, stress, trauma)
- Norepinephrine: > 100 mcg (24-hour urine collection) (infection, stress, trauma)
- Dopamine: < 65 or > 400 mcg (24-hour urine collection) (infection, stress, trauma)
- Normetanephrine: < 10 or > 80 mcg (24-hour urine collection) (infection, stress, trauma)
- Metanephrine: > 1.3 mg (24-hour urine collection) (pheochromocytoma)
- Vanillylmandelic acid: > 6.8 mg (24-hour urine collection) (pheochromocytoma)

- Cortisol: > 100 mcg (24-hour urine collection) (Cushing syndrome)
- Phosphate: < 0.9 or > 1.3 g (24-hour urine collection) (kidney disorder, hyperparathyroidism, osteomalacia)
- Potassium: < 25 or > 100 mEq/L (24-hour urine collection) (kidney disorder)
- Sodium: < 40 or > 220 mEq (24-hour urine collection) (indicate high blood pressure, heart disease, or kidney disorder)
- Microalbumin: > 30 mg (24-hour urine collection) (kidney disorder or diabetic nephropathy)

Teach the Patient

- Explain
  - Why the test is being performed.
  - What the patient will experience during the test.
  - That the patient will not feel any pain during the test.
  - How to perform the test.
  - That the patient should not exercise prior to the test.
  - That the patient should not take the test if she is menstruating.
  - That the patient should avoid eating blackberries, beets, or foods that might color urine.
  - That the patient should avoid usual exposure to sun.
  - That the patient should avoid extended bed rest.
  - That the patient should avoid ingesting nicotine or caffeine.
  - That the patient should keep warm during the test if catecholamine levels are being tested.
  - That the patient should avoid taking Dilantin, Pyridium, vitamin B, diuretics, rifampin, Trimpex, ascorbic acid, Probalan, Benemid, allopurinol, insulin, lithium, laxatives, steroids, antacids, NSAIDs, antibiotics, potassium supplements, growth hormones or parathyroid hormone, aspirin, antidepressants (including tricyclic), nitroglycerin, tetracycline, tricyclic, theophylline, cold and sinus medications, 2 weeks before the test.
  - That the patient should avoid taking sodium-based medication 2 weeks before the test.

22. Urine Culture and Sensitivity Test

A urine culture is ordered when the patient is suspected of having a urinary tract infection. A urine collection is placed in an environment conducive to the growth of microorganisms for 3 days. The urine is examined to identify the presence and the type of microorganism. Once the microorganism is identified, a sensitivity test is performed to determine the medication that kills the microorganism.

What Is Being Examined?

- Existence of microorganisms in urine

How Is the Procedure Performed?

- The patient washes hands.
- The patient opens the collection cup without touching the inside of the cup.
- Clean the urethral area with an antiseptic.
- Do not touch the cup to the urethra or any skin when collecting the sample.
- Do not contaminate the urine sample with feces, pubic hair, or other substances.
- If the sample becomes contaminated, then begin again with a new collection cup.
- Urinate for 5 seconds making sure no skin aside from the urethra touches the urine.
- Move the collection cup into the urine stream.
- Do not touch the collection cup to the urethra or any skin.
- Remove the collection cup and continue urinating.
- Place the lid on the collection cup.
- Refrigerate the collection cup until the sample is sent to the laboratory.

NURSING ALERT

A sterile sample may be taken from a Foley catheter.

Rationale for the Test

- To assess the existence and type of microorganism in a patient with a urinary tract infection.
- To assess the medication to use to treat the urinary tract infection.

Nursing Implications

- Determine if the patient
  - Has collected the urine properly
  - Has taken antibiotics, vitamin C, or diuretics

Understanding the Results

- The collection takes a few seconds. Results are known within 3 days.
- Normal (negative) test results indicate
  - No microorganism is present in the urine collection.
- Abnormal (positive) test results indicate
  - Microorganisms are present in the urine collection.

Teach the Patient

- Explain
  - Why the test is being performed.
  - What the patient will experience during the test.
  - That the patient will not feel any pain during the test.
  - How to perform the test.
  - Should not take antibiotics, vitamin C, or diuretics before the test.

Summary

When a patient reports abnormal feeling in the chest, abdomen, or urinary tract, the healthcare provider can hone in on the problem by performing one or more tests and procedures.

In this chapter, you learned about tests for the UGI tract, thyroid gland, liver, gallbladder, kidneys, spleen, urinary tract, and other organs in the upper part of the body.

You learned how the healthcare provider looks down the esophagus to examine the stomach, duodenum, and the bile and pancreatic ducts and how to take a biopsy or, in some cases, remove an obstruction.

There are several tests used to assess pulmonary function. These tests measure the carbon dioxide and oxygen exchange and the lungs' capability to expand and retract. In addition, these tests also examine blood flow to the lungs. Blood flow to the lungs is monitored by a lung scan and by performing a pulmonary angiogram to identify restriction or blockage of blood flow to the lungs.

You also learned there are a number of procedures that can be performed to restore pulmonary function or remove diseased tissue. For example, a bronchoscope is used to view the respiratory tract and remove obstructions or take tissue samples. A thoracotomy is a surgical procedure performed to remove a portion or the entire diseased lung. A thoracentesis is performed to drain excess pleural fluid from the pleural space enabling the patient's lungs to fully expand.

And you learned how scans of the liver, spleen, gallbladder, and kidney using contrast material highlight structural problems within the organ. You also learned about procedures that can temporarily or permanently repair a problem, whether it is removing a cancerous thyroid gland, or a tumor from the bladder, or fixing urinary incontinence.

QUIZ

1. **What is a V/Q scan?**
   A. A common lung scan in which a perfusion scan is performed and then a ventilation scan is performed
   B. A common lung scan in which a ventilation scan is performed and then a perfusion scan is performed
   C. A scan that measures the volume and quantity of a lung
   D. None of the above

2. **What test is performed if the healthcare provider suspects a pulmonary embolus?**
   A. Bronchoscopy
   B. Lung scan
   C. Pulmonary function test
   D. Thoracotomy

3. **What is the reason for administering the V/Q scan?**

   A. To assess for a pulmonary embolus

   B. To assess the capacity and function of the lung

   C. To assess vital capacity

   D. To assess for cardiac inflections

4. **What do normal results for a pulmonary function test depend on?**

   A. Patient's age, height, sex, weight, and race

   B. Laboratory standard

   C. If the patient wears dentures

   D. If the patient is a smoker

5. **During a 24-hour urine collection, urine from the first time the patient urinated should be**

   A. Refrigerated

   B. Stored in a gallon container

   C. Discarded

   D. All of the above

6. **Why might a whole body thyroid scan be ordered?**

   A. To assess for thyroid cancer metastasis

   B. To assess for hyperthyroidism

   C. To assess for hypothyroidism

   D. None of the above

7. **A total thyroxine test is used to determine**

   A. The total amount of thyroxine that is missing from the patient

   B. The amount of thyroxine that is not bound to globulin

   C. The amount of thyroxine that is attached to globulin and that is not bound to globulin

   D. All of the above

8. **How is the cause of xerostomia determined?**

   A. Using the thyroid gland scan

   B. Using the salivary gland scan

   C. Using the liver scan

   D. Using the bladder scan

9. **What is the purpose of the renin assay test?**

   A. To determine the underlying cause of hypertension

   B. To determine the underlying cause of hypotension

C. To determine the underlying cause of renal disease

D. To determine the underlying cause of liver disease

10. **Prior to taking the urine culture and sensitivity test the patient should**

    A. Take antibiotics

    B. Not take antibiotics

    C. Avoid eating for 48 hours prior to the test

    D. None of the above

ANSWERS

1. B. A common lung scan, in which a ventilation scan is performed and then a perfusion scan is performed.
2. B. Lung scan.
3. A. To assess for a pulmonary embolus.
4. A. Patient's age, height, sex, weight, and race.
5. C. Discarded.
6. A. To assess for thyroid cancer metastasis.
7. C. The amount of thyroxine that is attached to globulin and that is not bound to globulin.
8. B. Using the salivary gland scan.
9. A. To determine the underlying cause of hypertension.
10. B. Not take antibiotics.

Skin, Muscle, and Bone Tests

LEARNING OBJECTIVES

1. Allergy Skin Testing
2. Bone Mineral Density (BMD)
3. Bone Scan
4. Chemical Peel
5. Dermabrasion
6. Mantoux Skin Test
7. Wound Culture

KEY WORDS

Bacillus Calmette-Guérin (BCG) vaccination

Conductive velocity

Curettage

Dual-energy X-ray absorptiometry (DEXA)

Dual-photo absorptiometry (DPA)

Exfoliates

Glycolic acid

Intradermal test

Liquid nitrogen

Peripheral dual-energy X-ray absorptiometry (P-DEXA)

Phenol

Quantitative computed tomography (QCT)

Retin-A

Skin patch test

Skin prick test

Spinal stenosis

Tretinoin cream

Trichloroacetic acid (TCA)

T-score

Z-score

Skin is the largest and the most visible organ in the body and is susceptible to wrinkles, blemishes, growths including both nonmelanoma and melanoma, and infection. Healthcare providers perform an assortment of tests and procedures to diagnose and treat skin conditions.

Lesions, warts, and blemishes that make skin unsightly and unhealthy can be removed by performing one of a number of procedures. For example, undesired tissue can be frozen with cryosurgery and removed, or layers of skin can be peeled away using chemicals or micrographic surgery. Layers can also be removed using curettage, electrosurgery, or the dermabrasion procedure where a rotating burr scrapes scars and aging skin to encourage new skin growth.

Melanoma and nonmelanoma skin cancer affects many patients. The healthcare provider can cure or minimize discomfort of this condition by performing a skin excision where the tumor is surgically removed.

Infected skin can be treated once the microorganism that causes the infection is identified. The healthcare provider is able to identify the microorganism by performing a wound culture, where a sample of the infected tissue is placed in an environment that is favorable for the growth of microorganism (culture) which is then identified. Once the laboratory determines the medication which will fight the microorganism, the medication is administered to find out whether it actually kills the microorganism.

Skin is also a perfect site for testing of allergic reactions. There are several tests that healthcare providers administer to the skin to identify allergens that cause the patient to develop an allergic reaction. The skin is also the site of the Mantoux skin test to determine if the patient has ever been exposed to *Mycobacterium tuberculosis*.

Aching bones and muscles might be from a cause other than overexercising. It could be a sign of an underlying disorder that needs immediate medical attention. Healthcare providers are able to assess the reason for the patient's discomfort by testing his/her bones and muscles.

Healthcare providers have an assortment of tests and procedures that are used to investigate signs of a disorder. An image of the bone can be taken by using a bone scan where a radioactive tracer highlights the structure of the bone or a myelogram that uses contrast material to bring out the structure of the spine into view. An arthrogram is used to create an image of soft tissues and structures of a joint. A bone mineral density test is ordered to determine the thickness of bone, looking for the first sign of osteoporosis.

When X-ray, ultrasound, and other imaging technologies indicate something is abnormal, the healthcare provider may perform arthroscopy to look directly into the joint or a bone biopsy, or bone marrow aspiration to take samples of suspicious tissue.

Once a diagnosis is made, there are a number of procedures that the healthcare provider can perform to either fix the disorder or reduce the impact of the disorder on the patient's daily activities. If the patient has a herniated disc, the healthcare provider can perform a discectomy to remove all or part of the disc. The healthcare provider can fuse together bones or use arthroplasty to reconstruct a joint. Discomfort from spinal stenosis can be reduced by performing a decompressive laminectomy that removes the lamina that is causing pressure on the nerve.

You will learn about these tests and procedures in this chapter.

1. Allergy Skin Testing

An allergen is a substance that causes an immune reaction. Allergy skin testing is performed to identify allergens. There are three types of skin testing for allergens. These are

- Skin patch test: This test is used to identify allergens that cause contact dermatitis and requires the placement of a pad that contains an allergen solution on the skin for 72 hours. An allergic reaction occurs if the patient is allergic to the allergen.
- Skin prick test: This test requires that a drop of an allergen solution be placed on the patient's skin. The skin is scratched allowing the allergen solution to penetrate. A wheal occurs if the patient is allergic to the allergen.

- Intradermal test: This test requires that a small amount of an allergen solution be injected into the dermal layer of the skin. A wheal occurs if the patient is allergic to the allergen.

What Is Being Examined?

- Skin

How Is the Procedure Performed?

- The patient signs a consent form.
- The patient removes his/her clothes from the affected area.
- The patient lies on a table.
- The site is cleaned with an antiseptic.
- Skin prick test and intradermal test
  - The allergen is introduced into the skin.
  - The healthcare provider examines the site for wheals in 15 minutes.
- Skin patch test
  - The allergen-containing pad is applied to the site.
  - The pad is removed in 72 hours.
  - The site is assessed for redness and wheals.

Rationale for the Test

- To identify a source of a patient's allergic reaction

Nursing Implications

- Determine if the patient
  - Has signed a consent form
  - Has not been taking anticoagulant medication such as Plavix, Coumadin, heparin, or aspirin
  - Can lie still
  - Does not develop an itch at the site
  - Has not been taking antihistamines
  - Has not been taking antidepressants

Understanding the Results

- The procedure takes less than 1 hour. Result is immediate except for the skin patch test, which takes 72 hours.
- Normal (negative) test results indicate
  - No change to the site
- Abnormal (positive) test results indicate
  - Wheals appear at the site.

Teach the Patient

- Explain
  - Why the procedure is being performed.
  - What the patient will experience during the procedure.
  - That the patient will not feel any pain during the procedure except for a pinch if the intradermal test or the skin prick test is performed.
  - The patient must keep the site clean and dry until the site is assessed by the healthcare provider.
  - The patient should not scratch the site.
  - The patient should not take antihistamines 2 weeks prior to the test.
  - The patient should not take antidepressants 2 weeks prior to the test.

> **NURSING ALERT**
>
> The patient should call the healthcare provider if experiencing itchiness while the skin patch test is being performed.

2. Bone Mineral Density

The bone mineral density (BMD) test measures the density of bone to assess if the patient has osteopenia or osteoporosis. A low bone density might result in an increased risk for fracture. There are five ways to measure BMD. These are

- Ultrasound: This test uses sound waves to determine the density of bone. However, this method does not assess hip and the spine, which are bones that commonly fracture because of low BMD.

- Dual-photo absorptiometry (DPA): This method uses a low-dose radio-active tracer to measure bone density in all bones including the hip and spine.
- Quantitative computed tomography (QCT): This method measures the density of the vertebra; however, this is less accurate than the DPA, DEXA, and P-DEXA methods.
- Dual-energy X-ray absorptiometry (DEXA): This method uses two X-ray beams to measure bone density and can measure up to 2% bone loss, making it the most accurate way to measure BMD.
- Peripheral dual-energy X-ray absorptiometry (P-DEXA): This method measures bone density in arms and legs, but cannot be used to measure the bone density of the hip or spine.

What Is Being Examined?

- BMD

How Is the Procedure Performed?

- The patient signs a consent form.
- The patient lies on a table.
- The ultrasound, CT, or X-ray device scans the site.
- The insertion site is cleaned with an anesthetic.

Rationale for the Test

- To assess for osteoporosis
- To assess the progression of osteoporosis
- To assess the impact of long-term treatment with corticosteroids

Nursing Implications

- Determine if the patient
  - Has signed a consent form
  - Is pregnant
  - Is able to lie still
  - Has had broken bones

- Has arthritis
- Has had bone replacement
- Has had a barium test within 2 weeks of the test

Understanding the Results

- The procedure takes less than 1 hour. Results are ready within 2 weeks of the procedure.
- The patient is given a T-score.
  - The T-score compares the patient's BMD with the average healthy 30-year-old's T-score.
  - A negative T-score indicates that the patient's BMD is less than the T-score of the average healthy 30-year-old.
  - A positive T-score indicates that the patient's BMD is greater than the T-score of the average healthy 30-year-old.
- The patient is given a Z-score. The Z-score compares the patient to those of the same age, sex, and race.
  - A negative Z-score indicates that the patient's BMD is less than the Z-score of the average person of his/her age, sex, and race.
  - A positive Z-score indicates that the patient's BMD is greater than the Z-score of the average person of his/her age, sex, and race.
- Normal test results indicate
  - T-Score
    - Normal is within +/−1 T-score of the average healthy 30-year-old's T-score.
  - Z-Score
    - Normal is within +/−1 Z-score of the average person of his/her age, sex, and race.
- Abnormal test results indicate
  - T-Score
    - 2.5 or less than T-score of the average healthy 30-year-old's T-score indicates osteoporosis.
  - Z-Score
    - 2.5 or less than Z-score of the average person of his/her age, sex, and race.

Teach the Patient

- Explain
  - Why the procedure is being performed.
  - What the patient will experience during the procedure.
  - That the patient will not feel any pain.

3. Bone Scan

A bone scan assesses the infection, trauma, and metastasized cancer growth to the bone. A radioactive tracer is injected in the patient's vein. The tracer is removed from the blood into the bone. A gamma camera takes an image of the tracer as the tracer is absorbed. Lack of absorption indicates bone infarction and possibly cancer. Areas of high absorption might indicate an infection, tumor, or fracture.

What Is Being Examined?

- The bone

How Is the Procedure Performed?

- The patient signs a consent form.
- The patient removes his/her clothes.
- The patient lies on a table.
- The injection site is cleaned.
- The patient is injected with the radioactive tracer.
- The gamma camera is moved into position.
- Images are taken immediately, then periodically for up to 5 hours.
- The patient should drink lots of fluid to flush the tracer from his/her body.
- The patient should flush the toilet quickly after urinating and defecating since the tracer is excreted in urine and feces for 2 days following the test.

Rationale for the Test

- Determine if cancer has metastasized.
- Assess for bone infection.

Nursing Implications

- Determine if the patient
  - Has signed a consent form
  - Has emptied his/her bladder
  - Has allergies
  - Is pregnant
  - Is breast-feeding
  - Has recently had a barium test performed within 4 days prior to the test
  - Has not been taking anticoagulant medication such as Plavix, Coumadin, heparin, or aspirin for 2 weeks prior to the test
  - Has not taken Pepto-Bismol for 48 hours before the test

Understanding the Results

- The procedure takes less than 1 hour. Results are known within 2 days.
- Normal test results indicate
  - The bone is normal.
- Abnormal test results indicate
  - Cancer has metastasized to the bone.
  - The bone is inflamed.
  - A bone infarction is identified.

Teach the Patient

- Explain
  - Why the procedure is being performed.
  - What the patient will experience during the procedure.
  - That the patient will not feel any pain during the procedure except for a pinch when the tracer is injected into his/her vein.
  - That the patient must sign a consent form.
  - That the patient should not take anticoagulant medication such as Plavix, Coumadin, heparin, or aspirin for 2 weeks prior to the test.
  - That the patient should not take Pepto-Bismol for 48 hours before the test.

- That the patient must empty his/her bladder before the test.
- That the patient should drink lots of fluids to flush the tracer following the test.
- That the patient should flush the toilet immediately after urinating and defecating.
- That the patient should wash his/her hands thoroughly after urinating and defecating.
- That the patient should apply a warm compress to the injection site if there is swelling.
- If the patient is breast-feeding, breast milk must be discarded for 2 days after the scan.

4. Chemical Peel

A chemical peel is a procedure that exfoliates injured or dead skin, enabling new skin to replace it. There are three types of chemical peels. These are

- Superficial: This procedure removes the surface layer of the skin for a smoother, brighter appearance and uses glycolic acid or dry ice for the peel.
- Medium: This procedure is commonly used to smooth fine wrinkles, remove blemishes, and treat pigment problems. It uses trichloroacetic acid (TCA) for the peel.
- Deep: This procedure is commonly used to correct coarse wrinkles and blotches on the face only and uses phenol for the peel. New skin might be lighter in tone because the skin loses some ability to produce pigment.

> **NURSING ALERT**
>
> A chemical peel might change the patient's skin tone and result in scarring and cold sores. It might cause flaking and dryness.

What Is Being Examined?

- Skin

How Is the Procedure Performed?

- The patient moisturizes his/her skin twice a day for 3 weeks prior to the procedure.

- The patient is administered acyclovir 2 weeks prior to the procedure to prevent a viral infection.
- The patient signs a consent form.
- The patient removes his/her clothes from the affected area.
- The patient lies on a table.
- The healthcare provider may test the peel on skin at a less visible location.
- The site is cleaned with an antiseptic.
- Superficial peel
  - The chemical is applied on to the site using an applicator.
  - The chemical remains on the site for several minutes.
  - Alcohol or water is applied to the site to neutralize the chemical.
  - The chemical is removed by wiping the skin.
  - Discomfort is relieved by using a fan.
- Medium peel
  - The patient is administered a sedative.
  - The chemical is applied on to the site using an applicator.
  - The chemical remains on the site for several minutes longer than in a superficial peel.
  - Alcohol or water is applied to the site to neutralize the chemical.
  - The chemical is removed by wiping the skin.
  - Discomfort is relieved by using a cool compress.
- Deep peel
  - The patient is administered a general anesthetic.
  - The patient is connected to an ECG to monitor his/her heart.
  - The patient is connected to a pulse oximeter to monitor the oxygen level in the blood.
  - A breathing tube is inserted into the patient's mouth.
  - The chemical is applied on to a small area of the site using an applicator.
  - The chemical remains on the site for several minutes.
  - Alcohol or water is applied to the site to neutralize the chemical.
  - The chemical is removed by wiping the skin.
  - The healthcare provider waits 15 minutes before repeating treatment to another small area of the site in order to prevent the building of chemical on the skin.

- The healthcare provider may cover the area with an ointment or tape. The ointment is removed with water 24 hours following the procedure. The tape is removed 2 days following the procedure.
- The patient might be told to be administered Retin-A on the site after the peel to speed up healing.

Rationale for the Test

- Cosmetic improvement of the skin

Nursing Implications

- Determine if the patient
  - Has signed a consent form
  - Has not been taking anticoagulant medication such as Plavix, Coumadin, heparin, or aspirin
  - Can lie still
  - Has moisturized his/her skin twice a day for 3 weeks prior to the procedure
  - Has administered acyclovir 2 weeks prior to the procedure to prevent a viral infection

Understanding the Results

- The procedure takes less than 2 hours. Result is realized in 6 months following the procedure.
- Normal test results indicate
  - The wrinkle or the blemish is removed.
- Abnormal test results indicate
  - Scarring occurred

Teach the Patient

- Explain
  - Why the procedure is being performed.
  - What the patient will experience during the procedure.
  - That the patient will not feel any pain during the procedure.

- That the patient must moisturize his/her skin twice a day for 3 weeks prior to the procedure.
- That the patient must be administered acyclovir 2 weeks prior to the procedure to prevent a viral infection.
- That the patient might have to administer Retin-A on the site to encourage healing.
- That the patient must apply tretinoin cream every night on the site beginning 3 weeks following the procedure.
- That the patient must clean the site frequently following the procedure.
- That the patient must avoid exposure to the sun until the site heals.
- That the patient must use sun block every day since new skins can be damaged by the sun.
- For superficial peel, the skin is pink but eventually fades to your natural skin tone. Normal activities can be resumed immediately.
- For medium peel, it takes 7 days to heal during which the site is swollen and reddish. A crust forms over the site, which will fall off within 10 days following the procedure. Normal activities can resume in a week.
- For deep peel, it takes 2 weeks for regrowth to occur. The skin is reddening for 2 months. Healing takes less than 6 months. The patient will be prescribed pain medication for discomfort, antibiotics for infection, and corticosteroids for swelling. The patient can reduce crusting at the site by showering several times a day. Normal activities can resume in 2 weeks.

NURSING ALERT

The patient should call his/her healthcare provider if he/she has fever and drainage from the site following the procedure. The patient should also call his/her healthcare provider if the site remains red for longer than 2 months following the procedure.

5. Dermabrasion

Dermabrasion is a procedure that removes the upper layers of damaged skin caused by scars and aging to encourage new skin growth. The procedure is performed by using a rotating burr to remove damaged tissue.

What Is Being Examined?

- Skin

How Is the Procedure Performed?

- The patient signs a consent form.
- The patient removes his/her clothes from the affected area.
- The patient will lie on a table.
- The site is cleaned with an antiseptic.
- A local anesthetic is administered to the patient.
- The skin is then hardened by using liquid nitrogen or ice packs.
- A rotating burr is used to scrap the skin.
- An antibiotic-treated dressing is applied to the site.

Rationale for the Test

- To remove scars
- To remove growths from the upper layer of the skin
- To remove wrinkles

Nursing Implications

- Determine if the patient
  - Has signed a consent form
  - Has not been taking anticoagulant medication such as Plavix, Coumadin, heparin, or aspirin
  - Can lie still
  - Has not used isotretinoin
  - Has not had a face lift
  - Has not had active herpes
  - Has not had an immune disorder

Understanding the Results

- The procedure takes less than 1 hour. Result is immediate.
- Normal test results indicate
  - The skin is removed.

- Abnormal test results indicate
  - Not all of the skin is removed.

Teach the Patient

- Explain
  - Why the procedure is being performed.
  - What the patient will experience during the procedure.
  - That the patient will not feel any pain during the procedure except for a pinch when the local anesthetic is administered.
  - The patient must keep the site clean and dry until it heals.
  - The patient should not scratch or remove the scab that forms over the site.
  - The site will heal within 6 weeks following the procedure.
  - There might be a scar or skin tone change to the site.
  - The procedure may not produce the desired result.
  - Apply sunscreen every day.

> ### NURSING ALERT
>
> The patient should call his/her healthcare provider if he/she has fever and drainage from the site following the procedure.

6. Mantoux Skin Test

The Mantoux skin test determines if the patient has ever been exposed to *Mycobacterium tuberculosis*. The healthcare provider injects the purified protein derivative (PPD), with the *M tuberculosis* antigen, into the patient's forearm. If the patient develops a wheal within 48 hours indicating a positive immune response, then he/she either is or had been infected with *M tuberculosis*. A chest X-ray is taken to diagnose a current infection of *M tuberculosis* should there be a positive immune response to the test.

What Is Being Examined?

- Antibodies to the *M tuberculosis* antigen

How Is the Procedure Performed?

- The patient signs a consent form.
- The patient exposes his/her forearm.
- The site is cleaned with an antiseptic.
- A needle is inserted slightly under the upper layer of the skin.
- Purified protein derivative is injected.
- The site remains uncovered.

Rationale for the Test

- To identify if the patient is or was ever exposed to *M tuberculosis*

Nursing Implications

- Determine if the patient
  - Has signed a consent form.
  - Has not been taking anticoagulant medication such as Plavix, Coumadin, heparin, or aspirin.
  - Has not had the bacillus Calmette-Guérin (BCG) vaccination. Patients who have had this vaccination will likely test positive.
  - Has not taken corticosteroids.
  - Has not had an immune-compromised disease.
  - Has not had a measles, mumps, rubella, chickenpox, or polio vaccine 6 weeks prior to the test.
  - Is older than 3 months of age.
  - Has not had a prior positive PPD and should not have another PPD.

Understanding the Results

- The procedure takes less than 10 minutes. Result is known in 48 hours.
- Normal (negative) test results indicate
  - No change to the site
- Abnormal (positive) test results indicate
  - Wheals appear at the site.

> **NURSING ALERT**
>
> A negative test result does not mean that the patient is not infected with M tuberculosis. It can take up to 10 weeks following the infection for the immune system to develop antibodies.

Teach the Patient

- Explain
  - Why the procedure is being performed.
  - What the patient will experience during the procedure.
  - That the patient will not feel any pain during the procedure except for a pinch when the needle is inserted beneath the skin.
  - That the patient must keep the site clean and dry.
  - That the patient should not scratch the site.
  - The patient must return in 48 hours to have the healthcare provider assess the test results.

7. Wound Culture

A wound culture is ordered when the patient is suspected of having a skin infection. A tissue sample of the infected area is taken and placed in an environment conducive to the growth of microorganisms for 3 days. The tissue sample is then examined to identify the presence and the type of microorganism. Once the microorganism is identified, a sensitivity test is usually performed to determine the medication that kills the microorganism.

What Is Being Examined?

- Existence of microorganisms in infected skin

How Is the Procedure Performed?

- The healthcare provider swabs the wound with a sterile swab to collect a tissue sample. More than 1 sample might be taken if the healthcare provider suspects that the microorganism may be aerobic (grows in the presence of oxygen) or anaerobic (grows without the presence of oxygen) bacteria.

- The sterile swab is placed in either an aerobic or anaerobic culture tube and sent to the laboratory.
- The sample(s) is then placed in a culture dish in an environment conductive to growing microorganism.
- After 3 days, tests are performed to identify the microorganism.
- Medication is applied to a portion of the culture to determine which medication kills the microorganism. Preliminary results are known quickly, but final results can take 72 hours or longer.

Rationale for the Test

- To assess the existence and type of microorganism in a patient with a skin infection
- To assess the medication used to treat the skin infection

Nursing Implications

- Determine if the patient has not taken antibiotics or applied an antiseptic to the wound prior to the test.

Understanding the Results

- The collection takes a few seconds. Results are known within 3 days.
- Normal (negative) test results indicate
  - No microorganism present in the tissue sample
- Abnormal (positive) test results indicate
  - Microorganisms are present in the tissue sample.

Teach the Patient

- Explain
- Why the test is being performed.
- What the patient will experience during the test.
- That the patient will not feel any pain during the test.
- That the patient should not use antibiotics or apply antiseptic to the wound before the test.

Summary

Healthcare providers perform an assortment of tests and procedures to diagnose and treat skin conditions.

Undesired skin tissue can be frozen with cryosurgery and removed. Layers of skin can be peeled away using chemicals, Mohs micrographic surgery, curettage, electrosurgery, or by using the dermabrasion procedure where a rotating burr scrapes scars from aging skin to encourage new skin growth.

The healthcare provider can cure or minimize discomfort of melanoma and nonmelanoma skin cancer by performing a skin excision from where the tumor is surgically removed.

The microorganism that causes a skin infection is identified by performing a wound culture. In a wound culture, a sample of the infected tissue is placed in an environment conducive for growing microorganisms. The microorganism is then identified and medication is administered to the microorganism to determine which medication kills the microorganism.

Skin is used to test for allergic reactions. There are several tests that healthcare providers administer to the skin to identify allergens that cause the patient to develop an allergic reaction. The skin is also the site of the Mantoux skin test to determine if the patient has ever been exposed to *M tuberculosis*.

Practitioners have an assortment of tests and procedures that are used to investigate signs of a bone disorder. Initially they will order an image be taken of the suspected structure. These include a myelogram that uses contrast material to highlight structures in the spine, or a bone scan that uses a radioactive tracer to make the structure of the bone appear on a video screen. The healthcare provider may also order an arthrogram to visualize the soft tissues and structures of a joint.

The thickness of bone is a factor that determines the risk of spontaneous stress factors, especially with the elderly who are susceptible to osteoporosis. The healthcare provider assesses the thickness of bone by ordering a BMD test.

When imaging technology indicates something might be abnormal, the healthcare provider usually performs arthroscopy to look directly into the joint or a bone biopsy, or bone marrow aspiration to take samples of suspicious tissue.

The healthcare provider can perform procedures to either fix the disorder or reduce the impact of the disorder on the patient's daily activities. For example, a herniated disc is repaired by performing a discectomy to remove all or part of the disc. The healthcare provider can fuse together bones or use arthroplasty to reconstruct a joint. Discomfort from spinal stenosis can be reduced by performing a decompressive laminectomy that removes the lamina that is causing pressure on the nerve.

QUIZ

1. **What parts of the body are measured using P-DEXA?**

   A. Arms and legs

   B. Spine and arms

   C. Hip and spine

   D. Hip and legs

2. **What can produce a false-positive result in the bone mineral density (BMD) test?**

   A. The patient has arthritis.

   B. The patient has a T-score of 1.

   C. The patient has a Z-score of 1.

   D. The patient has an X-score of less than 1.

3. **Chemical peel changes skin tone.**

   A. True

   B. False

4. **How does the dermabrasion improve the appearance of skin?**

   A. It removes the outer layer of skin, enabling new skin to grow.

   B. It removes the inner layer of skin, enabling new skin to grow.

   C. It uses a chemical to remove the outer layer of skin, enabling new skin to grow.

   D. All of the above.

5. **Why is not the Mantoux skin test used to diagnose tuberculosis?**

   A. A positive result indicates that the patient has developed antibodies to *M tuberculosis* antigen possibly from a previous exposure to *M tuberculosis*.

   B. A negative result indicates that the patient has not developed antibodies to *M tuberculosis* antigen; however, the immune system can take up to 10 weeks to develop the antibodies following the infection.

   C. Diagnosis is made using an X-ray.

   D. All of the above.

6. **What allergy test requires that an allergen-containing pad be applied to the patient's skin?**

   A. Skin patch test

   B. Skin prick test

   C. Intradermal test

   D. The Q patch test

7. **Why the patient is usually administered acyclovir 2 weeks prior to a chemical peel?**
   A. To prevent a fungal infection
   B. To prevent a bacterial infection
   C. To prevent a viral infection
   D. To reduce bleeding during the procedure

8. **Why would a patient be administered Retin-A following a chemical peel?**
   A. To reduce bleeding following the procedure
   B. To prevent an infection
   C. To encourage healing
   D. None of the above

9. **What would you recommend if the site of a chemical peel remained red for 3 months following the procedure?**
   A. Rush the patient to the hospital.
   B. Contact the healthcare provider immediately.
   C. Place a topical antibiotic on the site.
   D. Do nothing.

10. **What is the allergy test called where a drop of allergen solution is placed on the skin and the skin is scratched?**
    A. Skin patch test
    B. Skin prick test
    C. Intradermal test
    D. The Q patch test

ANSWERS

1. A. Arms and legs.
2. A. The patient has arthritis.
3. A. True.
4. A. It removes the outer layer of skin, enabling new skin to grow.
5. D. All of the above.
6. A. Skin patch test.
7. C. To prevent a viral infection.
8. C. To encourage healing.
9. B. Contact the healthcare provider immediately.
10. B. Skin prick test.

chapter 20

Sinus, Ears, Nose, Throat (ENT) Tests and Procedures

LEARNING OBJECTIVES

1. Audiometric Testing
2. Electroencephalogram (EEG)
3. Sinus X-ray
4. Sputum Culture
5. Sputum Cytology
6. Throat Culture
7. Tympanometry

KEY WORDS

Acoustic immittance

Auditory brain stem response (ABR)

Otitis media

Otoacoustic emissions (OAE)

Pure-tone audiometry

Saliva

Speech reception/word recognition

Sputum

Tuning fork test

Tympanometer

Vestibular test

Whispered speech test

Snoring, headaches, frequent infections, and turning the volume on the TV high could be signs of an underlying problem that might be prevented or resolved by performing one of several procedures that you will learn about in this chapter.

Snoring is annoying to those who have to listen to it and can also be a symptom of something more ominous such as obstructed sleep apnea. The healthcare provider can fix this problem by performing an uvulopalatopharyngoplasty or radiofrequency palatoplasty that focus on the underlying cause of snoring.

There can be a number of reasons why a patient has a headache. One common cause is sinusitis. The healthcare provider can perform a number of tests to assess the sinus, including a sinus endoscopy, sinus X-ray, and a sinus aspiration where a sample of sinus is sent to the laboratory for a culture and sensitivity test. If problem is a blockage of the sinus rather than an infection, the healthcare provider might perform sinus surgery to remove the blockage.

The headache may be caused by something more involved than sinusitis. The healthcare provider might order an electroencephalogram, which records electrical activity in the brain and can help the healthcare provider diagnose the underlying cause of the headache and other neural symptoms.

Frequent infections can be challenging to resolve. The healthcare provider might order a throat culture, sputum culture, or sputum cytology study to identify the cause of the infection and the mediation that will kill the infecting microorganism. In addition, the healthcare provider may perform a procedure to prevent reinfection. The most common are a tonsillectomy tympanostomy tube and a tympanocentesis.

Decreased hearing can be caused by a number of factors, including a buildup of cerumen in the ear canal, disorders of the eardrum, or a neurological problem. The healthcare provider can perform tympanometry and audiometric tests to determine the cause of hearing loss.

These and other tests and procedures are discussed in this chapter.

1. Audiometric Testing

Audiometric testing determines the degree with which a patient can hear. Hearing loss is the patient's inability to hear or understand a range of sound frequencies due to either structural problems with the ear or neural problems preventing the brain from receiving impulses from the ear or properly interpreting those impulses. There are eight types of audiometric tests. These are

- Pure-tone audiometry: This test determines sound frequencies that can be heard by the patient.
- Whispered speech test: This test determines if the patient can hear low-volume sounds spoken behind him.
- Speech reception/word recognition: This test is used to identify sensorineural hearing loss.
- Tuning fork test: This test determines if the hearing problem is caused by sound being received by nerves in the ear or nerve problems.
- Auditory brain stem response (ABR): This test is used to detect sensorineural hearing problems.
- Otoacoustic emissions (OAE): This test identifies hearing problems in newborns.
- Vestibular test: This test identifies problems with the inner ear.
- Acoustic immittance: This test assesses the middle ear's ability to conduct sound.

What Is Being Examined?

- Hearing

How Is the Procedure Performed?

- The patient signs a consent form.
- Pure-tone audiometry
  - The patient wears headphones that are connected to an audiometer.
  - The audiometer produces a series of tones.
  - The patient indicates which tones are heard.
- Whispered speech test
  - The patient places his/her finger in the ear canal of one ear.

- The healthcare provider stands 2 ft behind the patient.
- The healthcare provider whispers words.
- The patient indicates if he/she can hear those words.
- The test is repeated using the opposite ear.
- Speech reception/word recognition
  - The healthcare provider speaks familiar two-syllable words at varied degrees of loudness.
  - The patient is asked to repeat those words.
  - The results are measured as the patient's spondee threshold.
- Tuning fork test
  - The healthcare provider places a vibrating tuning fork either behind the ear or on the patient's head.
  - The patient indicates when he/she hears the tuning fork.
- ABR
  - Electrodes are placed on the patient's ear lobe and scalp.
  - Earphones are placed in the patient's ears.
  - A clicking noise is sounded through the earphones.
  - The electrodes detect neural responses to the clicking noise and record the response on a graph.
- OAE
  - A microphone is placed in a newborn's ear.
  - A flexible probe is also placed in the baby's ear.
  - Sound is passed through the probe.
  - The microphone detects the response of inner ear to the sound.
- Vestibular test
  - The patient moves arms and legs, stands on one foot, walks heel-to-toe with his/her eyes open and then closed.
  - The patient's ability to keep his/her balance is assessed.
- Acoustic immittance
  - The ear canal is sealed closed using a soft-tip instrument.
  - Sound and air are directed toward the ear at different pressures.
  - A measurement is taken that registers how the middle ear relays sound.

Rationale for the Test

- To assess the patient's hearing
- To identify the underlying cause of hearing loss

Nursing Implications

- Determine if the patient
  - Has signed a consent form
  - Can sit still
  - Can respond to instructions
  - Can indicate if sound is heard

Understanding the Results

- The procedure takes less than 1 hour. Results are immediate.
- Normal test results indicate
  - Normal hearing
- Abnormal test results indicate
  - Structural or neurological problems cause reduced hearing ability.

Teach the Patient

- Explain
  - Why the procedure is being performed.
  - What the patient will experience during the procedure.
  - That the patient will not feel any pain during the procedure.

2. Electroencephalogram

Electroencephalogram (EEG) measures electrical activities of the brain using electrodes attached to the patient's head. Electrical activities are recorded and displayed on a video screen and stored in a computer.

> **NURSING ALERT**
>
> The healthcare provider may order an ambulatory EEG, which monitors electrical activities of the brain while the patient goes about normal daily activities.

What Is Being Examined?

- Electrical activities in the brain

How Is the Procedure Performed?

- The patient signs a consent form.
- The patient lies on a table.
- Twenty-five electrodes are attached to the patient's head using a paste.
- Wires connect the electrodes to the EEG.
- Electrical activity is measured.
- A strobe light might be displayed as the electrical activity is measured, if the stroboscopic simulation test is performed.
- Sleep might be induced with a sedative, if the sleep study is performed.
- The patient might be asked to hyperventilate.

Rationale for the Test

- To determine the underlying cause of narcolepsy
- To determine the underlying cause of seizures
- To assess if the patient has dementia
- To assess if the patient is brain-dead

Nursing Implications

- Determine if the patient
  - Has signed a consent form
  - Has taken tranquilizers, barbiturates, sedatives, seizure medication, or muscle relaxant prior to the test
  - Has ingested caffeine 8 hours before the test
  - Has not shampooed his/her hair the morning of the test
  - Has not applied creams, sprays, lotion, or oil on the scalp prior the test
  - Has not slept prior to the test, if the test is studying sleeping disorders
  - Has not moved during the test
  - Has normal body temperature

Understanding the Results

- The procedure takes less than 2 hours unless a sleep study is performed, which might take 8 hours. Results are available within 2 weeks.
- Normal test results indicate
  - Normal electrical activities
- Abnormal test results indicate
  - Abnormal electrical activities

Teach the Patient

- Explain
  - Why the procedure is being performed.
  - What the patient will experience during the procedure.
  - That the patient will not feel any pain during the procedure.
  - That the patient should not take tranquilizers, barbiturates, sedatives, seizure medication, or muscle relaxants prior to the test.
  - That the patient should not ingest caffeine 8 hours before the test.
  - That the patient should not shampoo his/her hair the morning of the test.
  - That the patient should not apply creams, sprays, lotion, or oil on the scalp prior the test.
  - That the patient should not sleep prior to the test, if the test is studying sleeping disorders.

3. Sinus X-ray

An X-ray of the sinus is ordered if the healthcare provider suspects that the patient has sinusitis or other conditions that might cause similar symptoms.

> **NURSING ALERT**
>
> The healthcare provider may also order a CT scan of the head, which provides clearer images of the sinus than an X-ray.

What Is Being Examined?

- Sinuses

How Is the Procedure Performed?

- The patient signs a consent form.
- The patient sits in front of the X-ray machine.
- Several X-rays are taken, each at a different angle.

Rationale for the Test

- To identify blockage in the sinus
- To diagnose sinusitis

Nursing Implications

- Determine if the patient
  - Has signed a consent form
  - Can sit still

Understanding the Results

- The procedure takes less than 30 minutes. Results are immediate.
- Normal test results indicate
  - Normal sinuses
- Abnormal test results indicate
  - A blockage is identified.
  - The patient has sinusitis.

Teach the Patient

- Explain
  - Why the test is being performed.
  - What the patient will experience during the test.
  - That the patient will not feel any pain during the test.

4. Sputum Culture

A sputum culture is ordered when the patient has a respiratory infection. A sample of sputum is collected in a sterile container and taken to the laboratory where the sample is placed in an environment conducive to the growth of microorganisms for 3 days. The sample is then examined to identify the presence and the type of microorganism. Once the microorganism is identified, a sensitivity test is usually performed to determine the medication that kills the microorganism.

> **NURSING ALERT**
>
> Sputum is not saliva. Sputum is produced in the respiratory system.

What Is Being Examined?

- Existence of microorganisms in the infected respiratory tract

How Is the Procedure Performed?

- The sample is taken immediately after the patient awakens from sleep.
- The patient removes dentures.
- The patient rinses his/her mouth with water.
- The patient coughs deeply to produce the sputum.
- If the patient is unable to produce the sputum, the healthcare provider may loosen sputum in the lungs by using a mist inhaler. If this does not produce the sputum, then the healthcare provider collects the sputum using a bronchoscope that is inserted into the patient's airway.
- The sample(s) is then placed in a culture dish in an environment conducive to growing microorganism.
- After 3 days, tests are performed to identify the microorganism.
- Medication is applied to a portion of the culture to determine which medication kills the microorganism.

Rationale for the Test

- To assess the existence and type of microorganism in a patient with a respiratory infection
- To assess the medication used to treat the respiratory infection

Nursing Implications

- Determine if the patient
  - Has not used mouthwash prior to collecting the sample

- Has not taken antibiotics prior to collecting the sample
- Has eaten or drunk 6 hours prior to collecting the sample, if the health-care provider is using a bronchoscope to collect the sample

Understanding the Results

- It takes a few seconds to collect the sample. Results are known within 3 days.
- Normal (negative) test results indicate
  - No microorganism is present in the sample.
- Abnormal (positive) test results indicate
  - Microorganisms are present in the sample.

Teach the Patient

- Explain
- Why the test is being performed.
- What the patient will experience during the test.
- That the patient will not feel any pain during the test.
- That the patient should not use antibiotics prior to the test.
- That the patient should not use mouthwash prior to collecting the sample.
- That the patient should cough deeply prior to taking the sample.
- That the patient should take the sample the first thing in the morning after awakening from sleeping.
- That the patient should make sure the sample is delivered to the laboratory immediately after it is collected.
- That sputum is different from saliva.

5. Sputum Cytology

Sputum cytology is a procedure that examines cells contained in a sputum sample to assess for asbestosis, pneumonia, respiratory infection, tuberculosis, and lung cancer.

> **NURSING ALERT**
>
> Sputum is not saliva. Sputum is produced in the respiratory system.

What Is Being Examined?

- Cells in the sputum

How Is the Procedure Performed?

- The sample is taken immediately after the patient awakens from sleep.
- The patient removes dentures.
- The patient rinses his/her mouth with water.
- The patient coughs deeply to produce the sputum.
- If the patient is unable to produce the sputum, the healthcare provider may loosen sputum in the lungs by using a mist inhaler. If this doesn't produce the sputum, then the healthcare provider collects the sputum using a bronchoscope that is inserted into the patient's airway.
- The sample(s) is then viewed with a microscope to identify cells contained in the sputum.

Rationale for the Test

- To assess for lung cancer
- To assess for pneumonia
- To assess for asbestosis

Nursing Implications

- Determine if the patient
  - Has used mouthwash prior to collecting the sample
  - Has taken antibiotics prior to collecting the sample
  - Has eaten or drunk 6 hours prior to collecting the sample, if the healthcare provider is using a bronchoscope to collect the sample

Understanding the Results

- It takes a few seconds to collect the sample. Results are known within 3 days.
- Normal (negative) test results indicate
  - Normal cells in the sample
- Abnormal (positive) test results indicate
  - No respiratory cells in the sample

Teach the Patient

- Explain
  - Why the test is being performed.
  - What the patient will experience during the test.
  - That the patient will not feel any pain during the test.
  - That the patient should not use antibiotics prior to the test.
  - That the patient should not use mouthwash prior to collecting the sample.
  - That the patient should cough deeply prior to taking the sample.
  - That the patient should take the sample the first thing in the morning after awakening from sleep.
  - That the patient should make sure the sample is delivered to the laboratory immediately after the sample is collected.
  - That sputum is different from saliva.

6. Throat Culture

A throat culture is ordered when the patient has a throat infection. A tissue sample of the infected area is taken and placed in an environment conducive to the growth of microorganisms for 3 days. The tissue sample is then examined to identify the presence and the type of microorganism. Once the microorganism is identified, a sensitivity test is usually performed to determine the medication that kills the microorganism.

What Is Being Examined?

- Existence of microorganisms in the infected throat

How Is the Procedure Performed?

- The healthcare provider swabs the throat with a sterile swab to collect a tissue sample. More than 1 sample might be taken.
- The sterile swab is placed in a culture tube and sent to the laboratory.
- The sample(s) is then placed in a culture dish in an environment conducive to growing microorganism.
- After 3 days, tests are performed to identify the microorganism.
- Medication is applied to a portion of the culture to determine which medication kills the microorganism.

Rationale for the Test

- To assess the existence and type of microorganism in a patient with a throat infection.
- To assess the medication to use to treat the throat infection.

Nursing Implications

- Determine if the patient has taken antibiotics or applied an antiseptic to the throat prior to the test.

Understanding the Results

- It takes a few seconds to collect the specimen. Results are known within 3 days.
- Normal (negative) test results indicate
  - No microorganism is present in the sample.
- Abnormal (positive) test results indicate
  - Microorganisms are present in the sample.

Teach the Patient

- Explain
  - Why the test is being performed.
  - What the patient will experience during the test.
  - That the patient will not feel any pain during the test.
  - That the patient should not use antibiotics or apply antiseptic to the throat before the test.

7. Tympanometry

The tympanometry is a test to measure the eardrum's response to pressure and sound and assess if there is fluid behind the eardrum. It is ordered if the patient is suspected of having otitis media, hearing loss, fluid behind the eardrum, or blocked Eustachian tube.

> **NURSING ALERT**
>
> This test is frequently performed in children.

What Is Being Examined?

- The eardrum

How Is the Procedure Performed?

- The tympanometer is placed into the ear canal.
- The tympanometer produces a tone that causes pressure change in the ear.
- The tympanometer measures the pressure change.

Rationale for the Test

- To identify fluid behind the eardrum
- To identify blockage of the Eustachian tube
- To assess for otitis media
- To assess hearing loss

Nursing Implications

- Determine if the patient can lie still.

Understanding the Results

- The procedure takes less than 5 minutes. Results are known immediately.
- Normal test results indicate
  - Normal pressure
- Abnormal test results indicate
  - Abnormal pressure

Teach The Patient

- Explain
  - Why the test is being performed.
  - What the patient will experience during the test.
  - That the patient will not feel any pain during the procedure.

Summary

In this chapter you learned that the underlying cause of snoring can be remedied by performing an uvulopalatopharyngoplasty that removes excess tissue and radiofrequency palatoplasty that inhibits tissue vibration.

Sinusitis might be diagnosed by performing a sinus endoscopy, sinus X-ray, or a sinus aspiration, where a sample of sinus is sent to the laboratory for a culture and sensitivity test. The healthcare provider might also perform sinus surgery if the sinus is blocked.

The healthcare provider might order an electroencephalogram to identify abnormal electrical activities in the brain that may be a symptom of a serious neurological disorder.

Frequent throat infections are challenging to resolve; however, the healthcare provider might order a throat culture, sputum culture, or sputum cytology to identify the cause of the infection and the medications that will kill the infecting microorganism. In addition, the healthcare provider may perform a procedure to prevent reinfection. The most common are a tonsillectomy tympanostomy tube and a tympanocentesis.

Hearing loss is caused by a number of factors, including a buildup of cerumen in the ear canal, disorders of the eardrum, or a neurological problem. The healthcare provider can perform tympanometry and audiometric tests to determine the cause of hearing loss.

QUIZ

1. **What a practitioner should order for a patient who experiences random seizures?**
    A. An ambulatory EEG
    B. A helmet
    C. Restraints
    D. OAE test

2. **A patient arrives for an EEG for sleep disorder tells you that she had a long nap before arriving for the test. What would you do?**
    A. Cancel the test, since the patient no longer has a sleeping disorder.
    B. Reschedule the test.
    C. Reschedule the test asking the patient not to sleep before the test.
    D. Wait 2 hours before conducting the test.

3. **You tell a patient take a deep cough to produce a sputum sample. Why do you give her this instruction?**

    A. A deep cough loosens sputum.

    B. Sputum is produced in the respiratory system.

    C. A deep cough brings sputum into the oral cavity.

    D. Sputum contains food particles.

4. **What is the difference between sputum cytology and a sputum culture?**

    A. A sputum cytology studies cells contained in the sputum, while a sputum culture identifies microorganism in the sputum.

    B. There is no difference.

    C. A sputum cytology identifies microorganism in the sputum, while a sputum culture studies cells contained in the sputum.

    D. All of the above.

5. **The patient asks why it takes more than 1 day to get the results of a throat culture. What is your best response?**

    A. The laboratory is backed up with other samples.

    B. Sufficient time must pass to allow the microorganism to grow.

    C. An outside laboratory is used.

    D. It takes time to determine what drug to use to kill the microorganism.

6. **What is your response if a patient tells you that he/she spit into the sterile container when you asked for a sputum culture?**

    A. Teach the patient how to properly produce a sputum sample.

    B. Sputum is not saliva.

    C. He/she contaminated the container.

    D. Take the sample to the laboratory quickly.

7. **What is the best time to collect a sputum sample?**

    A. Right before meals

    B. First thing in the morning

    C. Immediately after the patient awakens from sleep

    D. After the patient rinses his/her mouth with water

8. **What is the purpose of tympanometry?**

    A. To measure the eardrum's response to pressure and sound

    B. To identify the contents of fluid behind the eardrum

    C. To permit fluid behind the eardrum to drain

    D. To treat an ear infection

9. **What test is performed to determine if the patient has sensorineural hearing loss?**

   A. Pure-tone audiometry

   B. Speech reception/word recognition

   C. Whispered speech test

   D. Otoacoustic emissions test

10. **What test is performed to identify hearing problems in a newborn?**

    A. Pure-tone audiometry

    B. Speech reception/word recognition

    C. Whispered speech test

    D. Otoacoustic emissions test

ANSWERS

1. A. An ambulatory EEG.
2. C. Reschedule the test asking the patient not to sleep before the test.
3. D. Sputum contains food particles.
4. A. A sputum cytology studies cells contained in the sputum, while a sputum culture identifies microorganism in the sputum.
5. B. Sufficient time must pass to allow the microorganism to grow.
6. A. Teach the patient how to properly produce a sputum sample.
7. C. Immediately after the patient awakens from sleep.
8. A. To measure the eardrum's response to pressure and sound.
9. B. Speech reception/word recognition.
10. D. Otoacoustic emissions test.

chapter 21

Vision Tests and Procedures

LEARNING OBJECTIVES

1. Vision Tests
2. Tonometry
3. Electronystagmogram (ENG)

KEY WORDS

Amsler grid test
Applanation tonometry
Color vision test
Confrontation test
E-chart test
Electronic indentation tonometry
Fluorescein
Near test
Perimetry test

Pneumotonometry test
Refraction test
Schiotz tonometry
Snellen test
Tangent screen test
Tonometer
Trabecular meshwork
Vitreous hemorrhage

Light rays pass through the cornea, the pupil, and lenses which focus the ray of light on to the retina located at the back of the eye. When light rays are not properly focused on the retina, the patient is unable to see clearly.

Light rays focused in front of the retina cause myopia (nearsightedness), enabling patients to better see things near them than at a distance. Light rays focused behind the retina cause hyperopia (farsightedness), enabling patients to see things at a distance better than up close. When light rays are irregularly bent, images are blurred resulting in astigmatism.

In this chapter you will learn about tests that are used to diagnose problems with sight and disorders that can lead to loss of vision. You will also learn about procedures that can be performed to treat vision disorders.

A standard vision test is used to assess the patient's ability to see close-up and at a distance. It also determines if the patient is experiencing peripheral vision difficulty or might have macular degeneration. In addition, the test determines the refractive error of the patient's eye, which determines the corrective lenses needed to restore his/her eyesight.

Patients who have myopia might be able to have this condition fixed by having corneal ring implants or by reshaping with cornea using photorefractive keratectomy.

Glaucoma is caused by increased intraocular pressure. The healthcare provider assesses intraocular pressure by performing tonometry. If intraocular pressure is elevated, the healthcare provider may perform one of several procedures to relieve the pressure.

A trabeculectomy or a trabeculotomy can be performed to drain aqueous humor that might be backing up due to a blockage in the trabecular meshwork.

Seton glaucoma surgery might be performed to insert a drainage tube in the eye to drain the aqueous humor.

Blood flow in the eye can be assessed by performing an eye angiogram, which detects a vitreous hemorrhage. A vitreous hemorrhage is treated by performing a vitrectomy.

A detached retina is a common problem. It occurs when the retina is detached from the back wall of the eye. When this occurs, the healthcare provider can repair the problem by performing a sclera buckling to relieve traction on the retina. A pneumatic retinopexy might be performed to push the retina back into the position by using a gas bubble.

These and other tests and procedures are covered in this chapter.

1. Vision Tests

The healthcare provider examines the patient's peripheral vision and ability to see near and far distances, along with his/her ability to distinguish colors by performing nine vision tests. These are

- Confrontation test: This test assesses the patient's peripheral vision by gazing at the healthcare provider's nose.
- Amsler grid test: This test assesses for macular degeneration.
- Perimetry test: This test assesses the patient's peripheral vision by flashing lights randomly in a perimeter.
- Tangent screen test: This test assesses the patient's peripheral vision by gazing at a concentric circle image.
- Snellen test: This test assesses the patient's ability to see distances.
- E-chart test: This test assesses the patients' ability to see distances when they are unable to read.
- Near test: This test assesses the patient's ability to see near distances.
- Color vision test: This test assesses the patient's ability to distinguish colors.
- Refraction test: This test measures the refractive error of the patient's eyes to determine lens that corrects his/her eyesight.

What Is Being Examined?

- Eyesight

How Is the Procedure Performed?

- Confrontation test
  - The healthcare provider sits 3 ft from where the patient is sitting.
  - The patient covers one eye.
  - The patient stares at the healthcare provider's nose with the other eye.
  - The healthcare provider moves his/her finger from outside the visual field to the center of the visual field.
  - The healthcare provider moves his/her finger from the center of the visual field to opposite outside of the visual field.
  - The patient signals when he/she first sees the healthcare provider's finger.
  - The test is repeated using the other eye.
- Amsler grid test
  - The patient covers one eye.
  - A 4-in square chart containing straight lines and a grid with a black dot at the center is held 14 in from the patient.
  - The patient focuses his/her eye on black dot on the chart.
  - The patient tells the healthcare provider if he/she can see the black dot, sees a dark spot other than the black dot, or sees the straight lines.
  - The patient should see the black dot and the straight lines.
- Perimetry test
  - The patient looks into the perimeter, focusing on a dot in the center of the perimeter screen.
  - Lights randomly flash at various locations on the perimeter screen.
  - The patient presses a button each time he/she sees a light on the screen.
  - The perimeter generates a printout, showing areas in the patient's peripheral vision where he/she did not see the light.
- Tangent screen test
  - The patient sits 6 ft away from the black screen that contains concentric circles and lines.
  - The patient covers one eye.
  - The patient focuses the other eye on a center of the circle.
  - A wand containing an object is moved from the outside of the circle to the inside of the circle.

- The patient signals the healthcare provider when he/she sees the object.
- The test is repeated using different-sized objects on the wand.
- The test is repeated for the other eye.
- Snellen test
  - The patient is positioned 20 ft from the Snellen chart.
  - The patient covers one eye.
  - The patient reads the smallest row of letters on the chart.
  - Each row is designated with a visual acuity value.
  - A row designated as 20/20 visual acuity means a person with normal vision can read this line at a distance of 20 ft.
  - A row designated as 20/40 visual acuity means a person with normal vision can read this line at a distance of 40 ft.
- E-chart test
  - The patient covers one eye.
  - The patient reads the smallest E on the chart.
  - Each row is designated with a visual acuity value, the same as in the Snellen test.
- Near test
  - The patient is given a card that contains text.
  - The patient holds the card 14 in from his/her eyes.
  - The patient reads the text on the card.
  - The test is repeated with cards that have progressively smaller type size.
- Color vision test
  - The patient views pages that contain numbers, symbols, and paths that appear on a background of color dots.
  - The patient is asked to say out loud the number, symbol, or path.
  - The patient may have problems differentiating colors if he/she is unable to identify the number, symbol, or path correctly.
- Refraction test
  - The patient views the Snellen chart or E-chart and the cards used for the near test while looking through corrective lens.
  - The patient then notifies the healthcare provider when he/she can clearly read the chart and cards.
  - The healthcare provider then writes a prescription for those lenses.

Rationale for the Test

- To determine if the patient is color blind
- To correct the patient's vision with glasses or contact lenses
- To determine if the patient is losing his/her peripheral vision
- To determine if the patient has macular degeneration

Nursing Implications

- Determine if the patient
  - Has signed a consent form
  - Can sit still
  - Can read
  - Wears glasses or contact lenses
  - Has an eye infection
  - Can follow instructions
  - Has his/her glasses or contact lenses with them

Understanding the Results

- The procedure takes less than 1 hour. Results are immediate.
- Normal test results indicate
  - Normal eyesight
  - Normal peripheral vision
  - No macular degeneration
  - Can see all colors
- Abnormal test results indicate
  - Near sighted (can see near distances)
  - Far sighted (can see far distances)
  - Restricted peripheral vision
  - Possible macular degeneration
  - Color blind

Teach the Patient

- Explain
  - Why the procedure is being performed.
  - What the patient will experience during the procedure.

- That the patient will not feel any pain during the procedure.
- The patient should bring his/her glasses or contact lenses to the test.

2. Tonometry

Tonometry is a test for glaucoma that measures the intraocular pressure of the patient's eye by assessing the amount of pressure necessary to flatten the cornea. There are four methods used to perform tonometry. These are

- Pneumatonometry: This method uses a puff of air to measure intraocular pressure. No direct contact is made with the eye.
- Applanation tonometry: This method uses a tonometer to measure intra-ocular pressure.
- Electronic indentation tonometry: This method uses a tonometer that is connected to a computer to measure intraocular pressure.
- Schiotz tonometry: This method uses a plunger to measure intraocular pressure.

What Is Being Examined?

- Intraocular pressure

How Is the Test Performed?

- The patient removes contact lenses.
- Pneumatonometry
  - The patient sits.
  - The patient places his/her chin on a chin rest and forehead against a stabilizing bar of the slit lamp.
  - A light is shined into the eye.
  - A puff of air is blown into the eye.
  - The tonometer measures the change in the reflection of the light off the cornea when the puff of air strikes the eye.
  - Intraocular pressure is read from the tonometer.
- Applanation tonometry
  - The patient sits.
  - A local anesthetic is placed in the eye.
  - Fluorescein is administered to the eye to make the cornea visible.

- The patient places his/her chin on a chin rest and forehead against a stabilizing bar of the slit lamp.
- A tonometer is pressed against the cornea.
- The tension dial on the tonometer records the intraocular pressure.
- Electronic indentation tonometry
  - The patient sits.
  - A local anesthetic is placed in the eye.
  - The patient places his/her chin on a chin rest and forehead against a stabilizing bar of the slit lamp.
  - A tonometer is pressed against the cornea.
  - A click sounds when a reading is taken.
  - Four readings are taken.
  - Intraocular pressure is displayed on the computer screen.
- Schiotz tonometry
  - The patient lies on a table.
  - A local anesthetic is placed in the eye.
  - The patient stares at a fix point on the ceiling.
  - A tonometer is pressed against the cornea.
  - Intraocular pressure is displayed on the tonometer.

Rationale for the Procedure

- Assess for glaucoma

Nursing Implications

- Determine if the patient
  - Has not drunk alcohol 12 hours before the test
  - Has not drunk anything for 4 hours before the test
  - Can sit still
  - Has not smoked marijuana 24 hours before the test
  - Can respond to directions during the procedure
  - Can withstand a probe being directed at his/her eye
  - Has removed his/her contact lenses
  - Signed a consent form

Understanding the Results

- The procedure takes less than 30 minutes. Results are immediate.
- Normal test results indicate
  - Normal intraocular pressure
- Abnormal test results indicate
  - High intraocular pressure
  - Low intraocular pressure

Teach the Patient

- Explain
- Why procedure is being performed.
- How the procedure is performed.
- That the patient will not feel any pain during the procedure.
- That the patient should not insert contact lenses for 2 hours following the test.
- That the patient should not drink alcohol 12 hours before the test.
- That the patient should not drink anything for 4 hours before the test.
- That the patient should not smoke marijuana 24 hours before the test.
- That the patient should not rub his/her eyes for 30 minutes following the test.

3. Electronystagmogram

Electronystagmogram (ENG) is a test that measures eye movement, both voluntary eye movement and nystagmus, to assess the patient's balance and the underlying cause of vertigo.

What Is Being Examined?

- Balance

How Is the Test Performed?

- The patient signs a consent form.
- Any obstruction in the ear canal is removed.

- Five electrodes are pasted on the patient's face.
- The room is darkened.
- During each of the following, electrical activities from the electrodes are recorded.
- The patient follows a moving light with his/her eyes while holding his/her head still.
- The patient closes his/her eyes and is asked to perform mental arithmetic.
- The patient opens his/her eyes and follows the back and forth movement of a pendulum.
- The patient is asked to look at objects that are moved in front of him/her.
- The patient is asked to move his/her head up and down and side to side.
- Cold water is placed in the patient's ear.
- Warm water is placed in the patient's ear.

Rationale for the Procedure

- To assess the underlying cause of loss of balance and vertigo
- To assess the inner ear

Nursing Implications

- Determine if the patient
  - Has not taken tranquilizers 5 days before the test
  - Has not drunk alcohol 5 days before the test
  - Has not ingested caffeine 5 days before the test
  - Has not eaten 4 hours before the test
  - Is not wearing facial makeup
  - Has not had a back or neck disorder

Understanding the Results

- The procedure takes less than 2 hours. Results are known within 1 week.
- Normal test results indicate
  - Normal voluntary and involuntary eye movement
- Abnormal test results indicate
  - Abnormal involuntary eye movement

Teach the Patient

- Explain
  - Why procedure is being performed.
  - How the procedure is performed.
  - That the patient will not feel any pain during the procedure.
  - The patient should not take tranquilizers 5 days before the test.
  - The patient should not drink alcohol 5 days before the test.
  - The patient should not ingest caffeine 5 days before the test.
  - The patient should not eat 4 hours before the test.
  - The patient should not wear facial makeup during the test.

Summary

In this chapter you learned about tests that are used to diagnose problems with sight and disorders that can lead to loss of vision and about procedures that can be performed to treat vision disorders.

Patients undergo a standard vision test to assess their ability to see close-up, at a distance, and to assess their peripheral vision. During the test, the healthcare provider determines the patient's refractive error and then prescribes corrective lenses needed to restore his/her eyesight. Some patients who have myopia choose to have this condition fixed by having corneal ring implants or by reshaping the cornea using photorefractive keratectomy.

Increased intraocular pressure causes glaucoma. The tonometry test measures intraocular pressure and, if elevated, the healthcare provider may perform a trabeculectomy or a trabeculotomy (children only) to drain aqueous humor that might be backing up due to a blockage in the trabecular meshwork. Seton glaucoma surgery might be performed to insert a drainage tube in the eye to drain the aqueous humor.

An eye angiogram assesses blood flow in the eye and can detect a vitreous hemorrhage. A vitreous hemorrhage is treated by performing a vitrectomy.

The retina can become detached from the back wall of the eye. It can be repaired by performing a sclera buckling to relieve traction on the retina. A pneumatic retinopexy might be performed to push the retina back into the position using a gas bubble.

QUIZ

1. **What is an E-chart used for?**
    A. To assess the patient's ability to see distances when he/she is unable to read
    B. To assess the patient's ability to see distances
    C. To assess the patient's ability to see near him/her
    D. To assess the patient's ability to see near him/her when he/she is unable to read

2. **What is a confrontation test?**
    A. Examination of patient's peripheral vision by gazing at the healthcare provider's eyes
    B. Examination of patient's peripheral vision by gazing at the healthcare provider's nose
    C. Examination of patient's peripheral vision by gazing at the healthcare provider's hands
    D. None of the above

3. **What tests the patient's peripheral vision by flashing lights randomly in a perimeter?**
    A. Amsler grid test
    B. Perimetry test
    C. Tangent screen test
    D. Snellen test

4. **What tests the patient's peripheral vision by gazing at a concentric circle image?**
    A. Amsler grid test
    B. Perimetry test
    C. Tangent screen test
    D. Snellen test

5. **How is the pneumotonometry test performed?**
    A. It measures intraocular pressure directly on the eye.
    B. It uses a puff of air to measure intraocular pressure.
    C. It uses a probe to measure intraocular pressure.
    D. None of the above.

6. **During the Schiotz tonometry test a tonometer is pressed against the cornea.**
    A. True
    B. False

7. **What test measures for macular degeneration?**

   A. Amsler grid test
   B. Perimetry test
   C. Tangent screen test
   D. Snellen test

8. **Why should a patient not take tranquilizers 5 days before the electronystagmogram (ENG) test?**

   A. Tranquilizers might slow eye movement giving a false test result.
   B. Tranquilizers might increase eye movement giving a false test result.
   C. Tranquilizers might cause nausea and vomiting during the test.
   D. Tranquilizers might cause nausea and vomiting following the test.

9. **The near test assesses the patient's ability to see long distances.**

   A. True
   B. False

10. **What is the purpose of a refraction test?**

    A. To determine the corrective lens for prescribing to the patient
    B. To assess if the patient can see refracted light waves
    C. To assess if the patient can see refracted light waves at night
    D. All of the above

ANSWERS

1. A. To assess patient's ability to see distances when he/she is unable to read.
2. B. Examination of patient's peripheral vision by gazing at the healthcare provider's nose.
3. B. Perimetry test.
4. C. Tangent screen test.
5. B. It uses a puff of air to measure intraocular pressure.
6. A. True.
7. A. Amsler grid test.
8. A. Tranquilizers might slow eye movement giving a false test result.
9. B. False.
10. A. To determine the corrective lens to prescribe to the patient.

Medical Tests and Procedures Demystified

Final Exam

1. **What enzymes were found mostly in cardiac muscles?**

   A. Troponin and CPK-MB

   B. CPK and creatinine phosphokinase

   C. CK and creatinine phosphokinase

   D. CKB and creatinine phosphokinase

2. **Why should a blood sample for prolactin be taken 3 hours after the patient awakens?**

   A. The test should always be taken immediately prior to lunch

   B. The patient requires a good night sleep before the test

   C. Prolactin levels are normally high when the patient first awakens

   D. None of the above

3. **Why should you assess if the patient has taken antibiotics before testing for potassium?**
   A. Taking antibiotics indicates that the patient has a bacterial infection
   B. Some antibiotics contain potassium
   C. Patients who take antibiotics always have higher than normal levels of potassium
   D. Patients might vomit during the test

4. **The spirometry test measures**
   A. The amount of gasses that cross the alveoli per minute
   B. The patient's airway responses to allergens
   C. Volume and capacity of the lungs
   D. None of the above

5. **What is a transurethral biopsy?**
   A. A needle is inserted through the rectum to remove samples of the prostate tissue
   B. A needle is inserted through the urethra to remove samples of prostate tissue
   C. A needle is inserted in the skin between the anus and the scrotum to remove samples of the prostate tissue
   D. A needle is inserted between the third and fourth ribs to remove samples of lung tissue

6. **What is the purpose of administering tracer material in a lymph node biopsy?**
   A. To highlight cancer cells
   B. Tracer material helps map the route that cancer cells spread from the cancer site through the lymphatic system
   C. To highlight noncancerous cells
   D. An incident report

7. **What test is ordered to screen for malabsorption syndrome?**
   A. D-xylose absorption test
   B. Fasting blood glucose (FBG) test
   C. Two-hour postprandial blood sugar test
   D. Oral glucose tolerance test (OGTT)

8. **Why might a practitioner test for potassium levels?**
   A. The patient shows signs of arrhythmia
   B. The patient shows signs of muscle weakness
   C. The patient reports nausea and vomiting
   D. All of the above

9. **What is the potential risk if the patient is on aspirin therapy prior to drawing the arterial blood sample?**

   A. Inaccurate test results

   B. The patient must take a baby aspirin following the test

   C. Coagulation time may be longer than normal

   D. The test should not be performed

10. **Why might a practitioner order the ALT test if the patient has taken excessive amounts of acetaminophen?**

    A. To assess liver damage as a result of accidental or intentionally overdosing with acetaminophen

    B. To assess the ammonia level in the patient's blood

    C. To assess the effect lactulose has interrupting the effects of acetaminophen

    D. To assess if the patient intentionally overdose with acetaminophen

11. **What is a function of magnesium?**

    A. It is used to transfer potassium and sodium in and out of cells

    B. It is used in deactivated nerves

    C. It is used to relax the patient

    D. It is used to balance leukocytes and erythrocytes

12. **Why is not a cranial ultrasound performed after 18 months of age?**

    A. The fontanelles are closed

    B. The fontanelles remain open

    C. The test is too painful for the child to undergo

    D. Complications from a premature birth would have already manifested

13. **What is the purpose of the color duplex Doppler test in men?**

    A. To assess the velocity and direction of blood flowing through the penis

    B. To assess size of an erection

    C. To assess if the patient had an erection during sleep

    D. To assess if the patient has urine in his bladder

14. **What is used to hold the cervix in place during an endometrial biopsy?**

    A. Braca clamp

    B. Spectrum clamp

    C. Tenaculum clamp

    D. Braca2 clamp

15. **Why is the direct Coombs test administered?**

    A. On a patient to determine if an autoimmune response is occurring
    B. On a patient who received a blood transfusion to determine if there is a transfusion reaction
    C. On a newborn whose mother is Rh-negative to determine if the antibodies crossed the placenta into the newborn's blood
    D. All of the above

16. **Why should a patient with kidney disease avoid being administered contrast material prior to an MRI?**

    A. The patient might have difficulty excreting the contrast material
    B. The contrast material contains metallic elements
    C. Patients with kidney disease should never receive an MRI
    D. None of the above

17. **Why stop taking Coumadin before a bone biopsy?**

    A. Coumadin increases coagulation time, thereby increasing the risk of bleeding during the procedure
    B. Coumadin decreases coagulation time, thereby increasing the risk of bleeding during the procedure
    C. Coumadin has a negative reaction to anesthetic administered during the procedure
    D. Coumadin has a negative reaction to the antibiotic that is administered following the procedure

18. **What test measures the ejection fraction of the heart?**

    A. Cardiac blood pool scan
    B. Venogram
    C. Pericardiocentesis
    D. ABI

19. **What is the purpose of using pilocarpine during a sweat test?**

    A. Pilocarpine helps to draw sweat from the newborn
    B. Pilocarpine prevents the newborn from sweating
    C. Pilocarpine is not used in the sweat test
    D. Pilocarpine protects the skin from electrodes that are placed on the skin during the test

20. **What does a patient wear during an MRI?**

    A. The patient removes all clothing and wears a gown during the MRI
    B. The patient needs only to expose the area of the body that is being assessed
    C. The patient removes all clothing during the MRI
    D. The patient can remain in street clothes during the MRI

21. **What must you verify before the patient undergoes a transvaginal ultrasound?**

    A. A signed consent is received that acknowledges that conductive gel will be placed on the patient's abdomen

    B. That the patient is over 18 years of age

    C. That the patient is not allergic to latex

    D. A signed consent is received that acknowledges that the transducer will be pressed down on her abdomen

22. **During what type of X-ray might the patient be placed in a brace for the X-ray?**

    A. Facial X-ray

    B. Orthopantogram

    C. Periapical

    D. Occlusal

23. **Give three reasons for administering the CEA test**

    A. Screening for cancer, assessing cancer treatment, and identifying the location of the tumor for surgery

    B. Screening for cancer, assessing cancer treatment, and for diagnosing cancer

    C. Screening for cancer, assessing cancer treatment, and assessing for the success of surgery to remove the tumor

    D. None of the above

24. **What would you tell the patient whose ELISA test is positive?**

    A. You have a confirmed diagnosis of HIV

    B. You have a confirmed diagnosis of AIDS

    C. The test result does not mean that you are HIV positive. Further testing is necessary

    D. You do not have HIV

25. **What might the practitioner prescribe if the patient has a high level of ammonia?**

    A. Echinacea

    B. Lactulose

    C. Nonsteroidal anti-inflammatory drugs

    D. Valerian

26. **How does the snap gauge work?**

    A. It measures the size of an erection

    B. The snap gauge consisting of a film is placed around the penis. The film snaps when the patient has erection

    C. It measures the length of time of an erection

    D. All of the above

27. What is liquefaction time?

A. The time necessary for semen to liquefy

B. The time necessary for semen to dehydrate

C. The time necessary for sperm to liquefy

D. The time necessary for sperm to dehydrate

28. What can produce a false-positive result in the bone mineral density test?

A. The patient has arthritis

B. The patient has a T-score of 1

C. The patient has a Z-score of 1

D. The patient has an X-score of less than 1

29. A mastopexy is a

A. Breast augmentation

B. Breast reduction

C. Breast lift

D. None of the above

30. What test is performed before drawing an arterial blood sample?

A. Allen test

B. Collection test

C. Acid-alkaline test

D. None of the above

31. What might you suspect if the patient's urine is cloudy?

A. The patient is dehydrated

B. The patient has taken Pepto-Bismol

C. Bacterial infection

D. The patient is overhydrated

32. How does the dermabrasion improve the appearance of skin?

A. It removes the outer layer of skin enabling new skin to grow

B. It removes the inner layer of skin enabling new skin to grow

C. It uses a chemical to remove the outer layer of skin enabling new skin to grow

D. All of the above

33. What tests the patient's peripheral vision by flashing lights randomly in a perimeter?

A. Amsler grid test

B. Perimetry test

C. Tangent screen test

D. Snellen test

34. **What allergy test requires that an allergen-containing pad be applied to the patient's skin?**
    A. Skin patch test
    B. Skin prick test
    C. Intradermal test
    D. The Q patch test

35. **What might cause low sperm motility?**
    A. Sample not kept at body temperature
    B. Delay in delivering the sample to the laboratory
    C. Sample not kept away from direct sunlight
    D. All of the above

36. **Why is chorionic villus sampling preferred over amniocentesis?**
    A. Chorionic villus sampling can be performed earlier in the pregnancy than amniocentesis
    B. Chorionic villus sampling can be performed later in the pregnancy than amniocentesis
    C. Chorionic villus sampling is safer than amniocentesis
    D. None of the above

37. **Why would a woman who is positive for BRCA1 receive annual MRI scan?**
    A. The patient is at high risk for breast cancer and the MRI provides highly detailed views of the patient's breasts
    B. BRCA1 interferes a normal mammogram is necessary
    C. Only radiowaves can penetrate the BRCA1 so an MRI is not necessary
    D. A positive BRCA1 means that the patient is not at risk for cancer and does not need an MRI scan

38. **Why would you ask the patient to drink a large amount of water following a CT scan?**
    A. To disperse X-rays
    B. To flush the contrast material
    C. To avoid cramps
    D. To concentrate X-rays

39. **What test is the quickest and most sensitive test for Lyme disease?**
    A. ELISA
    B. Western blot test
    C. The POCkit tests
    D. *Helicobacter pylori* stool antigen test

40. **What conditions might affect the results of the PSA test?**
    A. A urinary tract infection
    B. Catheterized within the past 8 weeks
    C. Taking Avodart
    D. All of the above

41. **Why would a practitioner order the CD4+ count test?**
    A. To assess for T-lymphocytes
    B. To assess for T-cells
    C. To assess for T-helper cells
    D. All of the above

42. **What might be the results of high ammonia levels?**
    A. The patient may become confused
    B. The patient might experience hand tremors
    C. The patient might experience increased sleepiness
    D. All of the above

43. **What should you do if the patient ate breakfast before fasting blood glucose (FBG) test?**
    A. Postpone the test for 1 month
    B. Administer the test. Estimate the sugar content of the breakfast and subtract that amount from the test results
    C. Reschedule the test after 2 weeks
    D. Postpone the test for at least 8 hours

44. **During the biophysical profile test performed early in the trimester, the mother should**
    A. Have an empty bladder before the test
    B. Have a full bladder before the test
    C. Have a bowel movement prior the test
    D. None of the above

45. **The patient who is 8 months pregnant and is scheduled to receive a transabdominal ultrasound**
    A. Does not have to have a full bladder for the test
    B. Must have a full bladder for the test
    C. Cannot have their bladder filled using a urinary catheter
    D. Must have their bladder filled using a urinary catheter

46. **What is an orchiectomy?**
    A. A procedure performed to assess for testicular cancer
    B. A procedure performed to remove tissue samples of the ovaries

C. A procedure performed to remove tissue samples of the kidneys

D. A procedure performed to remove tissue samples of the lung

47. **What is a vaginal vault prolapse?**

A. The upper segment of the vagina collapses and extends outside the vagina

B. The pelvic wall collapses

C. The pelvic ligaments are stretched

D. The lower abdominal wall collapses

48. **What test measures creatinine in 24-hour urine sample?**

A. Creatinine clearance test

B. Creatinine level test

C. BUN:creatinine level test

D. None of the above

49. **What is an E-chart used for?**

A. It assesses the patients' ability to see distances when they are unable to read

B. It assesses the patients' ability to see distances

C. It assesses the patients' ability to see near them

D. It assesses the patients' ability to see near them when they are unable to read

50. **Why is a perfusion CT ordered?**

A. To determine osteoporosis

B. To assess the results of the KUB

C. To determine blood supply to the brain

D. None of the above

51. **What instructions would you give to a patient who is scheduled for the renin assay test?**

A. Relax 2 hours before the first blood sample is taken

B. Ambulate for 2 hours after the first blood sample is taken

C. Sit upright when blood samples are taken

D. All of the above

52. **What should the patient do before the homocysteine test?**

A. Avoid eating and drinking except for water 12 hours before the test is administered

B. Walk 10 blocks before the test is administered

C. Avoid walking

D. Avoid driving

53. **What is the purpose of tympanometry?**

    A. To measure the eardrum's response to pressure and sound
    B. To identify the contents of fluid behind the eardrum
    C. To permit fluid behind the eardrum to drain
    D. To treat an ear infection

54. **You tell a patient take a deep cough to produce a sputum sample. Why do you give her this instruction?**

    A. A deep cough loosens sputum
    B. Sputum is produced in the respiratory system
    C. A deep cough brings sputum into the oral cavity
    D. Sputum contains food particles

55. **What parts of the body are measured using P-DEXA?**

    A. Arms and legs
    B. Spine and arms
    C. Hip and spine
    D. Hip and legs

56. **What is the purpose of an intracavernosal injection?**

    A. To increase sperm count
    B. To prevent an erection
    C. To cause an erection
    D. None of the above

57. **What does it mean if a woman's husband has the BRCA1 and BRCA2 genes?**

    A. He can pass these genes to the woman during sexual intercourse
    B. The woman is at a high risk for cancer
    C. The couple should refrain from unprotected sexual intercourse
    D. The man might be at high risk for developing breast cancer and/or prostate cancer

58. **What test is used to assess changes in the brain chemistry caused by disease?**

    A. Magnetic resonance spectroscopy
    B. MRA
    C. Diffusion-perfusion imaging
    D. MRI

59. **What should the patient do if she experiences a seizure following the CT scan?**

    A. Call her healthcare provider immediately
    B. Call for emergency medical care immediately

    C. Lie down on her bed

    D. Keep her head elevated

60. **What should you tell the patient not to use prior to a mammogram?**

    A. Deodorant

    B. Ointments

    C. Powders

    D. All of the above

61. **What is the function of progesterone?**

    A. Prevents milk from ejecting

    B. Causes lactogenesis

    C. Increases the production of milk

    D. Eases the ability for the newborn to be feed

62. **Why the ACTH may be difficult to interpret?**

    A. ACTH levels vary by the minute

    B. ACTH levels are normally low

    C. ACTH levels are normally high

    D. ACTH levels cannot be calculated

63. **Why are blood samples taken every 12 hours for 2 days following a suspected myocardial infarction?**

    A. The patient may have multiple myocardial infarctions during that period

    B. It takes 6 hours for troponin levels to rise after a myocardial infarction

    C. It takes 2 days for troponin levels to rise after a myocardial infarction

    D. To confirm the test results

64. **Hyperventilation affects the arterial blood gas values and may result in which of the following?**

    A. Respiratory alkalosis

    B. Metabolic acidosis

    C. Metabolic alkalosis

    D. Respiratory acidosis

65. **What test is used to differentiate between Type 1 and Type 2 diabetes?**

    A. C-peptide

    B. Two-hour postprandial blood sugar test

    C. Fasting blood glucose (FBG) test

    D. Random blood glucose test

66. **What test is performed to determine if the patient has sensorineural hearing loss?**

    A. Pure-tone audiometry

    B. Speech reception/Word recognition

    C. Whispered speech test

    D. Otoacoustic emissions test

67. **What is a Z-score?**

    A. A score that compares the patient's conductive velocity with that of people of his/her own age, sex, and race

    B. A score that compares the patient's bone mineral density with that of a healthy 30 years old

    C. A score that compares the patient's bone mineral density with that of people of his/her own age, sex, and race

    D. None of the above

68. **What is the difference between sputum cytology and a sputum culture?**

    A. A sputum cytology studies cells contained in the sputum and a sputum culture identifies microorganism in the sputum

    B. There is no difference

    C. A sputum cytology identifies microorganism in the sputum and a sputum culture studies cells contained in the sputum

    D. None of the above

69. **What is the purpose of the VDRL test?**

    A. Identifies *Treponema pallidum* antibodies

    B. Identifies *T pallidum* antibodies

    C. Identifies the anti-cardiolipin antibodies

    D. Identifies the *T pallidum* bacterium

70. **Why would a healthcare provider order a transesophageal echocardiogram?**

    A. To assess cardiac contraction under stress

    B. To generate an image of the heart that is not obstructed by bone

    C. To assess cardiac blood flow to the extremities

    D. To assess cardiac blood flow to the lungs

71. **Why is not the Mantoux skin test used to diagnose tuberculosis?**

    A. A positive result indicates that the patient has developed antibodies to *Mycobacterium tuberculosis* antigen possibly from a previous exposure to *M tuberculosis*

    B. A negative result indicates that the patient has not developed antibodies to *M tuberculosis* antigen; however, the immune system can take up to 10 weeks to develop the antibodies following the infection

C. Diagnosis is made using an X-ray

D. All of the above

72. **Why would a patient be administered Retin-A following a chemical peel?**

A. To reduce bleeding following the procedure

B. To prevent an infection

C. To encourage healing

D. None of the above

73. **What hormone signals the adrenal glands to release aldosterone?**

A. Renin

B. Cortisol

C. Phenytoin

D. Dexamethasone

74. **What would you tell a patient who is about to undergo FBS test?**

A. The patient should fast for 8 hours before the test. All diabetes mellitus (DM) medications are withheld until the test is completed

B. The patient should eat a regular meal but refrain from ingesting sugar beverages

C. The patient should eat a regular meal, including ingesting sugar beverages

D. The patient should eat a bland meal and refrain from ingesting sugar beverages

75. **What may the healthcare provider suspect if a patient lacks hexosaminidase A enzyme?**

A. May have multiple sclerosis

B. May have Tay-Sachs disease

C. Is pregnant

D. Is infertile

76. **Why is the GHb test administered?**

A. To determine if the DM patient has maintained adequate blood glucose level for the previous 60 days

B. To determine if the DM patient has maintained adequate blood glucose level for the previous 120 days

C. To determine if the DM patient has maintained adequate blood glucose level for the previous 30 days

D. None of the above

77. **What allergy test requires that an allergen-containing pad be applied to the patient's skin?**

    A. Skin patch test
    B. Skin prick test
    C. Intradermal test
    D. Q patch test

78. **What microorganism causes a fishy odor in vaginosis?**

    A. *Candida albicans*
    B. *Trichomonas vaginalis*
    C. Bacterial vaginosis
    D. None of the above

79. **What test is performed if the healthcare provider suspects pulmonary emboli?**

    A. Bronchoscopy
    B. Lung scan
    C. Pulmonary function test
    D. Thoracotomy

80. **Why should a breast-feeding mother avoid undergoing a PET scan?**

    A. The mother's breasts will be tender 24 hours following the PET scan
    B. The tracer is likely to pass to the baby in breast milk
    C. The PET scan places the mother under extreme stress that decreases the volume of breast milk
    D. None of the above

81. **A PET scan helps the healthcare provider diagnose**

    A. Transient ischemic attack
    B. Multiple sclerosis
    C. Cancer
    D. All of the above

82. **Why would the uric acid blood test be ordered?**

    A. To assess treatment for hypouricemia
    B. To screen for uric acid kidney stones
    C. To assess for inflammation
    D. To assess for infection

83. **An elevated C-reactive protein level prior to surgery indicates**

    A. Higher risk of infection following surgery
    B. Lower risk of infection following surgery

    C. Surgery is no longer necessary

    D. All the above

84. **What might be suspected if the patient has increased leukocyte count but no signs of infection?**

    A. Polycythemia

    B. Risk of bleeding

    C. Anemia

    D. Leukemia

85. **When the patient arrives in the morning for the metabolic panel, the patient states that she arrived home at three in the morning following a bachelorette party. How should you reply?**

    A. When did the party begin

    B. When was the last time you drank alcohol

    C. How much alcohol did you drink

    D. Where was the party held

86. **What might a high level of carbon dioxide indicate?**

    A. Respiratory acidosis

    B. Metabolic acidosis

    C. Pneumonia

    D. All of the above

87. **If the ALT is high, then would you tell the patient that he has liver disease?**

    A. Yes. ALT is mainly found in the liver

    B. No. ALT is also found in muscle. Assess if the patient performed strenuous exercise before the test was administered

    C. Yes. No other tests need to be performed

    D. No. ALT is used to assess damage to the pancreas

88. **If a practitioner believes that the patient had a myocardial infarction 4 days ago, would the practitioner order a CPK-MB?**

    A. No. CPK-MB level returns to normal in 3 days

    B. No. Total creatine phosphokinase level is a better test

    C. Yes. CPK-MB level indicates cardiac muscle injury

    D. Yes. CPK-MB level returns to normal in 10 days

89. **Why is the ANA test ordered?**

    A. Screen for autoimmune diseases

    B. Screen for infection

    C. Screen for pregnancy

    D. Screen for HIV

90. **What happens when there is a high level of cortisol in blood?**

   A. Suppresses ACTH
   B. Increases Dexamethasone levels
   C. Increases ACTH
   D. Indicates that the patient is intoxicated

91. **What is antigen 125?**

   A. A protein attached to the ovarian cancer cells and other cancer cells
   B. An enzyme attached to the ovarian cancer cells and other cancer cells
   C. An enzyme attached to the colon cancer cells
   D. An enzyme attached to the liver cancer cells

92. **What should you tell a patient who has a positive CEA test result?**

   A. A positive result will require further tests
   B. The patient will undergo chemotherapy
   C. The patient will undergo radiation treatments
   D. The patient will be admitted to the hospital

93. **The presence of hCG in a blood sample may indicate**

   A. Pregnancy
   B. Ectopic pregnancy
   C. Testicular cancer
   D. All of the above

94. **What should you tell the patient who is undergoing the urea breath test?**

   A. Cold sores might develop 2 days following the test
   B. There will be slight blisterlike sores for a few days
   C. There is no long-term effect of swallowing a capsule or water containing radioactive material
   D. Test can produce a false-negative result

95. **What would you do if a patient who is breast-feeding is scheduled for a mammogram?**

   A. Cancel the mammogram since a mammogram is not administered if the patient is breast-feeding
   B. Procedure with the mammogram
   C. Cover the patient's breasts with a lead apron
   D. Make sure that the patient is finished breast-feeding for the day before taking the mammogram

96. **What would concern the practitioner if the patient is morbidly overweight before taking a spinal X-ray?**

    A. Details in the X-ray can be blurred by the additional weight
    B. The patient may break the X-ray machine
    C. The patient may not be able to withstand the test
    D. The patient is unable to be moved during the X-ray

97. **Should you ask a patient to stop taking Glucophage before being administered a CT scan?**

    A. Yes, Glucophage may react with contrast material
    B. Yes, Glucophage reacts to X-rays
    C. No, Glucophage reacts to MRI
    D. No, Glucophage has no effect on the test

98. **How do you increase conductivity of sound waves across the patient's skin?**

    A. Place gel on the patient's skin over the site of the test
    B. Place gel on the patient's body before conducting the test
    C. Increase ambient noise
    D. Decrease ambient noise

99. **The patient tells you he is feeling relax since smoking several cigarettes in the parking lot before coming in for a Doppler ultrasound. What should you do?**

    A. Notify the practitioner since nicotine constricts blood vessels and could result in a false test result
    B. Continue with the test as scheduled
    C. Tell the patient about the dangers of smoking
    D. Tell the patient it is good that he is relaxed before the test

100. **The patient tells you she is fearful that the tracer will destroy her tissues. How should you respond?**

    A. Explain that the tracer contains a very low dose of radiation that remains in the body for 24 days after the test and causes minor tissue damage
    B. Explain that the tracer contains a very low dose of radiation that is flushed from the body within 24 hours of the test and rarely causes any tissue damage
    C. Explain that the tracer contains the same amount of radiation as the sun and causes no more than a minor sunburn
    D. You won't feel anything

101. **What is the most common type of echocardiogram?**
    A. Transabdominal
    B. Transesophageal
    C. Stress
    D. Transthoracic

102. **Why is oxytocin administered during a contraction stress test?**
    A. To lower blood pressure of the fetus
    B. To stop contractions
    C. To induce contractions
    D. To keep the fetus from moving

103. **How would you respond if the patient who is scheduled for a Pap smear today mentions that her menstrual period ended 7 days ago?**
    A. Prepare the patient for the test
    B. Reschedule the test for the next day
    C. Reschedule the test for the next week
    D. Reschedule the test for 2 weeks

104. **What is liquefaction time?**
    A. The time necessary for semen to liquefy
    B. The time necessary for semen to dehydrate
    C. The time necessary for sperm to liquefy
    D. The time necessary for sperm to dehydrate

105. **What is the reason for administering the V/Q scan?**
    A. To assess for a pulmonary embolus
    B. To assess the capacity and function of the lung
    C. To assess vital capacity
    D. To assess for cardiac inflections

106. **A total thyroxine test is used to determine**
    A. The total amount of thyroxine that is missing from the patient
    B. The amount of thyroxine that is not bound to globulin
    C. The amount of thyroxine that is attached to globulin and that is not bound to globulin
    D. All of the above

107. **Chemical peel changes skin tone.**
    A. True
    B. False

108. **What is the allergy test called where a drop of allergen solution is placed on the skin and the skin is scratched?**

    A. Skin patch test
    B. Skin prick test
    C. Intradermal test
    D. The Q patch test

109. **The patient asks why it takes more than 1 day to get the results of a throat culture. What is your best response?**

    A. The laboratory is backed up with other samples
    B. Sufficient time must pass to allow the microorganism to grow
    C. An outside laboratory is used
    D. It takes time to determine what drug to use to kill the microorganism

110. **What does the urodynamic test measure?**

    A. Assesses bladder function
    B. Assesses the position of the urethra
    C. Assesses urethral pressure
    D. None of the above

111. **Why is the CEA test used to screen for cancer?**

    A. The carcinoembryonic antigen is normally present during fetal development and is terminated at birth. It is present if there is a tumor
    B. The carcinoembryonic antigen is excellent for diagnosing cancer
    C. The carcinoembryonic antigen is used for early detection of cancer
    D. None of the above

112. **What hormone does the renin cause to be released?**

    A. Aldosterone
    B. Cortisol
    C. Phenytoin
    D. Dexamethasone

113. **What is a stress echocardiogram?**

    A. A procedure that creates images of the heart
    B. A procedure that is performed after the patient has exercised
    C. A procedure that is performed when the patient's heart is placed under stressed using a medication
    D. All of the above

114. **What must be assessed before administering the BUN test?**

A. Age of the patient

B. If the patient has taken diuretics

C. If the patient has ingested meat

D. All of the above

115. **What kind of hysterectomy removes the uterus, cervix, ovaries, and fallopian tubes?**

A. Total hysterectomy

B. Radical hysterectomy

C. Total hysterectomy with bilateral salpingo-oophorectomy

D. Semi-hysterectomy

116. **What is an excision biopsy?**

A. The entire skin lesion is removed

B. A piece of the skin lesion is removed

C. A circular sample of skin is removed

D. A few cells are removed from the top of the lesion

117. **What test measure carboxyhemoglobin level in the blood?**

A. Carbon monoxide test

B. Total carbon dioxide test

C. Arterial blood gases

D. None of the above

118. **What is the purpose of the urea breath test?**

A. Determines the presence of *Helicobacter pylori* in stool

B. Determines the presence of *H pylori* in the blood

C. Determines the presence of *H pylori* in the stomach

D. Estimates the alcohol content of blood

119. **What is the purpose of using pilocarpine during a sweat test?**

A. Pilocarpine helps to draw sweat from the newborn

B. Pilocarpine prevents the newborn from sweating

C. Pilocarpine is not used in the sweat test

D. Pilocarpine protects the skin from electrodes that are placed on the skin during the test

120. **Why would the prothrombin time test be ordered?**

A. Risk for bleeding

B. Therapeutic level of Coumadin

C. Vitamin K deficiency

D. All of the above

121. **What should the nurse do if the patient drank a large cup of coffee the morning of the PET scan?**

A. Tell the patient this is unacceptable and continue with the PET scan

B. Notify the healthcare provider

C. Ask the patient to drink five cups of water prior to the PET scan

D. Take a sample of the patient's blood for testing

122. **What is the function of electrolytes?**

A. Maintains blood flow across cell membranes

B. Maintains voltage across cell membranes and carry electrical impulses within the body

C. Balances leukocytes and erythrocytes

D. Balances leukocytes and potassium

123. **Why is hemoglobin important to arterial blood gases test?**

A. Hemoglobin is used to measure the acidity of the blood that is used to calculate blood gases

B. Hemoglobin carries oxygen. A low level of hemoglobin may indicate a low blood oxygen level

C. Hemoglobin is used to measure the alkaline of the blood that is used to calculate blood gases

D. Low hemoglobin indicates respiratory disease

124. **How long must pressure be applied to the blood sample site after the needle is removed from the patient who is not taking anticoagulation medication?**

A. 3.5 minutes

B. 1 minute

C. 10 minutes

D. 20 minutes

125. **What is bilirubin?**

A. The reddish coloring in the eyes

B. The pigment formed by the breakdown of hemoglobin in the liver

C. Brown spots that appear on hands

D. The pigment formed by the breakdown of hemoglobin in the kidneys

126. **Why would the practitioner order an ECG if creatine phosphokinase and troponin are elevated?**

    A. To differentiate between right ventricle and left ventricle failure

    B. To differentiate between right and left heart failure

    C. To differentiate between heart muscle damage and other tissue damage

    D. To determine if the patient ate within 12 hours of the test

127. **Why would a practitioner order the immunoglobulin test?**

    A. To measure antibodies made by the patient's immune system

    B. To determine if the patient has an infection

    C. To determine if the patient has leukemia

    D. To assess if the patient has internal bleeding

128. **What is the seroconversion period?**

    A. The period when the HIV-2 infection is detectable in a patient

    B. The period when the HIV infection is detectable in a patient

    C. The period when the HIV infection is not detectable in a patient

    D. The period when the HIV-1 infection is detectable in a patient

129. **Renin signals the release of**

    A. Aldosterone

    B. Cortisol

    C. Phenytoin

    D. Dexamethasone

130. **The CA-125 test is used to**

    A. Screen for ovarian cancer

    B. Differentiate between benign or malignant ovarian tumor

    C. Screen for colon cancer

    D. None of the above

131. **What may affect the results of the CA-125 test?**

    A. Chemotherapy recently

    B. Menstruating

    C. Radioactive scan recently

    D. All of the above

132. **What how would you respond to a patient who reports that a home urine pregnancy test is positive?**

    A. You are pregnant

    B. Home pregnancy test assesses for hCG hormone

    C. Home pregnancy tests must be confirmed with other tests before the practitioner will know that you are pregnant

    D. Home pregnancy test is unreliable

133. What is the purpose of the urea breath test?

    A. To determine if the patient has the IgG antibody

    B. To determine if the blood sample has *H pylori* antibodies

    C. To determine the presence of *H pylori* antigens in feces

    D. To determine the presence of *H pylori* in the stomach

134. What would you do if the patient arrived for an X-ray wearing a cervical collar?

    A. Remove the cervical collar and take the X-ray

    B. Keep the cervical collar in place when taking the X-ray

    C. Reschedule the X-ray

    D. Ask the patient if the cervical collar can be removed

135. You are sending the patient for a CT scan and patient tells you she is allergic to shellfish. What do you do?

    A. Send the patient for the CT scan

    B. Reschedule the CT scan

    C. Notify the healthcare provider and radiologist

    D. Cancel the CT scan

136. How do you reposition the intestine prior to an abdominal ultrasound?

    A. Position the patient on her left side

    B. Fill the bladder with contrast

    C. Fill the bladder with water

    D. Position the patient on her right side

137. Can a patient with metal dental fillings undergo an MRI?

    A. No, the MRI metal alert alarm sounds

    B. Yes, but the patient may experience a tingling sensation in his/her mouth

    C. No, there is a risk that the fillings will be extracted by the MRI

    D. Yes, but a plastic cap must be placed over each filling

138. What should be done before the transesophageal echocardiogram?

    A. Make sure that the patient can talk

    B. Make sure that the patient can hold her breath for 5 seconds

    C. Arrange for a signal that the patient can give to the practitioner to indicate that the patient is uncomfortable during the procedure

    D. Arrange for the patient speak during the procedure

139. **What is meant by a score of 7 on the biophysical profile (BPP) test?**
    A. Undetermined results. The test should be repeated
    B. The fetus is normal
    C. There are possible problems with the fetus
    D. None of the above

140. **Why is transillumination performed?**
    A. To highlight growths found during a testicular examination
    B. To visualize the prostate gland through the urethra
    C. To scan the prostate gland
    D. To scan the bladder

141. **Why is the patient usually administered acyclovir 2 weeks prior to a chemical peel?**
    A. To prevent a fungal infection
    B. To prevent a bacterial infection
    C. To prevent a viral infection
    D. To reduce bleeding during the procedure

142. **What is the best time to collect a sputum sample?**
    A. Right before meals
    B. First thing in the morning
    C. Immediately after the patient awakens from sleep
    D. After the patient rinses his/her mouth with water

143. **During the Schiotz tonometry test a tonometer is pressed against the cornea.**
    A. True
    B. False

144. **What would you recommend if the site of a chemical peel remained red for 3 months following the procedure?**
    A. Rush the patient to the hospital
    B. Contact the healthcare provider immediately
    C. Place a topical antibiotic on the site
    D. Do nothing

145. **What is the purpose of the renin assay test?**
    A. To determine the underlying cause of hypertension
    B. To determine the underlying cause of hypotension
    C. To determine the underlying cause of renal disease
    D. To determine the underlying cause of liver disease

146. **What is a V/Q scan?**

    A. A common lung scan in which a perfusion scan is performed and then a ventilation scan is performed
    B. A common lung scan in which a ventilation scan is performed and then a perfusion scan is performed
    C. A scan that measures the volume and quantity of a lung
    D. None of the above

147. **Why would a practitioner order a MUGA?**

    A. To assess cardiac contraction
    B. To assess blood flow
    C. To assess blood flow to the extremities
    D. To assess blood flow to the lungs

148. **How are images taken in coordination with the patient's breathing?**

    A. Metal transducers are placed on the patient's body
    B. Plastic transducers are placed inside the patient's body
    C. A belt is placed around the patient's chest
    D. Plastic transducers are placed both on and inside the patient's body

149. **What should you tell a patient who is scheduled for thyroid ultrasound?**

    A. Remove all jewelry from the head and neck area
    B. The patient may be asked to remove all clothing from above the waist
    C. The patient lies on her back and a pillow is placed under the patient's shoulders
    D. All of the above

150. **What do you want the patient to do after a CT scan of the spine with contrast material?**

    A. Lie on the right side of her back
    B. Lie on her stomach with her head facing left
    C. Bend over with her head down
    D. Keep her head elevated

151. **What is the best way to avoid tenderness of the breasts in a mammogram?**

    A. Schedule the mammogram during the second week of patient's menstrual period
    B. Schedule the mammogram during the patient's menstrual period
    C. Schedule the mammogram for within 2 weeks after the end of the patient's menstrual period
    D. Schedule the mammogram for within 3 weeks after the end of the patient's menstrual period

152. **How is the Herpes virus antigen detection test performed?**

   A. A stool sample is taken

   B. Cells are scraped from the sore

   C. A urine sample is taken

   D. An arterial blood sample is taken

153. **Why is a quadruple screen test administered at the 20th week of gestation?**

   A. To determine the position of the number of fetuses

   B. To determine the position of the fetus

   C. To determine the gender of the fetus

   D. To determine if there is a risk of birth defects

154. **The CEA protein test is used to**

   A. Detect cancer early

   B. Diagnose cancer

   C. Assess the effectiveness of cancer treatment

   D. All of the above

155. **When is luteinizing hormone measured?**

   A. To assess for sarcoidosis

   B. To assess for the underlying cause of infertility

   C. To assess for pituitary gland tumor

   D. To assess for acromegaly

156. **What might a high level of IgM indicate?**

   A. RA

   B. Viral hepatitis

   C. Mononucleosis

   D. All of the above

157. **What causes increase secretion of the renin enzyme?**

   A. High blood pressure

   B. Low blood pressure

   C. Increase water intake

   D. Arterial sclerosis

158. **What would you say to the patient whose HAV test is negative?**

   A. You don't have Hepatitis A virus

   B. You've never been exposed to Hepatitis A virus

C. You don't have any HAV antibodies; however, it takes 2 weeks or more to develop antibodies

D. You don't have Hepatitis A virus or Hepatitis B virus

159. What might influence the level of calcium?

A. Corticosteroids

B. Estrogen

C. Albuterol

D. All of the above

160. Why would a practitioner order the total iron-binding capacity (TIBC) test?

A. To measure the amount of circulating iron in the blood

B. To measure the capacity of blood to carry iron

C. To assess the amount of vitamin B_{12} supplements taken by the patient

D. To determine if the patient has been taking St. John's wort

161. What is the purpose of a chemistry screen?

A. Assess the respiratory function only

B. Assess blood carrying capability of blood only

C. Assess blood serum only

D. Assess the patient's overall health

162. What happens if the patient is unable to drink a large volume of fluid before a transabdominal ultrasound?

A. The test is cancelled

B. An MRI is ordered

C. Sterile water is inserted into the bladder using a urinary catheter

D. A CT scan is ordered

163. What does the serum osmolality test measure?

A. The volume of blood in the body

B. Antidiuretic hormone

C. The number of particles of substances that are dissolved in the serum

D. The dose of a vasopressin

164. Alcoholism can result in

A. Respiratory alkalosis

B. Metabolic alkalosis

C. Metabolic acidosis

D. Respiratory acidosis

165. **Why is a pillow placed under the patient's shoulders during a thyroid gland biopsy?**

    A. This prevents the patient from moving during the procedure
    B. This causes the thyroid gland to be pushed backward
    C. This causes the thyroid gland to be pushed forward
    D. This assures that the patient's airway is open during the procedure

166. **What test is ordered to determine if the patient has a Borrelia burgdorferi bacteria infection?**

    A. Indirect fluorescent antibody
    B. Enzyme-linked immunosorbent assay
    C. ELISA
    D. All of the above

167. **Why should the patient avoid taking Coumadin prior to a cardiac procedure?**

    A. The patient's bleeding time increases
    B. There is a high risk of bleeding
    C. The healthcare provider will need to take precautions to control bleeding that might occur during the procedure
    D. All of the above

168. **Why would a patient be asked to refrain from taking a sedative prior to a pulmonary function test?**

    A. A sedative may invalidate the test results because it might slow down respiration
    B. The patient will fall asleep during the test
    C. The patient may vomit during the test
    D. None of the above

169. **What does the total thyroxine test measure?**

    A. The total amount of thyroxine that is missing from the patient
    B. The amount of thyroxine that is not bound to globulin
    C. The amount of thyroxine that is attached to globulin and that is not bound to globulin
    D. All of the above

170. **How do you assess the underlying cause of xerostomia?**

    A. By using the thyroid gland scan
    B. By using the salivary gland scan
    C. By using the liver scan
    D. By using the bladder scan

171. What negatively affects the immunoglobulins test?

A. Recent blood transfusion

B. Radioactive scan 3 days before the test is administered

C. Recent vaccination

D. All of the above

172. What test helps diagnose precocious puberty?

A. FSH test

B. AFP

C. hCG

D. Inhibin A

173. Aside from renal failure, what would a high BUN level indicate?

A. Shock

B. Urinary tract blockage

C. Respiratory tract bleeding

D. All of the above

174. What is the purpose of the monospot test?

A. This test identifies heterophil antibodies that form between 2 and 9 weeks after the patient becomes infected

B. This test identifies heterophil antibodies that form between 1 and 9 weeks after the patient becomes infected

C. This test identifies heterophil antibodies that form between 2 and 4 weeks after the patient becomes infected

D. This test identifies heterophil antibodies that form between 2 and 9 weeks before the patient becomes infected

175. Normal results for a pulmonary function test

A. Depend on the patient's age, height, sex, weight, and race

B. Depend on laboratory standard

C. Depend on if the patient wears dentures

D. Depend on if the patient is a smoker

176. What is the purpose of a cardiac blood pool scan?

A. Measures the ejection fraction of the heart

B. Measures the amount of blood that pools in the heart

C. Measures the amount of blood that pools on the extremities

D. Measures the amount of blood that pools in the coronary arteries

177. **What might an increase in bilirubin levels from an amniocentesis taken after the 20th week indicate?**

    A. The fetus is healthy
    B. Fetal blood cells are attacking the mother's antibodies
    C. Fetal blood cells are being attacked by the mother's antibodies
    D. The fetus' lungs have matured

178. **Why is the fructose level in semen measured?**

    A. Fructose prevents sperm motility
    B. Fructose provides energy for sperm
    C. Fructose reduces sperm count
    D. Fructose increase semen volume

179. **A fetal ultrasound produces a**

    A. Sonogram
    B. An X-ray of the fetus
    C. An X-ray of the mother
    D. None of the above

180. **Why should a patient take a deep cough to produce a sputum sample?**

    A. A deep cough loosens sputum
    B. Sputum is produced in the respiratory system
    C. A deep cough brings sputum into the oral cavity
    D. All of the above

181. **A low level of folic acid may indicate**

    A. Malabsorption
    B. Malnutrition
    C. Treatment of folic acid deficiency
    D. All of the above

182. **A high level of calcium may indicate**

    A. Addison disease
    B. Low magnesium
    C. Malabsorption syndrome
    D. Pancreatitis

183. **Potassium has an inverse relationship with**

    A. Sodium
    B. Magnesium

C. Phosphate

D. Chloride

184. Why should oxygen therapy be discontinued 20 minutes for the arterial blood gas test?

A. The test measures oxygen levels at room air

B. To determine if the patient has difficulty breathing

C. To make the patient more comfortable for the test

D. Supplemental oxygen will artificially decrease the results of the test

185. Which of the following conditions would you expect to find in a patient who is diagnosed with alcoholism?

A. Respiratory alkalosis

B. Metabolic alkalosis

C. Metabolic acidosis

D. Respiratory acidosis

186. Why would a practitioner not be concerned about elevated ALP if the patient was pregnant?

A. Prenatal vitamins negatively affect the ALP test

B. Pregnancy interferes with the patient's liver function

C. The placenta also makes ALP

D. The practitioner would be concerned because elevated ALP jeopardizes the pregnancy

187. Cardiac muscle is the only source of troponin.

A. True

B. False

188. What is IgE?

A. An immunoglobulin that forms when an infection occurs for the first time

B. An immunoglobulin that crosses the placenta

C. An immunoglobulin found on mucous membranes

D. An immunoglobulin found in tears

189. Why might the practitioner request a sample be taken from the inferior petrosal sinus near the pituitary gland for the ACTH test?

A. To determine if the pituitary gland is producing CRH

B. To determine if the pituitary gland is producing ACTH

C. To determine if the pituitary gland is producing cortisol

D. To determine if the adrenal gland is producing cortisol

190. **Why the CA-125 test ordered following treatment for cancer?**

    A. A low level of CA-125 might be found months before other diagnostic tests indicating the return of cancer

    B. A high level of CA-125 confirms that treatment is successful

    C. A high level of CA-125 might be found months before other diagnostic tests indicating the return of cancer

    D. A high level of CA-125 confirms that the tumor was benign

191. **Successful treatment of cancer may be indicated when the results in CEA level are**

    A. Normal within 6 weeks of treatment

    B. Normal within 4 weeks of treatment

    C. Normal within 2 weeks of treatment

    D. Elevated within 6 weeks of treatment

192. **Why is the AFP test administered?**

    A. Estimate the chances of birth defects

    B. Estimate the gender of the fetus

    C. Estimate the fetal liver function

    D. Estimate the uE3 level

193. **Why might the practitioner order a FSH test?**

    A. To assess the underlying cause of precocious puberty

    B. To assess the function of the pituitary gland

    C. To assess the underlying cause of abnormal menstrual periods

    D. All of the above

194. **What is autoimmune hemolytic anemia?**

    A. The patient's immune system creates antibodies against the patient's erythrocytes

    B. The patient's immune system creates antibodies against the patient's leucocytes

    C. The patient's immune system is unable to create antibodies

    D. The patient's immune system is unable to create leucocytes

195. **Why should the patient avoid taking Pepto-Bismol (bismuth) prior to an X-ray?**

    A. Bismuth might prevent the patient from remaining still during the X-ray

    B. Bismuth might absorb the X-ray beam

    C. Bismuth might obstruct the X-ray beam

    D. Bismuth might enhance the X-ray beam

196. Can a patient who is breast-feeding receive a CT scan?

A. Yes, however the patient should use formula instead of breast-feeding for 2 days following the CT scan if contrast material is administered

B. Yes, if a lead apron is placed over the patient's abdomen

C. No, The CT scan might affect the fetus

D. No, if contrast material is not administered

197. What test is used to indicate blood flow?

A. Doppler ultrasound

B. Continuous-wave Doppler

C. Color Doppler

D. All of the above

198. Why would a practitioner order a transabdominal ultrasound?

A. To assess the cause of urinary disorders

B. To assess pelvic inflammatory disease (PID)

C. To assess placement of intrauterine device (IUD)

D. All of the above

199. What is the purpose of cardiac calcium scoring?

A. To assess cardiac contractions

B. To stimulate cardiac contractions

C. To assess the buildup of plaque containing calcium on the walls of the coronary arteries

D. To assess the workload of the heart

200. Why is a cranial ultrasound not performed after 18 months of age?

A. The fontanelle is closed

B. The fontanelle remains open

C. The test is too painful for the baby to undergo

D. Complications from a premature birth would have already manifested

201. What is sperm morphology?

A. Liquefaction time

B. Semen volume

C. The number of normally shaped sperm

D. Fructose level

202. **What test is performed if the healthcare provider suspects a pulmonary embolus?**

    A. Bronchoscopy
    B. Lung scan
    C. Pulmonary function test
    D. Thoracotomy

203. **What can produce a false-positive result in the bone mineral density (BMD) test?**

    A. The patient has arthritis
    B. The patient has a T-score of 1
    C. The patient has a Z-score of 1
    D. The patient has an X-score of less than 1

204. **A patient arrives for an EEG for sleep disorder tells you that she had a long nap before arriving for the test. What would you do?**

    A. Cancel the test, since the patient no longer has a sleeping disorder
    B. Reschedule the test
    C. Reschedule the test asking the patient not to sleep before the test
    D. Wait 2 hours before conducting the test

205. **What test is performed to determine if the patient has sensorineural hearing loss?**

    A. Pure-tone audiometry
    B. Speech reception/word recognition
    C. Whispered speech test
    D. Otoacoustic emissions test

206. **What is an E-chart used for?**

    A. To assess the patient's ability to see distances when he/she is unable to read
    B. To assess the patient's ability to see distances
    C. To assess the patient's ability to see near him/her
    D. To assess the patient's ability to see near him/her when he/she is unable to read

207. **How does the dermabrasion improve the appearance of skin?**

    A. It removes the outer layer of skin, enabling new skin to grow
    B. It removes the inner layer of skin, enabling new skin to grow
    C. It uses a chemical to remove the outer layer of skin, enabling new skin to grow
    D. All of the above

208. What is the purpose of a refraction test?

A. To determine the corrective lens for prescribing to the patient
B. To assess if the patient can see refracted light waves
C. To assess if the patient can see refracted light waves at night
D. All of the above

209. What is a confrontation test?

A. Examination of patient's peripheral vision by gazing at the healthcare provider's eyes
B. Examination of patient's peripheral vision by gazing at the healthcare provider's nose
C. Examination of patient's peripheral vision by gazing at the healthcare provider's hands
D. None of the above

210. Prior to taking the urine culture and sensitivity test the patient should

A. Take antibiotics
B. Not take antibiotics
C. Avoid eating for 48 hours prior to the test
D. None of the above

211. What is the purpose of the Color duplex Doppler test?

A. To assess the velocity and direction of blood flowing through the penis
B. To assess size of an erection
C. To assess if the patient had an erection during sleep
D. To assess if the patient has urine in his bladder

212. What test measures if the patient has erections during sleep?

A. Intracavernosal injection
B. NPT
C. Color duplex Doppler
D. Liquefaction time

213. A common yeast infection that causes vaginosis is

A. *Candida albicans*
B. *Trichomonas vaginalis*
C. Bacterial vaginosis
D. None of the above

214. **What is the purpose of ankle-brachial index?**
    A. Assess for risk for stroke
    B. Blood pressure is taken in both arms and legs
    C. Screened for peripheral arterial disease (PAD)
    D. All of the above

215. **Can a patient who is claustrophobic undergo an MRI scan?**
    A. Yes, the patient can be given a sedative
    B. Yes, the patient can be scheduled for an open MRI
    C. Yes, the MRI should not be cancelled
    D. All of the above

216. **What should you tell the patient if the patient is unable to drink a large volume of fluid before a transabdominal ultrasound?**
    A. The test will be cancelled
    B. An MRI will be ordered
    C. Sterile water is inserted into the bladder using a urinary catheter
    D. The practitioner will order a CT scan

217. **What would you expect if the practitioner ordered a mammogram and the patient is pregnant?**
    A. Cancel the mammogram
    B. Reschedule the mammogram until the third trimester
    C. Reschedule the mammogram until the second trimester
    D. Place a lead apron over the patient's abdomen

218. **When would a practitioner order to detect EBV antibody test?**
    A. When the monospot test is negative
    B. When the patient shows symptoms of mononucleosis and the monospot test is negative
    C. When the patient shows symptoms of mononucleosis
    D. When the patient is diagnosed with mononucleosis

219. **What might also produce the hCG hormone besides the placenta?**
    A. Molar pregnancy
    B. Choriocarcinoma
    C. Testicular cancer
    D. All of the above

220. **Why would the prostate-specific antigen density (PSAD) test be ordered?**
    A. To diagnose prostate cancer
    B. To compare the PSA value to the prostate gland size

    C. To confirm the magnetic resonance imaging (MRI) diagnosis of prostate cancer

    D. None of the above

221. What is the reason for ordering the estrogen level test?

    A. To assess for estrogen-producing tumors

    B. To assess the effect of fertility therapy

    C. To assess for fetal birth defects

    D. All of the above

222. Why are T-lymphocytes, T-cells, and T-helper cells important?

    A. These are factors that spread HCV

    B. These are factors that cause rheumatoid arthritis

    C. These are factors that spread HAV

    D. These are three types of leukocytes important in fighting infection

223. When is the immunoglobulin test typically ordered?

    A. To diagnose pneumonia

    B. As a follow-up to an abnormal result from the total blood protein test or from the blood protein electrophoresis test

    C. To rollout pneumonia

    D. To measure erythrocytes levels

224. What would you tell the patient scheduled for the BNP test who is taking Echinacea and valerian?

    A. Stop taking Echinacea and valerian for a week before the test

    B. Reduce the amount of Echinacea and valerian for two days before the test

    C. You cannot take the test

    D. Tell the practitioner that you are taking Echinacea and valerian so the practitioner can adjust the test results accordingly

225. What might a high ammonia level indicate?

    A. The patient exercised before the ammonia test

    B. The liver is unable to convert ammonia to urea

    C. The liver is unable to convert heme to hemoglobin

    D. All of the above

226. Bicarbonate is a form of

    A. Carbon monoxide

    B. Oxygen

    C. Carbon dioxide

    D. Hemoglobin

227. **Why would phosphate levels be normally higher in children?**

   A. Bones are actively growing

   B. Children have more energy than adults

   C. Children are more likely to be injured than adults

   D. Children rarely eat a balanced diet

228. **Why would a practitioner order an INR test?**

   A. To assess the volume of blood in the body

   B. To assess the therapeutic level of heparin

   C. The INR is used to standardize the results of the prothrombin time disregarding the testing method

   D. To assess the dose of vasopressin

229. **When is a contraction stress test not performed?**

   A. The mother had a cesarean section

   B. The mother has placenta previa

   C. The mother has placenta abruptio

   D. All of the above

230. **A breast ultrasound is commonly ordered**

   A. In place of a mammogram

   B. If there is a suspicious result on a mammogram

   C. Always in combination with a mammogram

   D. Only when performing breast augmentation

231. **Diarrhea can result in**

   A. Respiratory alkalosis

   B. Metabolic alkalosis

   C. Metabolic acidosis

   D. Respiratory acidosis

232. **What should the patient avoid before taking the creatinine clearance test?**

   A. Strenuous exercise

   B. Eating meat

   C. Drinking coffee

   D. All of the above

233. **What is the most accurate method of measuring bone mineral density?**

   A. Dual-photo absorptiometry

   B. Quantitative computed tomography

    C. Dual-energy X-ray absorptiometry

    D. Ultrasound

234. What should be done with the first urine during a 24-hour urine collection?

    A. It should be refrigerated

    B. It should be stored in a gallon container

    C. It should be discarded

    D. All of the above

235. Why would a patient who is scheduled for a CT scan stop taking Glucophage?

    A. Glucophage may react with contrast material

    B. Glucophage reacts to X-rays

    C. Glucophage reacts to MRI

    D. There is no need to stop taking Glucophage if contrast material is administered before the CT scan

236. Before taking the prolactin test what must the patient do?

    A. Avoid the sun

    B. Rest for 30 minutes

    C. Exercise for 30 minutes

    D. Avoid alcohol

237. What can cause a false-positive result from the bone mineral density test?

    A. The patient has arthritis

    B. The patient has a T-score of 1

    C. The patient has a Z-score of 1

    D. The patient has an X-score of less than 1

238. What is a first-pass scan?

    A. Captures images of blood going through the heart and lungs for the first time

    B. A type of cardiac blood pool scan

    C. A procedure that uses a radioactive tracer

    D. All of the above

239. A patient with 20% carbon monoxide blood level

    A. Will show symptoms of carbon monoxide poisoning

    B. Will not show symptoms of carbon monoxide poisoning

    C. Will show slight symptoms of carbon monoxide poisoning

    D. None of the above

240. **What is Holter monitoring?**

    A. An ambulatory electrocardiogram
    B. Monitoring the patient's blood flow at rest
    C. Monitoring the patient's blood flow at sleep
    D. Monitoring the patient's blood flow after exercising

241. **What is the purpose of tympanometry?**

    A. To measure the eardrum's response to pressure and sound
    B. To identify the contents of fluid behind the eardrum
    C. To permit fluid behind the eardrum to drain
    D. To treat an ear infection

242. **A patient arrives for a gastrin level test and tells you he is feeling better since taken Prilosec this morning. What should you do?**

    A. Reschedule the test and tell the patient to refrain from taking Prilosec 12 hour before coming for the test
    B. Continue with the test
    C. Ask the patient to rest 30 minutes before the test
    D. Refrain from drinking water 1 hour before the test is administered

243. **What should be asked of the patient if the patient has high level potassium?**

    A. Do you have a bacterial infection
    B. Are you taking potassium supplements
    C. Do you usually have a high level of potassium
    D. Are you pregnant

244. **How does carbon monoxide impede blood oxygenation?**

    A. Carbon monoxide can result in instant death
    B. Carbon monoxide is a colorless, odorless gas
    C. Carbon monoxide attaches to hemoglobin replacing oxygen
    D. Carbon monoxide is irreversible

245. **What does the presence of the IgG anti-HAV mean?**

    A. The patient was recently infected with hepatitis A virus
    B. The patient at some point was infected with hepatitis A virus
    C. The patient was recently infected with hepatitis B virus
    D. The patient at some point was infected with hepatitis B virus

246. **Why would the practitioner order a BNP test?**

    A. BNP increases when the heart works harder for long periods
    B. BNP decreases if the patient has a myocardial infarction

C. BNP indicates if the patient has taken Echinacea

D. BNP will indicate if the patient will develop chronic obstructive pulmonary disease

247. **What forms ammonia in the body?**

A. Bacteria in the intestine break down protein

B. The heme causes the liver to create ammonia

C. The heme causes the kidneys to create ammonia

D. Ammonia is the results of breakdown of hemoglobin

248. **Why would strenuous exercise before the cardiac enzyme study influence the test results?**

A. Enzymes being studied are contained in other muscle cells that might be injured during exercising

B. The patient should be relaxed before taking the test

C. Exercise may cause the patient to have a myocardial infarction

D. Muscle pain caused by exercising might be misunderstood as cardiac pain

249. **What regulates sodium?**

A. Bone marrow

B. Aldosterone hormone

C. Leukocytes level

D. Erythrocytes level

250. **What is dexamethasone?**

A. Dexamethasone is medication that signals the pituitary gland to release ACTH

B. Dexamethasone is medication that signals the pituitary gland that there is no cortisol in the blood

C. Dexamethasone is medication that signals the pituitary gland that there is a high level of cortisol in the blood

D. Dexamethasone is medication that signals the pituitary gland that there is a low level of cortisol in the blood

251. **Why would some practitioners not order the antisperm antibody test?**

A. Infertility maybe caused by immunologic infertility

B. Treatment is the same regardless of the test results

C. There is no treatment

D. Sampling is unreliable

252. What is Tay-Sachs disease?

    A. Accumulation of fatty acid in the brain and nerve cells

    B. No accumulation of fatty acid in the brain and nerve cells

    C. The presence of HexosaminidaseA enzyme in the new born

    D. Accumulation of protien in the brain and nerve cells

253. Why is a sensitivity test ordered with a blood culture?

    A. The sensitivity test identifies the microorganism

    B. The sensitivity test identifies medication that kills the microorganism

    C. The sensitivity test identifies erythrocytes

    D. The sensitivity test identifies leucocytes

254. What would you tell a patient who is positive for the IgM antibody?

    A. You will also be at risk for exposure to the rubella virus

    B. You will never be exposed to the rubella virus

    C. You are immune to the rubella virus

    D. You currently have or recently had a rubella virus infection

255. What risk is there with *H pylori* Tests?

    A. A false-positive result if the *H pylori* count is low and undetectable

    B. Results are never conclusive

    C. A false-negative result if the *H pylori* count is low and undetectable

    D. The test will kill the microorganism

256. An X-ray not be ordered if

    A. The results of the X-ray would not alter the treatment

    B. The patient is older than 7 years

    C. The patient is older than 82 years

    D. The patient has not been diagnosed with a bone disorder

257. The patient asks why the practitioner ordered orthopantogram. What is your best response?

    A. To assess temporomandibular joints

    B. To assess sinuses

    C. To assess jaw

    D. All of the above

258. A patient anxious about a CT scan may be administered

    A. An amphetamine

    B. Adderall

    C. Dexedrine

    D. A sedative

MEDICAL TESTS AND PROCEDURES DEMYSTIFIED   603

259. **What would you tell the patient who asks you purpose of a perfusion CT?**
    A. Perfusion CT determines if the patient has osteoporosis
    B. Perfusion CT determines results of the KUB
    C. Perfusion CT assesses blood supply to the brain
    D. Perfusion CT assesses the function of the lymph system

260. **Why is the Shilling test ordered?**
    A. To assess the absorption of vitamin B_{12}
    B. Screen for pregnancy
    C. To assess the vitamin B_6 level
    D. To assess the vitamin folic acid level

261. **What does the transcutaneous bilirubin meter measure?**
    A. It is a handheld meter that helps determine if the newborn has jaundice
    B. It measures the level of bilirubin by being placed on the skin
    C. It measures the level of bilirubin in a newborn
    D. All of the above

262. **What is done if a patient is anxious about being placed in a CT scanner?**
    A. Administer a sedative per order
    B. Cancel the test
    C. Wait for a calmer moment to administer the test
    D. Tell the patient to behave like an adult

263. **What is the function of an MRA?**
    A. Assess the speed, direction, and flow of blood
    B. Assess fluid content of the brain
    C. Assess changes in the brain chemistry
    D. All of the above

264. **A perfusion scan involves**
    A. A radioactive tracer being injected into a blood vessel
    B. Contrast material being injected into a blood vessel
    C. The patient inhaling a gas
    D. None of the above

265. **Why is the reticulocyte count test ordered?**
    A. To screen for anemia
    B. To screen for risk of bleeding
    C. To assess the vitamin B_{12} level
    D. To assess the vitamin B_6 level

266. **What test is performed to identify hearing problems in a newborn?**

A. Pure-tone audiometry

B. Speech reception/Word recognition

C. Whispered speech test

D. Otoacoustic emissions test

267. **What is the purpose of the TSH test?**

A. To assess the underlying cause of hyperthyroidism

B. To assess the underlying cause of hypothyroidism

C. To assess the treatment of hypopituitarism

D. All of the above

268. **What would negatively effect the cardiac enzyme studies?**

A. Intramuscular injection

B. Recent surgery

C. Statins

D. All of the above

269. **What should occur after a positive saliva test?**

A. Results must be confirmed by the ANA test

B. Results must be confirmed by the Western blot test

C. Results must be confirmed by the immunoglobulins test

D. Results must be confirmed by the IgM test

270. **What might the practitioner do if the patient has a high cortisol level?**

A. Order a 24-hour urine free cortisol test

B. Diagnose the patient with Cushing syndrome

C. Diagnose the patient with hyperthyroidism

D. Diagnose the patient with uncontrolled diabetes

271. **What is the purpose of the parathyroid hormone?**

A. Converts vitamin D to an active form

B. Increases absorption of calcium by the intestine

C. Causes the kidneys to retain calcium

D. All of the above

272. **What does the practitioner do with the AFP test results if the ultrasound gestation age is different from the estimated gestation age?**

A. Multiply the test results by 10

B. Adjust the test results using the multiple of median (MoM) factor

C. Multiply the test results by 15

D. Repeat the test

273. **Where is contrast material administered in a CT myelogram?**

A. Muscle

B. In the intrathecal space

C. Nerve

D. Legs

274. **The patient reports weakness in the extremities following a CT scan. What should you do first?**

A. Call her practitioner

B. Call the radiologist

C. Ask the patient to lie down

D. Call for emergency medical help immediately

275. **What does a fetal ultrasound produce?**

A. A sonogram

B. A discogram

C. An angiogram

D. Dexagram

276. **What would you do if the patient feels short of breath during a transvaginal ultrasound?**

A. Reposition the patient or raise the head of the bed

B. Stop the test

C. Tell the patient to take deep breaths

D. Distract the patient by asking the patient about her children

277. **Can a patient receive an MRI with contrast if the patient is allergic to shellfish?**

A. No, the MRI must be cancelled

B. The practitioner will evaluate the benefit and risk of continuing with the MRI

C. Yes, the MRI continues as scheduled

D. Yes, but a crash-cart must be standing by before continuing with the MRI

278. **What can influence the test for carbon monoxide?**

A. The patient smokes before taking the test

B. The patient refuses to take deep breaths before the test is administered

C. The patient takes shallow breaths before the test is administered

D. The patient vomits before the test

279. **What other test might the practitioner orders along with the cardiac enzymes test?**

    A. Aspartate aminotransferase test
    B. Alanine aminotransferase test
    C. IgG anti-HAV test
    D. Myoglobin test

280. **Why might a whole body thyroid scan be ordered?**

    A. To assess for thyroid cancer metastasis
    B. To assess for hyperthyroidism
    C. To assess for hypothyroidism
    D. None of the above

281. **How is the pneumotonometry test performed?**

    A. It measures intraocular pressure directly on the eye
    B. It uses a puff of air to measure intraocular pressure
    C. It uses a probe to measure intraocular pressure
    D. None of the above

282. **Why should a patient not take tranquilizers 5 days before the electronystag-mogram (ENG) test?**

    A. Tranquilizers might slow eye movement giving a false test result
    B. Tranquilizers might increase eye movement giving a false test result
    C. Tranquilizers might cause nausea and vomiting during the test
    D. Tranquilizers might cause nausea and vomiting following the test

283. **What test is performed to identify hearing problems in a newborn?**

    A. Pure-tone audiometry
    B. Speech reception/word recognition
    C. Whispered speech test
    D. Otoacoustic emissions test

284. **What tests the patient's peripheral vision by gazing at a concentric circle image?**

    A. Amsler grid test
    B. Perimetry test
    C. Tangent screen test
    D. Snellen test

285. **What test measures for macular degeneration?**

    A. Amsler grid test
    B. Perimetry test
    C. Tangent screen test
    D. Snellen test

286. The near test assesses the patient's ability to see long distances.
  A. True
  B. False

287. What is an ambulatory electrocardiogram?
  A. Holter monitor
  B. ECC
  C. ABI
  D. PAD Monitor

288. What might the practitioner do if the patient is diagnosed with cardiac tamponade?
  A. Perform an echocardiogram
  B. Perform a pericardiocentesis
  C. Perform an ABI
  D. Perform Holter monitoring

289. Why would a practitioner order a venogram?
  A. To assess blood flow through the heart
  B. To assess blood flow through veins
  C. To assess blood flow through the brain
  D. To assess blood flow through the eyes

290. What might an increase in bilirubin levels from an amniocentesis taken after the 20th week indicate?
  A. The fetus is healthy
  B. Fetal blood cells are attacking the mother's antibodies
  C. Fetal blood cells are being attacked by the mother's antibodies
  D. The fetus's lungs have matured

291. What cause of vaginosis causes a fishy odor?
  A. *Candida albicans*
  B. *Trichomonas vaginalis*
  C. Bacterial vaginosis
  D. None of the above

292. How does the snap gauge work?
  A. It measures the size of an erection
  B. The snap gauge consisting of a film is placed around the penis. The film snaps when the patient has erection
  C. It measures the length of time of an erection
  D. All of the above

293. **What do normal results for a pulmonary function test depend on?**

   A. Patient's age, height, sex, weight, and race
   B. Laboratory standard
   C. If the patient wears dentures
   D. If the patient is a smoker

294. **During a 24-hour urine collection, urine from the first time the patient urinated should**

   A. Be refrigerated
   B. Be stored in a gallon container
   C. Be discarded
   D. All of the above

295. **How is the cause of xerostomia determined?**

   A. Using the thyroid gland scan
   B. Using the salivary gland scan
   C. Using the liver scan
   D. Using the bladder scan

296. **What a practitioner to order for a patient who experiences random seizures?**

   A. An ambulatory EEG
   B. A helmet
   C. Restraints
   D. OAE test

297. **What is your response if a patient tells you that he/she spit into the sterile container when you asked for a sputum culture?**

   A. Teach the patient how to properly produce a sputum sample
   B. Sputum is not saliva
   C. He/she contaminated the container
   D. Take the sample to the laboratory quickly

298. **Why is C-reactive protein (CRP) test used to test for inflammation?**

   A. C-reactive protein is leaked from damaged cells shortly after cells are injured increasing the amount of C-reactive protein in blood
   B. A low level of C-reactive protein indicates that the liver is responding to reduce the inflammation process
   C. C-reactive protein attaches to damaged cells or microorganism enhancing phagocytosis in the destruction of the microorganism or damaged cell shortly after cells are injured
   D. C-reactive protein attaches to the liver causing an increase of white blood cells in blood to enhance phagocytosis in the destruction of the microorganism or damaged cell shortly after cells are injured

Medical Tests and Procedures Demystified

Answers

1. A. Troponin and CPK-MB
2. C. Prolactin levels are normally high when the patient first awakens.
3. B. Some antibiotics contain potassium.
4. C. Volume and capacity of the lungs
5. B. A needle is inserted through the urethra to remove samples of prostate tissue
6. B. Tracer material helps map the route that cancer cells spread from the cancer site through the lymphatic system.
7. A. D-xylose absorption test
8. D. All of the above
9. C. Coagulation time may be longer than normal.
10. A. To assess liver damage as a result of accidental or intentionally overdosing with acetaminophen.
11. A. It is used to transfer potassium and sodium in and out of cells.
12. A. The fontanelles are closed.
13. A. To assess the velocity and direction of blood flowing through the penis
14. C. Tenaculum clamp

15. D. All of the above
16. A. The patient might have difficulty excreting the contrast material.
17. B. Coumadin decreases coagulation time, thereby increasing the risk of bleeding during the procedure.
18. A. Cardiac blood pool scan
19. A. Pilocarpine helps to draw sweat from the newborn.
20. A. The patient removes all clothing and wears a gown during the MRI.
21. C. That the patient is not allergic to latex.
22. A. Facial X-ray
23. C. Screening for cancer, assessing cancer treatment, and assessing for the success of surgery to remove the tumor
24. C. The test result does not mean that you are HIV positive. Further testing is necessary.
25. B. Lactulose
26. B. The snap gauge consisting of a film is placed around the penis. The film snaps when the patient has erection.
27. A. The time necessary for semen to liquefy
28. A. The patient has arthritis.
29. C. Breast lift
30. A. Allen test
31. C. Bacterial infection.
32. A. It removes the outer layer of skin enabling new skin to grow.
33. B. Perimetry test
34. A. Skin patch test
35. D. All of the above
36. A. Chorionic villus sampling can be performed earlier in the pregnancy than amniocentesis.
37. A. The patient is at high risk for breast cancer and the MRI provides highly detailed views of the patient's breasts.
38. B. To flush the contrast material
39. A. ELISA
40. D. All of the above
41. D. All of the above
42. D. All of the above
43. D. Postpone the test for at least 8 hours.
44. B. Have a full bladder before the test
45. A. Does not have to have a full bladder for the test
46. A. A procedure performed to assess for testicular cancer
47. A. The upper segment of the vagina collapses and extends outside the vagina
48. A. Creatinine clearance test
49. A. It assesses the patients' ability to see distances when they are unable to read.
50. C. To determine blood supply to the brain
51. D. All of the above.
52. A. Avoid eating and drinking except for water 12 hours before the test is administered.
53. A. To measure the eardrum's response to pressure and sound

54. d. Sputum contains food particles.
55. A. Arms and legs
56. C. To cause an erection
57. D. The man might be at high risk for developing breast cancer and/or prostate cancer.
58. A. Magnetic resonance spectroscopy
59. B. Call for emergency medical care immediately.
60. D. All of the above
61. A. Prevents milk from ejecting
62. A. ACTH levels vary by the minute.
63. B. It takes 6 hours for troponin levels to rise after a myocardial infarction.
64. A. Respiratory alkalosis
65. A. C-peptide
66. B. Speech reception/Word recognition
67. C. A score that compares the patient's bone mineral density with that of people of his/her own age, sex, and race
68. A. A sputum cytology studies cells contained in the sputum and a sputum culture identifies micro-organism in the sputum.
69. C. Identifies the anti-cardiolipin antibodies
70. B. To generate an image of the heart that is not obstructed by bone
71. D. All of the above.
72. C. To encourage healing
73. A. Renin
74. A. The patient should fast for 8 hours before the test. All diabetes mellitus (DM) medications are withheld until the test is completed.
75. B. May have Tay-Sachs disease
76. B. To determine if the DM patient has maintained adequate blood glucose level for the previous 120 days
77. A. Skin patch test
78. C. Bacterial vaginosis
79. B. Lung scan
80. B. The tracer is likely to pass to the baby in breast milk.
81. D. All of the above
82. B. To screen for uric acid kidney stones
83. A. Higher risk of infection following surgery
84. D. Leukemia.
85. B. When was the last time you drank alcohol?
86. D. All of the above
87. B. No. ALT is also found in muscle. Assess if the patient performed strenuous exercise before the test was administered.
88. A. No. CPK-MB level returns to normal in 3 days.
89. A. Screen for autoimmune diseases
90. A. Suppresses ACTH
91. A. A protein attached to the ovarian cancer cells and other cancer cells

92. A. A positive result will require further tests.
93. D. All of the above
94. C. There is no long-term effect of swallowing a capsule or water containing radioactive material.
95. A. Cancel the mammogram since a mammogram is not administered if the patient is breast-feeding.
96. A. Details in the X-ray can be blurred by the additional weight.
97. A. Yes, Glucophage may react with contrast material.
98. A. Place gel on the patient's skin over the site of the test.
99. A. Notify the practitioner since nicotine constricts blood vessels and could result in a false test result.
100. B. Explain that the tracer contains a very low dose of radiation that is flushed from the body within 24 hours of the test and rarely causes any tissue damage.
101. D. Transthoracic
102. C. To induce contractions
103. B. Reschedule the test for the next day.
104. A. The time necessary for semen to liquefy
105. A. To assess for a pulmonary embolus
106. C. The amount of thyroxine that is attached to globulin and that is not bound to globulin
107. A. True
108. B. Skin prick test
109. B. Sufficient time must pass to allow the microorganism to grow.
110. A. Assesses bladder function
111. A. The carcinoembryonic antigen is normally present during fetal development and is terminated at birth. It is present if there is a tumor.
112. A. Aldosterone
113. D. All of the above
114. D. All of the above
115. C. Total hysterectomy with bilateral salpingo-oophorectomy
116. A. The entire skin lesion is removed.
117. A. Carbon monoxide test
118. C. Determines the presence of *H pylori* in the stomach
119. A. Pilocarpine helps to draw sweat from the newborn.
120. D. All of the above
121. B. Notify the healthcare provider.
122. B. Maintains voltage across cell membranes and carry electrical impulses within the body
123. B. Hemoglobin carries oxygen. A low level of hemoglobin may indicate a low blood oxygen level.
124. C. 10 minutes
125. B. The pigment formed by the breakdown of hemoglobin in the liver
126. C. To differentiate between heart muscle damage and other tissue damage
127. A. To measure antibodies made by the patient's immune system
128. C. The period when the HIV infection is not detectable in a patient
129. A. Aldosterone
130. D. None of the above
131. D. All of the above

132. C. Home pregnancy tests must be confirmed with other tests before the practitioner will know that you are pregnant.
133. D. To determine the presence of *H pylori* in the stomach
134. B. Keep the cervical collar in place when taking the X-ray.
135. C. Notify the healthcare provider and radiologist.
136. C. Fill the bladder with water.
137. B. Yes, but the patient may experience a tingling sensation in his/her mouth.
138. C. Arrange for a signal that the patient can give to the practitioner to indicate that the patient is uncomfortable during the procedure.
139. A. Undetermined results. The test should be repeated.
140. A. To highlight growths found during a testicular examination
141. C. To prevent a viral infection
142. C. Immediately after the patient awakens from sleep
143. A. True
144. B. Contact the healthcare provider immediately.
145. A. To determine the underlying cause of hypertension
146. B. A common lung scan in which a ventilation scan is performed and then a perfusion scan is performed
147. A. To assess cardiac contraction
148. C. A belt is placed around the patient's chest
149. d. All of the above.
150. D. Keep her head elevated
151. C. Schedule the mammogram for within 2 weeks after the end of the patient's menstrual period.
152. B. Cells are scraped from the sore
153. D. To determine if there is a risk of birth defects
154. C. Assess the effectiveness of cancer treatment
155. B. To assess for the underlying cause of infertility
156. A. RA
157. B. Low blood pressure
158. C. You don't have any HAV antibodies; however, it takes 2 weeks or more to develop antibodies.
159. D. All of the above
160. B. To measure the capacity of blood to carry iron
161. D. Assess the patient's overall health
162. C. Sterile water is inserted into the bladder using a urinary catheter.
163. C. The number of particles of substances that are dissolved in the serum
164. C. Metabolic acidosis
165. C. This causes the thyroid gland to be pushed forward.
166. D. All of the above
167. D. All of the above.
168. A. A sedative may invalidate the test results because it might slow down respiration.
169. C. The amount of thyroxine that is attached to globulin and that is not bound to globulin
170. B. By using the salivary gland scan
171. D. All of the above.

172. A. FSH test
173. D. All of the above
174. A. This test identifies heterophil antibodies that form between 2 and 9 weeks after the patient becomes infected.
175. A. Depend on the patient's age, height, sex, weight, and race
176. A. Measures the ejection fraction of the heart
177. C. Fetal blood cells are being attacked by the mother's antibodies.
178. B. Fructose provides energy for sperm.
179. A. Sonogram
180. D. All of the above.
181. D. All of the above
182. A. Addison disease
183. A. Sodium
184. A. The test measures oxygen levels at room air
185. C. Metabolic acidosis
186. C. The placenta also makes ALP.
187. B. False
188. C. An immunoglobulin found on mucous membranes
189. B. To determine if the pituitary gland is producing ACTH
190. C. A high level of CA-125 might be found months before other diagnostic tests indicating the return of cancer.
191. A. Normal within 6 weeks of treatment
192. A. Estimate the chances of birth defects
193. D. All of the above
194. A. The patient's immune system creates antibodies against the patient's erythrocytes.
195. C. Bismuth might obstruct the X-ray beam.
196. A. Yes, however the patient should use formula instead of breast-feeding for 2 days following the CT scan if contrast material is administered.
197. D. All of the above
198. D. All of the above
199. C. To assess the buildup of plaque containing calcium on the walls of the coronary arteries
200. A. The fontanelle is closed.
201. C. The number of normally shaped sperm
202. B. Lung scan
203. A. The patient has arthritis.
204. C. Reschedule the test asking the patient not to sleep before the test.
205. B. Speech reception/word recognition
206. A. To assess the patient's ability to see distances when he/she is unable to read
207. A. It removes the outer layer of skin, enabling new skin to grow.
208. A. To determine the corrective lens for prescribing to the patient
209. B. Examination of patient's peripheral vision by gazing at the healthcare provider's nose
210. B. Not take antibiotics

211. A. To assess the velocity and direction of blood flowing through the penis
212. B. NPT
213. A. *Candida albicans*
214. D. All of the above
215. D. All of the above.
216. C. Sterile water is inserted into the bladder using a urinary catheter
217. D. Place a lead apron over the patient's abdomen.
218. B. when the patient shows symptoms of mononucleosis and the monospot test is negative
219. D. All of the above
220. B. To compare the PSA value to the prostate gland size
221. D. All of the above
222. D. These are three types of leukocytes important in fighting infection
223. B. As a follow-up to an abnormal result from the total blood protein test or from the blood protein electrophoresis test
224. A. Stop taking Echinacea and valerian for a week before the test.
225. B. The liver is unable to convert ammonia to urea.
226. C. Carbon dioxide
227. A. Bones are actively growing.
228. C. The INR is used to standardize the results of the prothrombin time disregarding the testing method.
229. D. All of the above.
230. B. If there is a suspicious result on a mammogram
231. B. Metabolic alkalosis
232. D. All of the above
233. C. Dual-energy X-ray absorptiometry
234. C. It should be discarded.
235. A. Glucophage may react with contrast material.
236. B. Rest for 30 minutes.
237. A. The patient has arthritis.
238. D. All of the above.
239. B. Will not show symptoms of carbon monoxide poisoning
240. A. An ambulatory electrocardiogram
241. A. To measure the eardrum's response to pressure and sound
242. A. Reschedule the test and tell the patient to refrain from taking Prilosec 12 hour before coming for the test.
243. B. Are you taking potassium supplements?
244. C. Carbon monoxide attaches to hemoglobin replacing oxygen.
245. B. The patient at some point was infected with hepatitis A virus.
246. A. BNP increases when the heart works harder for long periods.
247. A. Bacteria in the intestine break down protein.
248. A. Enzymes being studied are contained in other muscle cells that might be injured during exercising.

249. B. Aldosterone hormone
250. C. Dexamethasone is medication that signals the pituitary gland that there is a high level of corti-sol in the blood.
251. B. Treatment is the same regardless of the test results.
252. A. Accumulation of fatty acid in the brain and nerve cells
253. B. The sensitivity test identifies medication that kills the microorganism.
254. D. You currently have or recently had a rubella virus infection.
255. C. A false-negative result if the *H pylori* count is low and undetectable.
256. A. The results of the X-ray would not alter the treatment.
257. D. All of the above
258. D. A sedative
259. C. Perfusion CT assesses blood supply to the brain.
260. A. To assess the absorption of vitamin B_{12}
261. D. All of the above.
262. A. Administer a sedative per order.
263. A. Assess the speed, direction, and flow of blood
264. A. A radioactive tracer being injected into a blood vessel
265. A. To screen for anemia
266. D. Otoacoustic emissions test
267. D. All of the above
268. D. All of the above
269. B. Results must be confirmed by the Western blot test
270. D. Diagnose the patient with uncontrolled diabetes.
271. D. All of the above.
272. B. Adjust the test results using the multiple of median (MoM) factor.
273. B. In the intrathecal space
274. C. Ask the patient to lie down
275. A. A sonogram
276. A. Reposition the patient or raise the head of the bed.
277. B. The practitioner will evaluate the benefit and risk of continuing with the MRI.
278. A. The patient smokes before taking the test.
279. D. Myoglobin test
280. A. To assess for thyroid cancer metastasis
281. B. It uses a puff of air to measure intraocular pressure.
282. A. Tranquilizers might slow eye movement giving a false test result.
283. D. Otoacoustic emissions test
284. C. Tangent screen test
285. A. Amsler grid test
286. B. False
287. A. Holter monitor
288. B. Perform a pericardiocentesis
289. B. To assess blood flow through veins

290. C. Fetal blood cells are being attacked by the mother's antibodies.
291. C. Bacterial vaginosis
292. B. The snap gauge consisting of a film is placed around the penis. The film snaps when the patient has erection.
293. A. Patient's age, height, sex, weight, and race
294. C. Be discarded
295. B. Using the salivary gland scan
296. A. An ambulatory EEG
297. A. Teach the patient how to properly produce a sputum sample.
298. C. C-reactive protein attaches to damaged cells or microorganism enhancing phagocytosis in the destruction of the microorganism or damaged cell shortly after cells are injured.

Appendix A

How to Collect Blood Specimen

1. How to Collect Blood Specimen From a Vein

Healthcare facilities provide training for collection of blood specimen. Here are the basic steps that are necessary to collect a blood sample.

1. Wrap a tourniquet around the patient's upper arm to stop blood flow, making veins easier to identify.

2. Clean the puncture site with alcohol.

3. Insert the needle into the vein with the bevel up.

4. Attach the appropriate test tube to the needle. Allow the blood to fill the test tube.

5. Remove the tourniquet to restore blood flow.

6. Place a gauze pad over the site while withdrawing the needle.

7. Apply firm pressure to the site until bleeding has stopped.

619

Teach the Patient

- Explain that
  - The tourniquet may feel tight.
  - The patient may feel a pinch or nothing at all when the needle is inserted into the vein.
  - There might be a small bruise at the site. Keeping pressure on the site reduces the chance of bruising.
  - Taking anticoagulants (aspirin, Coumadin) may require keeping pressure on the site for more than 10 minutes to stop the bleeding.
  - The vein may become swollen after the test (phlebitis). The patient should call their healthcare provider and apply a warm compress to reduce the swelling.

2. How to Collect Blood Specimen From a Heel Stick

Several drops of blood are collected from the heel of a baby.

1. Clean the heel with alcohol.
2. Puncture the heel with a small sterile lancer.
3. Collect several drops of blood in a small test tube.
4. Place a gauze pad over the site.
5. Maintain pressure until bleeding stops.
6. Apply a small bandage.

Teach the Parent

- Explain
  - That the patient may feel a pinch or nothing at all when the lancer punctures the skin.
  - There will be a bandage on the site for a short-time period.
  - That a small bruise might appear at the site.

3. How to Collect Blood Specimen From a Finger Stick

Several drops of blood are collected from the finger.

1. Clean the finger with alcohol.
2. Puncture the finger with a small sterile lancer.
3. Collect several drops in a small test tube.
4. Place a gauze pad over the site.
5. Maintain pressure until bleeding stops.
6. Apply a small bandage.

Teach the Patient

- Explain
  - That the patient may feel a pinch or nothing at all when the lancer punctures the skin.
  - There will be a bandage on the site for a short-time period.
  - A small bruise might appear at the site.

Index

patient teaching for, 181

rationale for, 179

results of, 180

antisperm antibody test, 256–288

implementation of, 257

nursing implications, 257

patient teaching for, 258

rationale for, 257

results of, 258

applanation tonometry, 553–554

arterial blood gases, 128

arterial blood gases test, 128–131

implementation of, 129

nursing implications, 129–130

patient teaching for, 131

rationale for, 129

results of, 130–131

aspartate aminotransferase (AST) test, 9, 152–155

implementation of, 152

nursing implications, 153

patient teaching for, 154–155

rationale for, 153

results of, 153–154

audiometric testing, 531–533

implementation of, 531–532

nursing implications, 533

patient teaching for, 533

rationale for, 533

results of, 533

auditory brain stem response (ABR), 531, 532

autoimmune hemolytic anemia, 177

B

bacterial vaginosis, 430

base (alkaline), 16

basic metabolic panel (BMP), 4, 39

basophils, 6

bDNA (branched DNA) test, 205

benign prostatic hyperplasia (BPH) ultrasound, 344–346

implementation of, 345

nursing implications, 346

patient teaching for, 346

rationale for, 345

results of, 346

beta globulins, 94, 96

bicarbonate (HCO_3), 128, 130

bilirubin, 9

bilirubin test, 155–158

implementation of, 155

nursing implications, 156

patient teaching for, 157

rationale for, 155–156

results of, 156–157

biophysical profile test (BPP), 404–406

implementation of, 404–405

nursing implications, 406

patient teaching for, 406

rationale for, 405–406

results of, 406

bitewing X-ray, 295

blood, elements of, 5. *See also* complete blood count (CBC)

blood alcohol test, 27–30

nursing implications, 28–30

patient teaching for, 30

rationale for, 28

results of, 30

blood creatinine level test, 54

high, 56–57

low, 57

normal, 56

blood culture, 181–182

implementation of, 181

nursing implications, 182

patient teaching for, 182

rationale for, 182

results of, 182

SPE. *See* serum protein electrophoresis (SPE)
SPECT (single photon emission computed
    tomography), 331
speech reception/word recognition test, 531, 532
sperm count, 441, 443
sperm morphology, 441
sperm motility, 441
sperm penetration tests, 426–428
    implementation of, 426–427
    nursing implications, 427
    patient teaching for, 428
    rationale for, 427
    results of, 428
spinal fluid sample, for syphilis test, 203
spine
    computed tomography scan of, 310–312
        implementation of, 311
        nursing implications, 312
        patient teaching for, 312
        rationale for, 311
        results of, 312
    magnetic resonance imaging of, 336–339
        implementation of, 336–337
        nursing implications, 337–338
        patient teaching for, 338–339
        rationale for, 337
        results of, 338
    X-ray of, 288–291
        implementation of, 289
        nursing implications, 290
        patient teaching for, 290–291
        rationale for, 289–290
        results of, 290
        types of, 288
spirometry, 472, 473–474
spleen scan, 466–468
    implementation of, 466–467
    nursing implications, 467

patient teaching for, 468
rationale for, 467
results of, 467
sputum culture, 536–538
    implementation of, 537
    nursing implications, 537–538
    patient teaching for, 538
    rationale for, 537
    results of, 538
sputum cytology, 538–540
    implementation of, 539
    nursing implications, 539
    patient teaching for, 540
    rationale for, 539
    results of, 539
SR. *See* sedimentation rate (SR)
stomach biopsy, 185
stool analysis, 480–482
    implementation of, 480
    nursing implications, 481
    patient teaching for, 481–482
    rationale for, 480
    results of, 481
stool culture, 482–484
    implementation of, 482–483
    nursing implications, 483
    patient teaching for, 483–484
    rationale for, 483
    results of, 483
stool sample, 460
stress echocardiogram, 386
SVC (slow vital capacity), 473
sweat test, 428–430
    implementation of, 428–429
    nursing implications, 429
    patient teaching for, 430
    rationale for, 429
    results of, 430